The Great Pain Deception

Faulty Medical Advice Is Making Us Worse

Steven Ray Ozanich

ISBN 978-1-949-00389-5

FIRST EDITION

Designed by Steven Ray Ozanich
Cover Photo: Michael Stephen
Illustrator: Mark Bush

Publisher: Silver Cord Records, Inc.
PO Box 8513
Warren, OH 44484

In partnership with
Waterside Productions
2055 Oxford Avenue
Cardiff by the Sea, CA. 92007

SteveOzanich.com
TMS Consulting, Inc.

(Steve is available for TMS consulting at info@SteveOzanich.com)

Library of Congress Control Number: 2011909722

Printed on acid-free paper

We can only take the great truths in little doses
Probably why God draws our life out over 70 or 80 years
The big truths are simply too much for the psyche
...at any one moment.

— Richard Rohr, OFM, *Portrait of a Radical*

Some of our current beliefs in our truths about medicine are actually not very correct at all—there's a revolution going on in the healthcare area, but it's at the leading edge of research... it really should come down to the people.... We've really been messed up by some ideas that are not absolutely correct... nature is simple in how she does everything—once I explain this, then you really start to see how powerful you have been, but how limited you have been because of alterations in our belief about how powerful we've been. You're not controlled by genes— you're actually controlled by perceptions of the environment— perceptions being beliefs.

— Bruce Lipton, PhD,
The New Biology—Where Mind and Matter Meet

The Truth is a fire burning brightly
Behind egos—within shadows.
If we face it, feel it, and accept it
We become part of its brilliance
And we too shine.

— Steven Ray Ozanich

Life Is Relationship

Life is pulling the other person back to you, pulling them toward your heart, pulling the separated hearts back together, that once beat as One.

Everyone needs to be heard in life—to be joined—their stories told, or relationship cannot survive. Those feeling isolated remain lost, life is void, fear and anger are generated by the separation—guilt and self-punishment follow.

Some hearts cut by separation will try to pull the Other back through acquiescence, others will try to pull the One back to them by taking the "opposing side" of the One that separated from them, yet others will seek neutral refuge within themselves—disappearing into routine and self-accomplishment.

The human mind will resort to infinite possibilities in order to gain an advantage in the effort to fulfill this most basic need—to pull the Others back to themselves, closing any separation, in order to avoid the fear of isolation, once again.

*Happiness surrounds the need for measured approval, unrequited self-acceptance, and the avoidance of rejection, as **Self** becomes unto itself; through the pain of each new separation comes a re-birth.*

— Steven Ray Ozanich

For my Dad, Mike

The most unpretentious man I have ever known. Who worked multiple jobs to keep his family fed and clothed. Who taught me when I was a little boy to never back down from what I knew to be true—words that I have lived by—giving me both strength and direction.

Table of Contents

A Philosophy on Life: Acting on New Knowledge and Healing

Foreword

There is an absolute epidemic of mindbody disorders in our society, yet the overwhelming majority of people fail to recognize this. It is not just the general public that is in the dark; most physicians and other health practitioners remain ignorant. What they all have in common is a lack of awareness of the prominent role of psychological factors in physical health. While most understand that stress can affect how we feel, few acknowledge that stress is often the sole cause for a multitude of unpleasant symptoms. In explanations to my patients, I like to say that psychology affects physiology.

John Sarno, MD, has been a pioneer in this field, attempting to educate the world about TMS (Tension Myositis Syndrome or The Mindbody Syndrome) in his books and in his efforts to reduce pain and suffering. Dr. Sarno's work initially focused on back pain, which has certainly become an epidemic in our culture, affecting large segments of the population at one time or another, at enormous cost. The great cost is due to time lost from the workplace, rising health care expenditures, disability claims, worker's compensation claims, etc. In the decades since he published *Mind Over Back Pain*, he has not only helped thousands eliminate their pain, but recognized that TMS can take many forms, causing pain and unpleasant symptoms affecting every part of the body. This insight has come from his extensive experience, and the experience of physicians like me, who have embraced TMS concepts and integrated them into the care of patients of all ages.

We have been conditioned to believe that physical symptoms must have a physical or structural cause, that our bodies are fragile and susceptible to breakdown or degeneration. Modern medicine does offer us remarkable insights into disease and wonderful therapeutic options. However, an entire mythology has also been created to explain why we have so many aches and pains, so many unpleasant symptoms. Who has conditioned us to think this way? The traditional medical establishment gets some credit. But the blame can also be shared by the alternative health fields; chiropractors, naturopaths, homeopaths and others have created what I sometimes call "alternate realities." They disregard what we do understand about human physiology and foist upon the desperate public their own explanation for what is occurring in the body, and people turn to them precisely because mainstream medicine may not be offering successful approaches for their symptoms. The media is also culpable, as they spread the mythology, trumpeting every charlatan's claim.

So if mainstream medicine is often off-base and the alternative remedies nonsense, what does the TMS approach offer? What do Dr. Sarno and other TMS practitioners have to offer? The answer is simple: knowledge. This is the core of psychosomatic medicine, understanding how the accumulated stress of life becomes a collective rage in the unconscious. Rage is not acceptable, but physical symptoms are, so the brain (unconscious) creates pain to distract us. It is an effective strategy, but one that can be defeated by the application of conscious thought, by understanding and accepting the process. Knowledge.

In this book, Steve tells his compelling story in an effort to impart this knowledge and help others to be well. It takes great courage to share the details of his 27-year journey through the darkness of pain into the light of wellness. From his perspective as a layman and former sufferer, he has done an excellent job exploring the realm of mindbody medicine, making this an excellent resource for those who are still looking for answers. The beautiful thing, as I like to tell my patients, is that there are no side effects from reading. So, read on.

Marc Sopher, MD

Acknowledgments

I want to first thank John E. Sarno, MD, who has improved the quality of countless lives through the time and effort he put forth in writing down his observations in healing. Who stood side-by-side with the truth in the face of cynical criticism among sufferers and colleagues alike. Who epitomizes the most basic concept of a true healer, placing the patient above all else. I am also very appreciative of him taking his personal time to read and approve my manuscript, as well as, providing his endorsement.

My deep appreciation also goes to Marc Sopher, MD, for taking the time from his medical practice and his family to help ease the suffering of many people, including myself. A special thanks to Dr. Sopher for taking even more time to review and add value to my manuscript from a clinical-medical aspect, without whose help I could not have even begun.

To Emmett Miller, MD, one of the earlier pioneers in mindbody healing whose publications helped me when I was stuck in the midst of healing, who gave me direction and who also took time from his life and schedule to review my manuscript.

A deep gratitude to Christiane Northrup, MD, Ken Pelletier, PhD, MD (hc), and Scott Anderson, MD, who took the time from their busy schedules to review my manuscript—for their kind words of support, and for their ringing endorsements.

A special thanks to John W. Travis, MD, and Meryn G. Callander for their friendship, guidance and support. I couldn't have pulled this project together without their help and extra efforts—they helped me make it a reality. Dr. Travis taught me a great deal throughout the book process and stuck with me to make certain my message got out there. Our work together led to a new friendship.

My gratitude also to those who helped me begin: Deborah Schuster, Graham Tuffee, Michael Lapmardo, Clancy McKenzie, MD, Russell A. Dewey, PhD, Robert Sapolsky, PhD, Gerald G. Jampolsky, MD, William Acar, PhD, Jeffrey S. Cramer, and Bernard Suzanne. Thank you Karen V. Kibler, PhD, for your support, advice, and tremendous effort to help out a fellow author achieve his goal.

A big thank you to Eric Fletcher for steering me back on course through his inscrutable knowledge of Word, and his experience in the book-formatting process.

Last and therefore first, the loves of my life, Matthew Steven and Kelsey Eileen, whom I admire more than I can possibly express, who give me strength, hope and purpose to face each new day.

Inside illustrations: Edward F. Smolko and Jessica Russo
YinYangOborous cover concept: Steven R. Ozanich
Original cover layout: Edward F. Smolko
Cover illustrator: Mark Bush
Cover designer: Doug Distel
Final cover design: Tom Ross
Photography: Michael Stephen and Anna Aulizia

Prologue

I began having severe back pain in my early teens. Its sudden appearance was a mystery, since I was a healthy kid at the time. I did the right thing by going to see a physician for a physical examination. He did the wrong thing by telling me that my pain was due to abnormalities in my back's structure, and that I would eventually need to be operated on. I would discover several decades and much pain later that this was never true. I accepted the new reality that the physician formed for me, and the pain that accompanied it. After all, he was an authority on the matter. I accepted his diagnosis, that I was physically flawed—for life.

And—so it was that for the next three decades as I visited pain clinics, chiropractors, surgeons, and many other health practitioners who gave me various diagnoses, from constantly slipping discs, and herniated discs, to fibromyalgia, arthritis, and spinal narrowing—on and on. Nothing they did ever helped much. The pain waxed and waned, until tragedy struck my family—an act of medical negligence rarely seen in medicine. Life would change forever and more physical symptoms suddenly appeared.

At the time I wasn't conscious of the correlation between the tragedy and my intensifying pain—as it did—to unbearable levels. My pain became so intense that I was finally convinced by several surgeons that I needed spinal surgery. However, miracle of miracles, shortly before the surgery, I was introduced to the work of a physician who specialized in healing pain, John E. Sarno, MD, Professor of Clinical Rehabilitation Medicine, New York University School of Medicine.

Dr. Sarno had shown, through decades of research and tremendous clinical success, that pain was rarely ever the result of structural abnormalities—whether it was in the spine or other body areas—pain came from a reduction in oxygen flow to muscles and nerves due to unconscious tension, which he refers to as TMS—Tension Myoneural Syndrome, or Tension Psychogenic Syndrome, TPS. This tension is the result of unknown, unfelt, repressed anger—more specifically, repressed rage.

I simply didn't believe Dr. Sarno at first. Not only did I not consider myself an angry person but, also, too many people in the realm of medicine had shown me visual "proof" that my pain was the result of structural defects. Dr. Sarno had to be wrong. He just had to be! But he wasn't.

After being repeatedly warned that I needed spinal surgery, all my pain disappeared after following Dr. Sarno's advice. In time, I was to learn that tension primarily derived from perfectionistic tendencies. Perfection being a most enraging personality characteristic that many perfectionists cannot consciously observe within themselves. They are also constantly angry, but they cannot sense it.

After three decades of pain, I went through the same healing process that tens of thousands before me had. After fully understanding Dr. Sarno's work, and **acting upon it**, my pain ended.

Hearing of my healing, people began writing, emailing, and calling me for help with their pain, anxiety, and other physical symptoms. I tried my best to help as many people as I could, but there were simply many more than I could respond to—so I began to write down how I healed. This book is for them—the suffering.

My first hope is that through this book, more people will learn of this healing process, will have their questions answered, and be moved to a deeper level of awareness; relieved of their pain and other symptoms—forever. My second hope is to be able to work with medical doctors and medical students to help them understand this process so they can integrate it into their practices, and educations.

Healing often takes much repetition of new information into the frontal association of the brain for full integration, since healing comes through deepening awareness. Therefore, many themes are purposefully reiterated throughout this book from many different angles—a manual for healing, if you will—or an act of extended meditation. The answer to healing most of our health problems is **knowledge**, and if it keeps getting offered, suffering will fade into the background, as good health and vitality replace it.

"If you bring forth what is within you, what you bring forth will save you. If you do not bring forth what is within you, what you do not bring forth will destroy you."
— *St. Thomas*, Verse 70

1

T M S—The Mindbody Syndrome

All truth passes through three stages. First, it is ridiculed, second it is violently opposed, and third, it is accepted as self-evident.

— Arthur Schopenhauer, German philosopher,
animal rights activist (1788-1860)

What Is TMS?

TMS was originally an acronym for Tension Myositis Syndrome, that through expanding awareness became the much more inclusive term, Tension Myoneural Syndrome, or Tension Psychogenic Syndrome, which includes acute and chronic nerve pain as well as muscular pain and a wide variety of other physical symptoms:

> **T** = Tension (the result of anger buried in the body)
> **M** = Myoneural (muscles and nerves)
> **S** = Syndrome (a collection of symptoms)

TMS is the cause of the current pandemic of back pain, neck pain, shoulder pain, migraine, hip pain, knee pain, wrist and hand pain, carpal tunnel pain, mouth and jaw pain, foot pain, fibromyalgia, chronic fatigue, so-called repetitive-stress "injuries," GERD and other stomach disorders, skin disorders, allergies, many eye problems, ulcerative colitis*—and an infinite variety of other pain equivalents. TMS is also the major cause of non-physical phenomena such as anxiety, addictions, and depression. The roots of our health problems are most often planted in childhood, through early separation anxiety—tension from trauma causing a lack of connection or attunement—forming a specific personality that is more conducive to these disorders.

It took many years of communicating with thousands of sufferers, but most importantly my own experience, to fully understand that it was the **loss of awareness**

---

* All these symptoms have a common tension-denominator, as we will discover throughout this book. They are designed by the brain to serve as **distractions**. From Andrew E. Weil, MD, "Ulcerative colitis (and its relative, Crohn's disease) is a complex problem with genetic, autoimmune, and psychosomatic components." [*Spontaneous Healing*, p. 233] There is a high reverse-correlation between smoking and ulcerative colitis. Smoking tends to reduce the symptoms of UC. But as Dr. Weil insightfully points out regarding TMS, "If you work from the premise that ulcerative colitis is psychosomatic, it does not take a great deal of intelligence to surmise that smoking is an effective outlet for stress and that if you shut that outlet, the stress is going to go somewhere else." [*Spontaneous Healing*, p. 90]

of negative emotions that was the culprit behind pain and most ill-health. Pain wasn't the only result of this lack of awareness either—other symptoms included fatigue, sleeplessness, sinus infections, digestive tract, and skin disorders. However, when I first read about this TMS concept, I thought it was absurd—totally preposterous—but I was wrong.

We have all been inundated with the false notion that our back pain, knee pain, foot pain, hip pain, repetitive stress syndrome—whatever—is due to either genetic flaws or a flaw in the human design—that sustained healing is not possible. This is not true. Some of the more common and fallacious back pain deceptions coming from the medical machine today are, "you need to strengthen your body's core to heal," or "you need to lose weight to heal," and the worst, "you need surgery within six weeks." If there's a problem, why isn't the surgery necessary now? These are archaic—antiquated concepts.

Most people believe, as I did, that they have "real" back injuries, and that they need "real" medical intervention. They have been conditioned by modern medicine's **faulty advice** to feel broken, and so they are broken, because they don't yet understand that unconscious activity causes "real" pain and very real symptoms. The mind and the body are one single unit—inseparable. What desperately desires to be known in the mind always reveals itself through the body.

> **Separation = Panic = Denial = Repression = Internal Conflict =**
> **Anger = Tension = Symptoms = Distractions = Messages**

The concept that tension is the primary cause of most chronic pain and many other symptoms has been clinically established by John E. Sarno, MD, former professor of rehabilitation medicine at the New York University School of Medicine. From Dr. Sarno's work we now understand that the demands of trying to maintain a false image of self in order to be accepted by, connect with, or control others, generates tremendous internal strife that is buried or repressed as rage—but is completely unfelt. It is this internalized energy that causes pain and a vast array of other symptoms, for a very specific purpose.

Pain and other chronic symptoms are physical manifestations of unresolved internal conflict. Symptoms surface as an instinctual mechanism for self-survival. They are messages from the inner self wanting to be heard, but ego takes center-stage, and hides the truth within the shadows of the unconscious mind: which is **the body.***

---

* "However, in the 1990s, neuroscientist Candice Pert, PhD, shared her discovery that the body, not the brain, is the subconscious mind, and that it communicates via neuropeptides, which are molecules that are produced by every thought we have. Pert discovered that thoughts have a biochemical component: While thoughts are real, neuropeptides are real, and the brain is real, what we think of as mind, is actually just the ego in disguise." [Alberto Villoldo: *The Four Insights: Wisdom, Power, and Grace of the Earthkeepers*, p. 164]

One purpose of these physical symptoms is to keep the individual focused on his physical body, and away from surfacing emotions.

Setting the Stage for Pain

Pain's stage was set when we were physically or emotionally abandoned by an important caretaker (or we feared we would be), when we were very young. The earlier in life the fear of abandonment is experienced, the greater the potential harm later in life—leading to more powerful and dangerous health problems. When unmet, this need for connection surfaces in the form of anxiety and tension, and the never-ending anger that results from trying to be all, take care of all, control all, and do all—to avoid any further rejection. It is the fear of separation that generates the greatest anger because it reminds us of our first rejection. The primal yearning for connection comes at great emotional and physical cost if the fears of separation are never eased or even recognized, and the **Self*** is never realized.

> Our most basic need in life is to **Tracordify**
> **Trac**(t) (Latin, "to pull")   **Cor** (Latin, "heart")
> *To pull another's heart toward ours—to reconnect—returning to wholeness*
> **Oneness ≡ Love**

We all need to feel connected and heard and accepted—flaws and all. We also need to express ourselves, our feelings, and our position in relationships—the position of our hearts known. When this basic need to tracordify is stifled, it generates tremendous amounts of rage within the unconscious—whether we are infants, children, or adults.

Experiences at an early age when we are completely or somewhat helpless and dependent on others can continue to replay throughout our life. Any stressful emotional or physical trigger like a twist or turn, birthday, retirement, or financial worry, may reactivate these old abandonment wounds and fuel the fires of **separation rage**, which then begin to manifest in the form of symptoms. You don't have a bad back (or hip, knees, or chronic fatigue disease), you are re-experiencing the fear and anger of the separation you experienced at a very early age—even from birth. Your symptoms, as experienced in adulthood, are simply an expression of how you have learned to handle the sensation of helplessness and anxiety.

---

* The self (Old English, "same, one's own person") is the individual as she currently sees herself in all her conflict with ego, but the **Self** (capitalized) is the ultimate archetype, who she truly is, beyond her ego and conflict.

These abandonment issues do not always need to be resolved in order to heal. Knowledge of them and how they are involved in the symptom process—and full belief in TMS—can free the person of suffering in the majority of cases.

As we will see, the emotional pain born of separation can be healed in a variety of ways, and built-up tension OR the build-up from the internal conflict can be reduced to healthy levels. But first, let's learn more about TMS itself.

What Is the Patho-Physiology of TMS?

The autonomic (involuntary) nervous system (ANS)* regulates organs such as the intestines, stomach, and heart, as well as a host of processes from the pace of breathing, to visual acuity, the rate and strength of cardiac contractions (heart rate), and the dilation and constriction of blood vessels. Emotions such as anxiety, guilt, depression, anger, rage, and resentment are processed through the ANS. Dr. Sarno has proven through decades of clinical work that when this repressed rage-tension reaches a certain level, the autonomic nervous system kicks in and produces physiologic alterations—various physical symptoms including pain—in the body. Simply put, when anger from various sources reaches a certain threshold, and deeply repressed emotions are forced to consciousness, the autonomic system creates a symptom. The energy from the conflict expresses itself through the body. Regarding pain, the cause is reduced bloodflow. In a fraction of a second you feel the pain of the emotions that you could never allow to surface—as the pain distracts your mind's eye from unwanted emotions.

Your boss, Jake Hass, informs you that you now have to begin working on Sundays; your knee begins to hurt. Your husband, Ira Tate, has left his shoes in the doorway again; your neck spasms.

If Jake's own boss is riding Jake's back for deadlines to meet, his back may begin to hurt. If Jake can no longer "stomach" his neighbor, Jake's ulcer may act up. Intellectually, Jake simply buries his conflict inside his body because he can't act out his violent or threatening thoughts. His body tells him exactly the level that something is bothering him—the more powerful the internal conflict, the more painful the physical distraction that is necessary. Thus, TMS is an avoidance mechanism, or distractionary technique—a deception by the brain to avoid facing sad, or socially unacceptable thoughts. Once the brain creates a pain or illness through the limbic system (the emotional center), the self no longer needs to face those pesky unwanted emotional shadows since there is now a more urgent need to attend to, which is the physical symptom itself.

---

* More detail on the autonomic nervous system's involvement in Chapter 2.

Dr. Sarno postulates that the pain is due to **mild oxygen deprivation** and he supports his clinical findings with rheumatology studies. He makes the case that decreased oxygen flow is the culprit by citing two separate studies, as well as his own clinical observations.[1] He has shown that TMS pain, as well as fibromyalgia and many other modern pain labels, are caused by this autonomic constriction of the oxygen-carrying blood vessels. He has also shown that fibromyalgia is merely a more severe form of myoneuralgia and is synonymous with TMS.

Pain—The Great Deception—Diverter of Awareness

TMS pain is a deception by the brain—an act of psychological subterfuge. Once in pain, the sufferer has no choice but to focus on his pain and away from his unconscious rage, along with the reason behind it. This is why Dr. Sarno believes TMS pain is a purposeful distraction created by the brain as a favor to the mindbody which enables the self to avoid having to think about darker, morbid, resentful, vengeful, and selfish thoughts. Life continues—emotions buried alive. When we don't get what we want, or don't like what we see in ourselves, the mind sets upon the flesh.

I have a friend who worked at the local emergency center and saw many people complaining of chest pains. These people most often were, or had recently been, under high-level stress. She told me on many occasions that when results came back negative for heart attack, they were sent home with the diagnosis of ischemia (from vasoconstriction, a reduction of the inflow of blood, which is TMS). They were under great relationship, financial, or work-related stress, and so their minds had utilized an avoidance mechanism as a distraction in order to glue their attention to their bodies. Anyone who has ever had chest pain knows that it will indeed hold one's attention. Things are not always great back at the farmhouse, and so repression is a highly efficient process for surviving tense family and job environments. It's quite ingenious of the mindbody to accomplish such a covert task.

Dr. Sarno says many people sit in his office and tell him that they would rather deal with their deeply hidden emotional conflict, than to suffer physically. The individual consciously feels that attending to her emotions would be easier than having severe symptoms, but her **ego** "thinks" otherwise. The emotional conflict is such that the ego understands it cannot handle it all. TMS symptoms are a kind of slap to the back of the head to say, "wake up, you're not truly happy with your situation." So the brain, being directed by ego, forces attention away from its own thoughts. For reasons of conscious image, the mind prioritizes physical pain over emotional pain, in the need to fit in or to silently rebel against societal and familial taboos and expectations.

Pain: An Emotional Barometer

Dr. Sarno believes that TMS is an emotional barometer that physically reveals the individual's hidden tension level. He has found that once the sufferer realizes that his pain is actually a distraction—and that he is fine physically—his pain more often disappears, because a distraction is only a distraction if one does not know it is a distraction. He calls this **knowledge therapy:** healing that occurs once the sufferer is told what is actually occurring within his mindbody—**he accepts this information** and integrates it deeply without a shadow of doubt, altering his body's physiology. Sometimes healing occurs instantly, and sometimes it's very difficult due to deeply ingrained beliefs. Dr. Sarno conducted a follow-up study in 1987 for a 3-year period of people who had gone through his TMS program utilizing knowledge therapy as the healing tool. The follow-up showed 88 percent were successful, 10 percent were improved, and 2 percent were unchanged.

Travis John is a dishwasher repairman who has communication problems with his 16-year-old son. He develops prolonged lower back pain, which he believes is from moving some equipment three years earlier. However, after he is given a book on TMS, he comes to understand that his pain is from relationship problems with his son, and in three weeks he is pain-free.* While the news that TMS is harmless is often enough to make the pain go away in most sufferers, it does not in all people, at all times, since modern medicine has thoroughly conditioned people to believe they are forever broken.

A tendency for many sufferers to deny TMS as the cause behind their pain and illness has currently forced knowledgeable mindbody doctors into a **dual-healing modality.** Some sufferers, who cannot be persuaded that their symptoms are coming from conflict within themselves, persistently demand medical intervention procedures from their physicians. Knowledgeable physicians have had to discreetly ascertain which mode of healing to pursue or to recommend to their patients. Will he be willing to look inward for the true cause of his pain and heal, or will he demand advanced medical procedures to focus outside of himself for something physical to blame—to maintain a false sense of image, denial, or control?

> Physical Pain Is Not "In the Head" of the Sufferer (unless it's a headache)

It's important to mention this early on because it is by far **the most misunderstood aspect in understanding pain.** Even after carefully explaining TMS in great detail, I still get that chicken-eyed stare from sufferers, and that all-too-caustic question, "So you're trying to tell me that my pain is all in my head?" No—it is not—it is very real. What is "in the head" is also in the body.

---

* This example was provided by TMS author Fred Amir.

The pain, stiffness, burning, pressure, numbness, tingling, and weakness were caused by mild oxygen deprivation in the muscles, nerves, or tendons involved in each case. In itself this was harmless. Although it could produce more severe pain than anything else I knew of in clinical medicine, you would not be left with residual damage when your symptoms disappeared.

— John E. Sarno, MD, *The Mindbody Prescription*[2]

I can personally attest to the reality and severity of TMS pain. It can knock you out when the blood withdraws to bury any surfacing conflict.

So Dr. Sarno has demonstrated that repression leads to emotions of anger and anxiety, which are the cause of most pain and other unpleasant symptoms. Many people have all the pain symptoms, but no pain. Some experience migraine tunnel vision but no headache, tingling and buzzing in legs, but no low back pain, foot drop, but no back pain or sciatica. One would think this is a blessing, but it frightens these people nonetheless, and the symptoms can interfere with their daily lives. In these cases the symptoms are still TMS, in that they serve the same distracting purpose, but fortunately there is no pain. The fear and focus remain, however.

So is the TMS pain real? Yes, it is. Does the TMS process begin in the mind? Yes, it does. Is TMS pain all in your head? No, it is not. It is a real physical mindbody phenomenon. The entire process is emotion-driven, and emotions are only experienced (felt) through the body.

What's in a Name?

For years, I had been using an all-encompassing term for TMS pain which I called tensionalgia. "Algia" simply means pain, and tension we know arises from psychological processes. It was a term that I felt made the complexity of the whole process more palpable. But tension causes more problems than just pain, and so TMS, or The Mindbody Syndrome, is a better all-encompassing acronym for describing the entire process. But as to not confuse people even more, the terms below all mean the same thing and are currently being interchangeably used:

TMS	= Tensionalgia
	= Tension Myositis Syndrome
	= Tension Myoneural Syndrome
	= Psychogenic Neural Pain Syndrome, PNPS
	= Tension Psychoneural Syndrome, TPS
	= **The Mindbody Syndrome**

Just Say No! Surgery: It Is Rarely a Solution

Pain is a mindbody manifestation. Any attempts to "cure" the pain via medical and therapeutic intervention merely prolong the pain and suffering. Although such interventions may temporarily relieve symptoms for various reasons, they usually fail in the longer term because pain must be addressed at its source, which is within **the shadows** of the unconscious mind. Heal the mind and the body will follow.

TMS is identified as a syndrome. A syndrome, as defined in Merriam-Webster, is "a group of signs and symptoms that occur together and characterize a particular abnormality." Thus, a syndrome is a multivariate problem, often difficult to qualify because of the complexity of the mindbody relationship.

Through decades of working with many thousands of patients, Dr. Sarno became acutely aware that surgery was not healing the vast majority of back pain sufferers: **it was never the solution.** So he wisely began looking for another reason behind the pain. It was obviously not due to the structural changes or so-called abnormalities of the spine and joints that were shown in medical imaging. "Obviously not" because sufferers' pain problems were not being corrected by surgeries and therapy, and because the wear and tear as seen on the x-rays and MRIs "couldn't in a million years produce the level of pain that people get with this syndrome (TMS)."[3] He concluded that disc degeneration, herniation, arthritis, and all the other hosts of spinal abnormalities were "normal abnormalities" and were nothing more than the body aging and transforming and healing itself as it had since the beginning of life's creation.* By its own nature, the body heals itself as a means of self-survival within reasonable time frames. As Dr. Sarno rightfully points out, even the femur, the largest bone in the human body heals within about six weeks. Why would a person's back pain take 30 months or 30 years to heal?

Deep massage, heat and ultrasound have been clinically shown to act as temporary relievers of pain, and are all known to temporarily increase local oxygen levels in the afflicted area—further evidence of the connection between pain and oxygen deficit. These therapies increase the bloodflow in the peripheral vasculature. The mere relief of pain for a short time may be all the soothing that some sufferers need to calm the fires of rage within them, allowing their pain to dissipate. But if their rage is too overwhelming, the therapy, massage, and manipulations will not be lasting—relief is short-lived, because the core cause, the emotional undercurrents of the pain, are never addressed. Over the years I was constantly having my back "put back in place" by chiropractors, but it was my **thought process** that needed resetting, never my back.

---

* Unfortunately, and for good reason, it must be clarified that in extreme cases a herniated disc or stenosis may cause pain. But this opens the door for anyone reading this to think that they are the extreme case when they are not as unique as they think they are. People often desperately need to feel that they are the extreme case in order to stay focused on their bodies. But this is the very purpose of the symptoms, **to keep them believing they are indeed somehow injured.** Physical symptoms provide a socially acceptable excuse or safe haven in which to bury socially unacceptable emotions and to avoid unwanted responsibilities, and so I write with extreme caution that those conditions can occasionally be a source of pain. After this cautionary statement, many people may now be breathing an unwarranted sigh of relief thinking they are that anomaly—stopping the healing process.

So, physical therapy and chiropractic manipulations should be discouraged if permanent healing is the goal.

Through understanding TMS and how pain manifests, the pain or fatigue sufferer **can** be relieved forever. Thus, there is no need for therapeutic intervention unless the pain is so severe that the person cannot live their daily life in the manner that they desire. I can personally attest to this after spending the majority of my life in pain, and now being pain-free. You, too, can be pain-free. But you must learn, and open your mind to something that your ego will certainly rebel against.

Herniated discs	→	Do not cause back pain
Degenerated discs	→	Do not cause back pain
Stenosis	→	Does not cause back pain
Arthritis	→	Does not cause back pain*

MRI Technology: The Double-Edged Sword of Damocles

The presence of a disc abnormality is a stumbling block to many patients who are not aware that this is a demonstration of the cleverness and ingenuity of the mind when it wishes to create a physical distraction. The mind is aware of everything that goes on in the body, including the site of herniated discs, meniscus tears in the knee joints, and tears of the rotator cuff at the shoulder… experience makes it clear that the brain will initiate TMS pain where a structural abnormality exists, the better to impress you and more firmly keep your attention on your body, just as it will induce pain at the site of an old injury.
— John E. Sarno, MD, *The Mindbody Prescription*[4]

Advanced technologies that allow us to look more deeply into the body have become a double-edged sword. MRI technology with its tremendous ability to look at miniscule changes inside the body has indeed improved countless lives through more accurate diagnoses. However, on the other edge of the blade, these new imaging procedures are also revealing natural wear and tear that has always existed. The catastrophe is that scientists are now routinely and erroneously attributing pain to these sites. But the degeneration seen in these discs and joints is normal. It can be seen beginning in most everyone by the late teens or early twenties.

As Rutherford D. Rogers, noted Yale librarian stated, "We're drowning in information and starving for knowledge."[5] A radiologist may see a tear or arthritic change in the back or knee or shoulder and by default assume that the pain is from that change because the pain is sometimes located within those areas.

This is yet another major stumbling block in understanding and believing that TMS exists, and in healing. Dr. Sarno refers to this hurdle as "the clever mind," knowing

---

* Some types of arthritis are very painful, such as gout and rheumatoid arthritis. The type I refer to here is post traumatic arthritis, PTA, or arthritis from aging.

where all the physiological changes have occurred within the body. The old football player and his "trick" knee: the great error in thought. His knee only bothers him when he doesn't want to do something, if he hates his situation, or if his anger suddenly rises to consciousness. He has been conditioned to believe that there is an inherent weakness there at that site that causes him pain, and so it often does, on and off in perpetuity. When we are truly injured, our bodies heal.* The old injury site is merely a trigger for the pain. The brain chooses to focus on that site because it remembers there was once a problem there, and so it is now an anticipated and socially acceptable safe haven for anxiety and tension to hide—whenever needed.

When I hear people say that their back pain is due to arthritis, it never fails to make me shake my head and smile because I also once believed this to be true, as my pain often found the arthritis in my back and hip and ankle. I now know this is not true.

Fortunately for millions of pain sufferers, Dr. Sarno has discovered that repressed emotion is most often the cause behind chronic pain and is now healing many, many people, while many other physicians, surgeons, and therapists "studiously ignore" his work. After all, there is nothing lucrative in skipping surgery and therapy and drugs. There's no money to be made in merely changing beliefs. What incentive does a physician have to accept Dr. Sarno's clinical findings? It all depends on his or her motive for becoming a healer. A primary reason the truth of TMS is ignored by many within the medical industry is that of the grueling hours spent studying pain from the wrong direction. It's not always easy to admit having made a mistake, ego will rarely allow it. Modern medicine has tragically taken the patient out of the healing equation because many doctors want quick mon$y and many patients want **quick avoidance-fixes**. It's a perfect match for failure.

Where Does TMS Occur?

Tension can find its way into any and every system of the mindbody; however, TMS tension as originally characterized by Dr. Sarno focuses on three types of soft tissue: muscles, nerves, and/or tendons.[6] Any one or any combination of these may be involved. If pain is present in multiple areas, TMS is labeled as fibromyalgia or myofascial pain syndrome (MPS).†

TMS pain currently strikes most often in the lower back, and leg pain is often involved. Two TMS examples, currently gaining popularity, are foot pain neuropathy

---

* Some nerves and cartilage cannot regenerate, but the pain eventually ends with a dead nerve as well as with non-regenerative cartilage—the pain does not continue for years.

† Fibromyalgia sufferers have pain in more localities and have higher tendencies toward characteristics of insomnia and chronic fatigue than most TMS sufferers. However, many patients Dr. Sarno has seen that have been previously diagnosed with fibromyalgia have been treated by him and recovered completely. Fibromyalgia is TMS—a mindbody myoneural syndrome.

and repetitive stress injuries (RSI), such as carpal tunnel syndrome. Both are tension-based, **tension-induced hypoxia** (hypoxia being lack of oxygen), and can be "cured" through mindbody healing.

Hidden tension can strike any organ in the body, from the heart to the epidermis; and any system in the body, from the immune to the digestive systems. Why tension chooses to express or appear in a particular area is not fully understood; however, what we do know is that:

- Tension often hides in old injuries or sites of herniation, and arthritic areas and sites of disc narrowing (foraminal stenosis).
- TMS can affect an area where there is no visual physical damage or wear and tear, but where it has been suggested the body is vulnerable to problems.
- The area or system involved often has symbolic connotations. I can't "stomach" the workload given me, so my ulcer acts up.

The Ulcer

Ulcers were the first identified stress-related disorder. Dr. Sarno commented, in *Healing Back Pain*, about an article posing the question, "Where Have All the Ulcers Gone?" We just don't hear much about ulcers anymore. At one time, ulcers were believed to be the result of actual physical/structural defects in the stomach, just as in the case of back pain today. However, over the years, the consensus of **collective thinking** began to understand that ulcers were directly caused by tension from stress—"**stension**." Ulcers then began to fade from the forefront once society came to understand their purpose. The distraction no longer worked as well.

Simply put, the areas afflicted by tension will always be **whatever is in vogue—popularized and focused on at any time in society**, defined as THE new fashionable disorder. This is the term of "in vogue" (voguer, Old French, "to sway"). Importantly, however, the body areas that are being afflicted must first be popularly preordained. Only tomorrow knows how today's thoughts will manifest physically—because the people haven't decided what to worry about yet.

Drug companies, medical supply companies, and many doctors are among the medical field's pushers that are seducing the next need for the next area to be afflicted, by suggesting to people what they will need to be well. If one watches enough television commercials, he will likely begin requesting more back pain medicine, anti-depression medicine, acid reflux medicine, anti-asthma medicine, peripheral artery disease medicine, harder mattresses, softer mattresses, blood pressure medicine, dry eye medicine, joint renewal products, cholesterol medicine, on and on ad naseum (I would add nausea medicine as well). The dire warnings in these commercials are planting the idea into the collective unconscious, targeting consumers' fears, and creating the next place of concern for the externalization of unconscious rage. This suggestive process is exacerbated by the individual's family beliefs, as well as self-doubt, and always by the most basic need to pull others back to self. To a worrier, a planner, a controller, a perfectionistic personality, there is a compulsion to always be ready to head-off the next disaster by pushing ahead of the light. Since worrying warriors often believe that they can worry a problem away, they can take an external suggestion and run with it, or in the case of TMS pain, lie down with it.

Sadly, the medical industry spends its time, effort, and money attacking the symptoms and not the source (emotions). Disorders will continue to pop up to hold the attention of people who cannot reduce their tension—the natural byproduct of their personalities.

Chicken Little or a Little Chicken?

After thousands of years of humankind having no recorded pandemic of back, knee, hand, and foot problems, societies around the world are now being inundated with the concept that the spine and limbs are now crumbling. It's like Chicken Little exclaiming the "sky is falling" in such a manner that people have begun to buy umbrellas. Even though body and mind are one, the body always follows the mind's lead. If the mind is headed in the wrong direction, the body will be as well, because the body is the passenger on the train of life and the brain is the conductor.

As noted, the new great horizon for psychosomatic response appears to be repetitive stress injuries (RSI) such as carpal tunnel syndrome and foot pain. It is currently being suggested that after many thousands of years of working with our hands, these same hands are suddenly failing us. The concept would be laughable if it weren't so pathetic. I read a report a few years back that correlated RSI with the rise of computer use. It was suggested in the report that there were dramatic increases in RSI because people now sit and work at computers. But what happened when people sat for eight to ten hours at a typewriter? A typewriter must have been much harder on the wrists and hands than a modern keyboard. But there was no epidemic of repetitive stress injury then. The entire notion is erroneous. *Ladies and gentlemen across the lands, there's nothing wrong with your feet and hands.*

Paradoxically, it is society's diminished use of the wrist and hands and backs that is a large part of the problem. Society has become more sedentary. This inactivity allows tension to rise. People sit more and are less active with their backs and hands and feet, which further restrict bloodflow, allowing tension to slither into the immobilized areas as **unwanted emotions seek shadows.**

The next popular body area or system that tensionalgia may attack may be a moot point. In Dr. Sarno's words, "It is my impression that virtually any organ or system in the body can be used by the mind as a defense mechanism against repressed emotionality."[7] So, it will be whatever the guy next to you has, since we all long to be connected. It will be whatever area is being legitimized by the medical machinery and perpetuated by society's ignorance and compliance.* Until societies understand that the body's health is directed by the individual's history, thoughts, and emotional processes, individuals worldwide will become increasingly crippled within recurring healthcare catastrophes.

Fortunately, today heralds a new era of **quantum healing.** Quantum healing is simply "healing from within," using the body's own natural healing capabilities. It is being popularized and practiced successfully by physicians: Deepak Chopra, John Sarno, Andrew Weil, Emmett Miller, David Schechter, Don Colbert, Mehmet Oz, Marc Sopher, and Clancy McKenzie, among others. Sadly, where there is ego and mon$y involved, there will always be deep pockets of apathy and steadfast resistance.

How Does TMS Work?

Matilda—There's a tornado spotted nearby. Matilda begins to panic from the news, but to visibly show panic at the level of fear she's experiencing is not acceptable to her. She unwittingly, reflexively, turns her fear inward—represses it. The autonomic function of the accommodating brain then constricts a blood vessel in her brain, which causes a severe headache (distraction). This pain enables her to avoid facing her hysterical fear. This all happens automatically. It can happen very quickly; and may leave when the tension, or tornado passes. The blood vessels can constrict as fast as a human can blush when embarrassed. She doesn't deny or ignore her fear, she doesn't know she has it or fully understand its magnitude; she has successfully repressed it due to the automatic nature of repression. The automatic feature of the TMS process is another major hurdle for many in the understanding of how pain occurs.†

Sadly, if unexpressed emotion is mentioned as the culprit behind their pain, many sufferers see this as a weakness in themselves. They don't realize that they are repressing, and that they have no direct control over it. Therefore, it's only a weakness to the extent that the individual does not know that there is a mindbody process constantly occurring within him. On the contrary, controlling anxiety, panic, and all unwanted emotion is a great strength, not a weakness. It is much easier to act out aggression than it is to reason it out or to intellectualize it away.

---

* "Lipton (Bruce Lipton, PhD, cell biologist) links the current high incidence of colon and rectal cancer with the fact that there is a lot of information around that says there is a high incidence of colon and rectal cancer. It's a case of self-fulfilling prophecy." [Anna Spencer, PhD, "Cell Consciousness—Proves Mind over Matter," Infinity Institute]
† Most people cannot consciously control constriction of blood vessels, or any of the other processes of the autonomic nervous system. Autonomic functions are mostly reflexive by nature, without conscious awareness.

I have heard it said that people get stress-induced pain because they can't cope. It is quite the opposite; TMS occurs because they cope too well.
— John E. Sarno, MD, *Healing Back Pain*[8]

Estefania—Estefania has a dinner to prepare but her children are yelling and screaming and jumping all over and calling to her, "mOm, Mom, moM, MOM, MAAAWWM!!" She loves her children more than her own life, but their demands of her enrages her so intensely that she could never follow through with what she is unconsciously thinking about doing to them (through her undeveloped-self). She could NEVER harm them because of her love for them, and so—she over copes and freezes emotionally, as her brain does her, and her kids, a favor by narrowing down a blood vessel carrying oxygen to her lower back, or hands or neck. This creates a painful distraction from her **unthinkable** thoughts. TMS pain arrives to save the day. The unthinkable can never become thinkable, and so TMS exists as a shield between true-self and idealized-self, as well as between mother and child. So, Estefania internalizes the energy created through the repression of her true desires, and it manifests physically in her body as a necessary diversion. The symptom indirectly tells her how she really feels inside, because she is unable to recognize it directly.

> Therefore, TMS is an early warning alert that imminent danger may be ahead. The emotions have become so overwhelming that they threaten to erupt into consciousness. But societal values do not allow people to act out their aggression, so the mindbody goes into what I have called **hyper-flight**, or **freeze**. In order to survive, the sufferer over-adapts—freezes—in order to obey or "be good." This safety mechanism, which allows for self-image to be maintained and for value systems to remain intact while rage is being automatically compartmentalized, is repression. **Repression is a part of the freeze response**, regarding the fight/flight/freeze survival mechanism. It is an invaluable tool in human survival when it's not unknowingly abused.

What Does TMS Feel Like?

From those who have suffered, and have healed, I've heard adjectives, nouns, and verbs such as: hell, burning, tingling, thumping, stiffness, electrical snapping, coldness, buzzing, stabbing, pins and needles, numbness, pressure, throbbing, weakness, and of course, painful.

When she can finally understand that TMS pain is her brain's way of saying, **look over here**, then she will truly understand and will begin to heal, just as I healed, as have tens of thousands of others who also understood how the mind and body work in tandem to create chronic pain and illness, both of which serve as the **shadow's messengers**.

That Which We Call a Rose by any Other Name Would Smell as *Sour*

Words like rage and anger and anxiety and guilt and resentment are nothing more than labels. It has been estimated that there are approximately 600 shades of emotions that people can experience. However, the mindbody doesn't understand labels, it only understands physical effects. Feelings are different from emotions in that they are born of cognitive functions and are considered evaluating functions such as weighing different values subjectively, based on what is, or is not, important. Emotions distinctively belong to our most primal and mysterious experiences and are physiological effects. These emotions like rage and anxiety and happiness generate energy within the body; so there are truly only two types of emotions: it is either a good one or a bad one, with varying shades of each color. Symptoms occur due to an energy overload of the more negative and darkest emotions. But from where do these negative emotions come? They come from negative thoughts.

TMS occurs within the freeze side (or hyper-flight) of the fight/flight/freeze survival response mechanism. At some point earlier in the individual's life, he survived a perceived threat, embarrassment, or even shame, by not fighting to express himself—or was unable to escape his situation due to helplessness. He then necessarily freezes to avoid the emotional pain—hardwiring false memories that are forever stored in his survival brain unless properly discharged—or recognized. His brain now has a new procedural conditioned response on how to handle future threatening scenarios because he feels continually helpless—with the help of the medical industry. The problem is that it is a false, conditioned response—not necessary. The individual suffering from any host of chronic symptoms has never purged an early perceived trauma from his memory bank. With each new conflict or trauma throughout his life, he screens the new threat through his false or corrupted memory and re-experiences helplessness—forever stuck in his own past, reacting the same way each time, as with OCD.

> If a gazelle escapes the attack of a lion, the next time a lion attacks, it had better do exactly what it did to survive the first time. This mechanism helps us survive more often than not.
>
> — Clancy McKenzie, MD, author of *Babies Need Mothers*

A lack of expression or of being heard results in an internalization of energy through this freeze mechanism and an interesting personality is born. **This is the genesis of TMS.** If self internalizes—turns emotions inward—or even "off" to persevere: then self will default to freeze repeatedly as a mechanism of survival (more on this in Chapter 2). This is hyper-adapting or **hyper-coping.** This is one way a TMSer is created. The other way a TMSer is created is if two TMSers breed.

So—without expressing self there is no release valve for the energy to dissipate, and the reservoir fills until it finally overflows into the body as symptoms, or more precisely, until the body can no longer contain the increase in energy.

REPRESSION → ENERGY INCREASE → IMBALANCE → SYMPTOMS

Repression generates potential energy. If enough energy is pent-up, it will begin to create havoc within the mindbody as the system futilely attempts to maintain homeostasis. As we will later see, increased physical activity reduces the fear of pain, as well as the potential energy held in the mindbody as tension.

Those Sons-of-a Disc—Spinal Scapegoats

It has been my experience that herniated disc material is rarely responsible for pain or any other neurological symptoms.... My conclusion that most disc herniations are harmless is based on 17 years of treating such patients* with a high degree of success, leading to the impression that the extruded material is not hurting anything; it's just there.

— John E. Sarno, MD, *Healing Back Pain*[9]

The Battle of the Bulge

There is no subject more controversial in the explanation of back pain than herniated discs. We know from several well-researched studies that most people have herniated, degenerated discs and often spinal narrowing, and have no pain. But in many cases these "normal abnormalities" are deemed to be causing the pain, even if the pain is nowhere near the site of the abnormality.

Why does a disc bulge or herniate? What is nature's purpose for a spinal disc? The logical explanation would be to keep the individual from experiencing pain from bone moving against bone and to give added flexibility to the spine for survival purposes. But "so what" if these discs bulge, or herniate, or rupture? Should we then conclude that the individual's pain is coming from these changes? We should not. Isn't this what the disc is supposed to do? To police the spine—bulge and protect? But what is normal bulging or "OK/okay" bulging? The entire process can be a confusing dilemma unless you look closely at the work of Dr. Sarno and begin to see that these herniations are usually incidental findings on MRI images. But the patients remain confused because the majority of physicians routinely attribute the pain to the appearance of bulging or ruptured discs.

Dr. Sarno points out in *Healing Back Pain* that a disc rupture is more commonly referred to as a herniation. The bulge is a herniation is a rupture. So they are one and the same, except that sometimes the pulpy material contained within the spinal disc

---

* It has been 18 years since the publication of the above statement—over 35 years of clinical experience—that has strongly reinforced Dr. Sarno's position that **disc material rarely causes pain**, and that the disc material is simply "there."

will simply bulge out the disc wall and sometimes it will break through the disc wall. So, can we assume then that it is only when the disc is fragmented that pain will ensue? Not necessarily. Not if it isn't compressing a nerve, and we know that a nerve cannot be compressed or it will "stop transmitting pain messages after a short time."[10] The same holds true for knee or shoulder abnormalities, etc. A nerve interfered with will cause more than pain, and the "more than pain" is a lack of pain ...*and the yin chases the yang... as this becomes that....* People are healing by the masses from their pain—armed with the knowledge of the TMS process, regardless of bulges and changes in the integrity and structure of the spine and joints.

The discs themselves are normally described as being similar to jelly-filled donuts, or a tube of toothpaste, that when compressed too hard, can fragment, which would certainly cause pain, wouldn't it? Not necessarily.

Ethan

Andrew Weil, MD, describes a patient of his, Ethan, in his book *Spontaneous Healing*. Ethan was suffering from such severe back pain and was so heavily medicated that Dr. Weil had trouble conversing with him. Ethan's "MRI showed two ruptured discs, one of them 'shattered into multiple fragments'" and unfortunately, and naturally, his orthopedist urged immediate surgery. However, in order to avoid surgery, Dr. Weil recommended that Ethan read Dr. Sarno's *Healing Back Pain*, but Ethan didn't want to hear "anything about his problem being psychosomatic."[11] Ethan opted for a second opinion. Again, the imaging revealed a "shattered disc," and immediate surgery was, again, recommended.

However, Ethan then wisely decided to forego the surgery and read *Healing Back Pain*. He reported, "Dr. Sarno presented a very compelling analysis and argument."[12] While Ethan's surgeon pressed for surgery, Ethan reflected on Dr. Sarno's statement that "herniated discs by themselves do not cause pain" and he eventually went to see Dr. Sarno.

Ethan remarked later, "Sarno wasn't very interested in the MRI... only in the results of muscle testing in the leg, which showed no nerve dysfunction. He did a quick physical exam and told me it was a clear case of TMS, that I should get off the painkillers because I didn't need them. And he told me I would definitely get better and would be playing basketball again. All I had to do was accept his diagnosis."[13]

During Sarno's evening lecture, Ethan's pain "subsided," and around dinnertime, he had no pain despite having a ruptured/shattered/fragmented disc. Dr. Sarno advised Ethan to stop physical therapy, but like many of us who experienced TMS healing, Ethan was unable to abruptly give up some sort of physical treatment, so he sought out an osteopath who told him Sarno was only partially correct—that he still needed physical therapy. Ethan decided not to go to therapy, as his pain lessened overnight after having a dream where the osteopath was arguing with Sarno over physical therapy.

When the diagnosis of TMS is accepted, the symptoms often begin to move around the body as the brain frantically tries to find another place in the body that the brain can focus on. Later, Ethan's brain attempted to make him think he was getting an ulcer in his stomach, but he recognized it as TMS and it, too, went away.

Ethan was also adhering to Dr. Sarno's advice of perusing the possible psychological factors involved in the production of his pain, which he realized was mainly his failing marriage. A month later his pain was gone and he returned to lifting weights and playing basketball "without worries."

Now, Ethan's brother is a physician, who of course does not believe that Ethan's pain left from TMS healing. Ethan's brother believed—as many doctors do—that it was the cortisone injection that relieved his pain. But it was not. It was Ethan's recognition and acceptance that his pain was from the stress of school, work, and relationship. He has remained pain-free despite having a shattered disc.

So do ruptured, shattered, and herniated discs cause pain? Not necessarily. The extruded disc material is often simply "there."

Dr. Weil describes listening to a lecturer at the *North American Academy of Musculoskeletal Pain* at which Weil was the keynote speaker. The lecturer described the current data on the lack of correlation between back pain and the abnormalities as seen on MRIs and x-rays. Weil states, "He showed x-rays and scans of patients that looked so awful you could not believe these people could stand or walk, yet they were free of pain and had normal mobility. In other cases, people were immobilized by pain, yet their spines looked normal. To my mind, all of this information was consistent with Dr. Sarno's philosophy."[14]

Abnormality Shmabnormality

In my experience structural abnormalities of the spine rarely cause back pain.
— John E. Sarno, MD, *Healing Back Pain*[15]

Its been well-documented that arthritis, bulging discs, herniated discs, degenerated discs actually don't cause pain. They're not a source of pain.
— David Hanscom, MD, orthopedic spine surgeon[16]

> The **ruptured** or **prolapsed** disc will rarely "pinch a nerve." If it did so, it would render the nerve painless through "objective numbness," which is the absence of pain during examination.
> Discs cannot **slip**, and so pain cannot come from a slipped disc.*

---

* "The popular term 'slipped disc' is misleading, as an intervertebral disc, being tightly sandwiched between two vertebrae to which the disc is attached, cannot actually 'slip,' 'slide,' or even get 'out of place.' The disc is actually grown together with the adjacent vertebrae and can be squeezed, stretched

Degeneration of the disc (most especially the last intervertebral disc) "is more or less degenerated in most people by the age of **twenty**."[17] So this, too, would rarely be the cause of pain.

Stenosis is the narrowing of the spinal canal, often from the buildup of bone called osteophytes. This, too, rarely causes pain but is often attributed as the factor in the manifestation of pain. Dr. Sarno writes, "My reaction to this abnormality is based on experience with patients. Most of those I have seen, regardless of age, were found to have TMS, which allowed me to disregard the x-ray diagnosis."[18]

The Four Phases of TMS—Timing of the Symptoms

Phase 1: Acute Threshold TMS:
Current high tension levels—No Physical Incident, Acute Rapid Onset.

This is the most easily understood manifestation of tension, which is characterized by sudden onslaught of pain during times of overstimulation and high anxiety, rejection, or personal loss (separation), with no apparent physical trigger for the initiation of the pain.

Phase 2: Blood in the Water TMS:
Current high tension levels—Physical Trigger Involved with Lingering Pain.

This is pain resulting from a supposed "injury" during frustrating or anxiety-filled time periods or times of financial insecurity. The individual lifts or bends or pulls and there is a sudden sharp pain as the bloodflow is suddenly cut off. This is blood-in-the-water-TMS, as emotions desperately seek an outlet like a shark seeks blood. The rage is so intense that the emotions are trolling for opportunity—an outlet—an **anger salt-lick**. Any movement deemed to be harmful to the body allows for anxiety and anger to come pouring out of the body. This TMS manifestation often results from conditioning through foolish admonitions and warnings "to be careful."

Phase 3: Back-door TMS:
Current high tension levels—Old Injury Seemingly Resurfaces.

This is characterized by sudden pain that revisits an old injury site. The area of pain is often the site of an injury that occurred many years ago. This is **back-door** TMS. It creates the illusion that somehow the old injury has suddenly resurfaced: but that particular injury has long since healed. This enables the mind to focus on the old injury as a possible cause for the pain, and leads the sufferer away from what is emotionally bothering him. The pain is merely hiding in the old injury site, since the cynical mind

---

and twisted, all in small degrees. It can also be torn, ripped, herniated, and degenerated, but it cannot 'slip.' The term 'slipped disc' may be harmful as it leads to a false idea of what is happening and therefore of the likely outcome." [Source: Wikipedia]

never forgets. This phase of TMS often manifests by moving around to other areas as the pain yearns for attention. The movement of the pain is elusive, in that, it often fools people into believing they have rid themselves of TMS, but that a brand new "real injury" has appeared. But it is only the brain seeking a new place to fear.

This phase of TMS found me in my severely arthritic ankle after I was informed that I "should be in great pain." The body holds all past images in the cells as memory.

Phase 4: After-the-Storm TMS:
Pain following a period of high tension levels—The Storm after the Calm.

This is the **most common manifestation** of TMS and follows periods of high tension, personal loss, or goal-achievement. This timing of TMS waits until everything has calmed down. The stressful period is over—the soldier has been removed from the battlefield. During the downtime (after prolonged periods of stress) this expression of TMS reveals the emotions that had been pushed aside, emotions that were previously compartmentalized into the body in order to persevere through the stressful period. Emotions lie in wait for opportune moments, which downtime provides. Pain, or depression, in this appearance can follow "on the heels" of good news or after successful accomplishment. Phase 4 found me after a very long and stressful period ended.

> There are not different "categorical types" of TMS, only varying phases or times in which tension can manifest and incarnate.

How Long Will It Take to Go Away?

A person suffering from chronic pain cannot buy his pain away with surgery or cortisone shots or physical therapy. His pain will only leave him when he finally **learns** it away or processes it away. I have only met a few who have been healed through the "simple" knowledge of the TMS process. The reasons for this are varied and complex and they all have to do with lingering doubt in the process. But first, what is a reasonable time frame for the pain to go away?

From the thousand people, or so, I've communicated with regarding TMS, it has taken an average of about five months to two years to heal. Mindbody physician Marc Sopher believes that it is highly variable but takes about 2 to 6 months, on average. Holding fast to a certain time frame only prolongs the healing time. Asking a doctor how long something will take to heal is like asking him how hard you will try, or how strong your beliefs and fears are. He has no idea of your unconscious motivations for success or failure because you don't either. My own healing took approximately 15 months, but healing can occur in just a few hours. It's difficult to recall exact time frames when the pain finally ceases because it's only when one stops focusing on the pain that the pain finally leaves. The pain levels also become very erratic toward the end, as it waxes and wanes—and finally disappears.

Dr. Sarno wrote in *Healing Back Pain* that, "experience has shown that the majority will have resolution of most of their symptoms in two to six weeks after the lectures."[19] The lectures on the TMS process follow the examination by Dr. Sarno, and on occasion, precede further follow-up if the patient hasn't progressed satisfactorily.

I believe that a primary reason some people don't heal within normal time frames or simple knowledge therapy is that there is a power of authority missing in their diagnosis of TMS. That is, they have not been "rubber stamped" with the TMS mark on their foreheads by a TMS expert, and so they **doubt** whether they actually have it, and so pain lingers. Visiting a mindbody physician can expedite recovery because it raises confidence by adding authority to the information, and affords them a desperately needed dose of compassion. Whatever people in authoritative positions say is more likely to be powerfully integrated into the unconscious process.

Would You Like Some More Real Examples, Billy? Sure Ya Would.

Zoltan has had three back surgeries. He doesn't believe that tension is causing his back pain of 40 years. He reluctantly reads *Healing Back Pain* and in two weeks he is pain-free.

Tiberius is a young boy who experiences knee pain before every track meet. His physician tells him he has "tendonitis," but this was never true. He suffers from TMS due to unconscious self-imposed pressures to "do well," and to never fail in the eyes of others. His anger (a social reaction to his fear) surfaces in the form of knee pain to distract his mind's eye. TMS is explained to him, he listens, he believes, and his pain never returns.

On rare occasions, people visit TMS-trained physicians but still don't heal within reasonable time frames. This may be because people need to "be heard," or tracordify. They may sense that the physician is not listening to them. People who don't cry or won't cry, or were taught as children not to cry, are far more susceptible to pain and disease because self-expression has been stifled. Repression isolates self and is a form of self-rejection. When a physician arrives late to see a patient, and then does not listen to her, appears apathetic, and spends only seven minutes with her, he exacerbates an existing problem. A listening ear and an open heart are some of the most valuable tools a physician can carry in his medical bag.

The opposite of repression is **expression**. So talking to a doctor about our thoughts, or anyone who will listen and understand and allow us to "be heard," is a great emotional catharsis (catharsis, Greek, defined as "cleansing"). Studies like James Pennebaker's at Southern Methodist University[20] confirm this. From Pennebaker's book, *Opening Up: The Healing Power of Confiding in Others*, "The observations of these people, and everyone else who participated in these studies, are almost breathtaking. They are telling us that our thought processes can heal."[21] Fear of the pain, and elevated levels of hidden anxiety, can further delay healing, and are symptoms of a deeper need.

> *Pain is, has been and always will be a symptom. If it becomes severe and chronic, it is because that which is causing it is severe and has gone unrecognized. Chronicity, in the case of these pain syndromes, is a function of faulty diagnosis.*
> — John E. Sarno, MD, *Healing Back Pain*[22]

Who Gets TMS? Or Better Yet, Who Doesn't?

I have never met anyone who has not had a mindbody-related problem. Everybody who lives in a modern society experiences emotional overload and pays a price for it psychologically, and by default, physically. I've spoken with thousands of people who have agreed with the concept of TMS; however, only a handful felt that it related to them. To most, it is always the "other person" that carries emotional baggage and has psychosomatic responses.* Ironically, it is these people who are exhibiting some of the most neurotic behavior. Remember, it's the repression that is the underlying cause of the physical manifestations. Thus, reason would dictate that sufferers who feel they are beyond emotional responses are the ones who are burying their feelings the most deeply since, as sentient beings, we all generate emotions. We all have fears and therefore anger. We behave in odd ways in order to cope with that which we fear. The more phobic and anxious she is, the more prone she is to tension-related symptoms, and the more likely she is to suffer from pain, since anxiety is simply unexpressed anger.

So who gets TMS? The answer is everybody. No one individual can express all that he feels all the time and so repression is inevitable. For this reason, Dr. Sarno calls TMS a "cradle-to-grave disorder"[23] because it can affect any age group from very young children to older adults. A survey he conducted in 1982 found that 77 percent of his patients with TMS were between the ages of 30 and 60. Only four percent were in their seventies. Now if pain is caused from structural decay within the musculoskeletal system, why aren't most of the back pain patients in their 70s, 80s, and 90s? The older a person gets the less likely he will be generating as much tension as he did in what Dr. Sarno calls the "years of responsibility," or "middle life."[24] Within these years there is more stress regarding family and career and relationship. But this isn't always the case. TMS respects no age. In fact, TMS quite often occurs because people **are** aging. Aging is one of the most enraging thoughts because it is the recognition that there will soon be the ultimate separation.

---

* Many mindbody insiders feel that Georg Walther Groddeck, MD, began the movement of psychosomatic enlightenment but Martin Charcot, Franz Alexander, and Josef Breuer, among others, were certainly major contributors in their own right. No matter how deep the original roots are buried, it was O. Spurgeon English, MD, and Edward Weiss, MD, who initiated the modern movement in the 1940s with a book called *Psychosomatic Medicine*.

The Myth of Growing Pains

Children can and do become very anxious and experience a wide variety of symptoms because they are dependent on others—their world is more confusing and frightening, and therefore enraging to them. What was once called growing pains in the legs and arms of children we now know is TMS from anxiety-induced reduction in bloodflow.

Ultimately, it comes down to the psyche or personality of the individual. TMS is primarily personality-driven, so its intensity depends on many factors in the individual's personal life. Normally a pain such as a headache, cramping, or a sore foot or shoulder will resolve itself quickly. Severe forms of TMS, however, can be life-altering and debilitating. It can occur after tragedy or separation, or fear of separation, and although it may appear to be genetic, its effects run through family lines as a result of environmental influences, or conditioned responses.

Through conversations with them, Dr. Sarno discovered that many TMS sufferers were perfectionists, worriers, or highly driven people who were unknowingly repressing unwanted emotions. This personality type experiences TMS in its most severe chronic forms—and has been referred to as a **Type T** personality by modern quantum healers, T referring to tension.* Even though all people everywhere suffer from psychosomatic pains and illness, the Type T is the perfect paragon of the pain process (PPPP).

Dr. Sarno's Cure

Dr. Sarno's treatment program for healing from chronic pain "rests on two pillars:"

1. The acquisition of knowledge, of insight into the nature of the disorder;
2. The ability to act on that knowledge and thereby change the brain's behavior.[25]

He states that: "the most important (but most difficult) thing that patients must do is to resume all physical activity, including the most vigorous."[26] I found this to be the sine qua non in my own recovery process. It also flies in the face of everything that many doctors are telling sufferers not to do when they have back and joint pain. If one is to heal from pain, he must forget everything he has been taught regarding

---

* Note, that while psychologist Frank Farley at Temple University, former president of the *American Psychological Association,* had earlier defined the personality characteristic of Type T as a risk-taker, it is the complete opposite of the Type T characterization used in this writing and by current TMS physicians. Farley had coined the usage of "T" to stand for "thrill seeker personality," or a thrill-seeking personality type with high energy levels, and a sense that they alone control their own destinies. The usage of the letter "T" regarding mindbody in this book, is diametrically opposite to Farley's earlier characterization.

healing and protecting his body or back. By protecting, I mean accommodating, or trying to sit, walk, bend, or sleep a certain way—we are not frail objects.

> *In the long run, fear and the preoccupation with physical restrictions are more effective as a psychological defense than pain.*
>
> — John E. Sarno, MD, *Healing Back Pain*[27]

I hope you understood the above quote because it is critical to healing. Your **fear of activity** because you are afraid of your pain keeps you more crippled than the actual sensation of the pain itself. Walking with a limp, the fear of lifting something, or sitting certain ways to avoid pain, instills deeply in the mind that there is a structural problem within the body itself. These are all **accommodations** to the pain, which keep the fear of structural defects alive, and the pain ongoing. In healing, a prime requisite is in the repudiation of the structural diagnosis, because this will begin to reduce the fear of hurting yourself. If she cannot get to the point of understanding and believing at a very deep level that her body is not falling apart, she will not be able to move to the next level of healing. Her trips to the chiropractor will increase, her drug intake will increase, and her pain will continue.

Another aspect of Dr. Sarno's healing pillars involves beginning to think psychologically, or introspectively. This means attempting to identify the **events** that one is involuntarily repressing. Some write out a checklist of all the possible underlying emotions they may be holding inside. Others talk out their problems, while others sit back and reflect on all the events that led up to the onset of their pain. Still others are wise enough to seek counseling in an attempt to **back track** in life and to hopefully expose the emotional wound that is the culprit behind their pain. Several sufferers have told me that the "power therapies," such as EMDR* have helped them resolve childhood issues. And so the end of the journey has many paths.

A Third Pillar: Letting Go—Forgiving

Here, I add a third pillar. Besides acquiring knowledge and acting on it, I would advise not only to stop obsessing about the body, but also to stop obsessing about the underlying reasons for the pain. Look, think, and ponder, but don't generate even more anger through the obsessive act of trying to find all answers, perfectly. Relax, you are OK. The relentless search for anger generates more anger. It's not always vital to find what precise separation was the culprit. Besides, the fear behind the rage could very well be life's stresses and rejections in general, and not one lone separation event.

Constant reflecting as to what may be wrong, or what the underlying emotions may be, can make the sufferer believe that his problems are unfixable. I've been asked, "Won't the cause remain if it is not dealt with?" Not necessarily. There is another

---

* EMDR—eye movement desensitization and reprocessing—is a form of psychotherapy that serves to finalize the escape freeze-response—completing the escape by walking the individual through the trauma.

healing panacea called **letting go**. Letting go of the past through forgiveness and understanding **releases** the grip of pent-up rage, past and present. So regarding finding that panacea-ic emotion, just understand that unwanted emotions are present, have a general idea of how one "got to this point" and confidently begin to allow the healing process to take place. Flow with confidence!

However, having said this, it may be the case that a person has a hidden whopper of an emotional experience that they may need to get a handle on, and it takes two hands to handle a whopper. A deep relationship wound that will not heal, that cannot be let go—**needs to be heard,** and so healing may only come through the revelations of insight, or psychotherapy.

Checking and rechecking progress maintains focus on the body, which is the point of the existence of the pain and so counterproductive. So again—relax—let go—stop trying so hard. People recover faster when not under pressure to do so.

Relaxation and healing are explained well in *Rapid Recovery from Back and Neck Pain*, by Fred Amir. Fred healed rapidly from approximately two years of disability due to TMS-induced pain. Fred writes, "Mental tasks are accomplished much better and more quickly if we are relaxed and enjoy the process. So in the same way that we can think, learn, and remember better and more rapidly when we are relaxed and enjoy the process, I knew that my recovery would be more rapid if I made it a fun and relaxing experience."[28]

Visual Spatial Learning

For many, it is enough to know that there is nothing wrong and that they can go back to living a normal life without fear. The issues may remain but don't necessarily need to be resolved in order to heal. This is the good news.

Knowledge therapy helped me when I began to become very physical once again. The knowledge that I could not hurt myself, no matter how bad the pain became (and it did!), was of great comfort to me. Thank you, John Sarno. Merely understanding what was happening to me did not cause my pain to diminish quickly, because I still was integrating the truth slowly—clinging to old beliefs—but knowledge did give me courage to push on.

While not all the above steps were of help to me in my healing, they have been to many others. Since I happen to be a **visual spatial learner** (VSL), I found it maddening to try to search for something that I could not pinpoint the details on, or could not feel. Once I decided to forget about the entire process of reflection, I began to forget about the pain at the same time. In my own healing, I skipped to the back of the book and read the ending first… *and he lived happily ever after… after he had read the ending first and discovered that he would live happily ever after.*

Old versus New

You never change things by changing the existing reality. To change something, build a new model that makes the existing model obsolete.

— Buckminster Fuller, architect and futurist (1895-1983)

Still don't believe this? TMS is a proposition that is *a posteriori*—that is—it is known to be true because experience has shown it to be. The tens of thousands who have healed from TMS pain are testimonials to its truth. I am one of those who has waded into the new paradigm and am living pain-free.

One final note before we delve deeper: as I said, Dr. Sarno has coined the phrase "knowledge therapy" in healing since the majority of sufferers heal once they fully understand the psychophysiological process happening within them—embrace the new information, integrate it—and uproot old beliefs. But it's important to note that this **new knowledge is a change**. It is a change in thinking, from what is perceived as happening structurally, to the understanding of what is truly occurring within. This healing is rooted deeply in Freudian psychology, and even more deeply in the personal shadow of Jungian psychology. We give ourselves symptoms to cope with our situations—a process of which we are not aware because we are riveted to our symptoms. Let's dig more deeply into the mindbody process... and into the roots of suffering.

2

The Mind's 👁 Witnesses

What happens in the mind of man is always reflected in the disease of his body.
— René Dubos, microbiologist (1901-1982)

An understanding of the rudimentary aspects of the **inner workings of the mind** was central to my healing—and may well be to yours, too. And so I urge you to take the time to stay with me through this very basic introduction into the human psyche—where pain and illness begin. It's not as daunting to understand as it may first appear. It may exercise your brain more than you would like, but exercise is GOOD! The reading will become more fun soon, when you see all the pain I went through—I promise. I know from personal experience that in severe pain it can be difficult to be patient enough to learn—but you must learn to heal. However, if you are suffering greatly, you can jump to Chapter 3 and read my story first and then return here for a deeper understanding. But if you are able, grind through the next 14 pages or so; it gets easier as I pull this material together into my own story. Hunker down....

Shadows 101

Pain is an effect, the surfacing expression of who you are, and how you react to life, based on your environment, conditioning, life experiences, and beliefs. Your emotions arise in response to the sensory and experiential information you receive from the world around and within you, which becomes your personal reality. While reality may appear to be very "real" to you, it may well be based on a misconception.

There is a hidden side of you that is unknown to you—it is undeveloped—and so it is rejected by your ego and cast outside of your awareness. Swiss psychiatrist Carl Jung called it **the shadow**—"the thing a person has no wish to be." Rejected thoughts are cast into the physical body itself where they create emotions—which are physiologic effects. Simply put, your sneaky little ego hides information from you in your body—things that it doesn't even want you to know—and so you don't. It is unconscious to you.

Although there are many insightful philosophies on the behavior of the human psyche, here I focus on the work of psychiatrists Sigmund Schlomo Freud and Carl Gustav Jung. Both Freud and Jung understood that certain psychic events take place beneath the surface of our conscious awareness—within our unconscious.* Psychic events are life itself; the Greek word psyche even means *spirit* or *soul*. So the study of psychiatry is the study of the **inner self**, and its relationship to the personality. Our health is a direct result of our personality, thinking process, and deep beliefs—not our physical body.

Dr. Sarno's clinical findings are supported by the concept of an unconscious process, best known as Freudian **repression**. From my own healing experience, I expanded the role of the unconscious in the understanding of pain to include Jung's concepts of **archetypes** and the **personal unconscious**. Freud's mainstreaming of the esoteric concept of an "unconscious mind" may have been his most brilliant contribution to health. His contemporary, Carl Jung, went on to expand Freud's concept of the unconscious. As a result of their work, millions of people have healed by simply peering into their unconscious, that part of their consciousness that lies below everyday awareness, yet makes them "tick."

The healing discoveries of Freud and Jung are **ego-based,** or based on the understanding that what we allow others to see of us is managed by our ego. The ego is at the very center of consciousness. Many unsavory aspects and riches of our true nature and feelings are cast away into the body by the ego, never to be revealed again, or so we naïvely believe; but the mindbody is a storehouse of memory that never forgets. Any effect of internal conflict such as pain or illness comes from the ego clashing with truth, or Self. Ego is the counteracting mechanism that prevents our conflict from coming out—from being exposed to the public's eye, preventing healing. It is this conflict that lies at the root of pain and symptoms, and so now we will look more closely at the key brain-characters in this conflict—not only the ego, but ego's head-mates—the **id** and the **superego**. It is the interaction between these three um-egos that shapes your personality. So, let's get inside your head and meet 'em.

Freud's ego-world

The **id** represents the most basic primitive urges within the psyche. Sex, thirst, hunger, anger, and the avoidance of pain are fundamental instincts of the id. The id is the selfish child inside that never grew up or matured, and id never will. Comprised of aggressive impulses and instincts, id is immutable and everlasting.

---

* Unconscious is very different from unconsciousness, which is a physical state of existence. In this text the lexical phrases "unconscious mind" and "subconscious mind" are the same thing, and used interchangeably, meaning: "unaware."

Freud's structural theory of the human psyche, a.k.a., personality*

Our personality is a function of our [id + ego + superego + outer world]

The Face Presented To The World

ID The Child	EGO The Adult *The repressing referee*	SUPEREGO The Moral Parent
OPERATES ON: The pleasure principle.	**OPERATES ON:** The reality principle.	**OPERATES ON:** The morals and values principle, <u>solely</u> to repress ID.
AWARENESS: Only in the unconscious.	**AWARENESS:** Mainly in the conscious, but also at the unconscious.	**AWARENESS:** Mainly in the conscious, but also at the unconscious.
MOTTO: *I want pleasure.*	**MOTTO:** *I will use what others want, to get what I want.*	**MOTTO:** *I will do what my parents, family, friends, and society want.*
DEVELOPS: At birth. All babies are Ids. First aspect of the psyche to develop.	**DEVELOPS:** In first few years of life.	**DEVELOPS:** Develops last, 5 years old or late preschool.
FUNCTION: Does what it wants.	**FUNCTION:** Does what is necessary to survive.	**FUNCTION:** Does solely what <u>others</u> want.

* Freud conceptually divided the psyche's structure (or personality) into id, ego, and superego.

Superego: The Mask in Front of the Man

The greatest happiness is to vanquish your enemies, to chase them before you, to rob them of their wealth, to see those dear to them bathed in tears, to clasp to your bosom their wives and daughters.

— Ghengis Khan (Temüjin) 1226

Temüjin didn't play well with others. He acted out of pure id-ian pleasure, unaccountable to everyone. He accommodated id and therefore enjoyed himself at the cost of the outer world. This is anti-Type T behavior. Temüjin would never need to suffer from primal conflict because he took immediate pleasure whenever he desired, regardless of others. But most of us must deal with others and delay the desires of id, increasing tension.

The **superego** is the antithesis to id. It synthesizes what it believes are expected patterns of behavior to provide "conscience" or moral direction over one's conduct. Poet and essayist, Sir Henry Taylor, wrote, "Conscience is, in most men, an anticipation of the opinion of others."[29] This is extremely important to our understanding of TMS, since anticipation generates anxiety, tension, and body symptoms. So, superego follows the norms, and counterbalances the primitive urges of the id. It can be likened to the "parent" within the individual that overrides (and sometimes punishes) the childlike id for id's selfish and socially unacceptable urges. TMS conflict then ensues as the superego pushes the id's needs and desires onto the back burner because superego wants to do what is "right" in the eyes of others. If you ignore your id's needs by cozying up to your self-created superego, your body will let you know, by giving you symptoms to attend to, that deep needs are not being nurtured.

> The superego, according to Freud, is the "advocate of a striving towards perfection"[30] that punishes id for its incessant pleasurable desires. This punishment manifests in the form of tension, guilt, inferiority, and low self-esteem. So, the kid in us simply wants things—but our superego parent says no—and TMS forms.

The superego is a false self that each of us has designed, based upon what we believe others want to see in us—to stay connected. The more demanding our people-pleasing superego is, the greater our internal conflict is, as we simply can't match or forever maintain such a false image. This conflict between superego and id is a key component in the formation of TMS—especially pertaining to relationships.

Our most primal instincts and impulses, from the id, constantly seek pleasure over pain—and id becomes fiercely incensed whenever superego stifles its basic desires—and tension rises because the pleasure has now been pushed aside, and by default, forever diminished.

But the story doesn't end here, there is a gremlin inside each individual, a parasite that feeds off both sides and calls both friend—but serves only itself. Freud called it **ego**.

Ego

Son—your ego is writing checks your body can't cash.
— Stinger to Maverick, *Top Gun*, 1986

The **ego** buffers the id and the superego in order to balance "primitive belief and primal desires" with moral and ethical beliefs. Therefore, the ego ultimately provides the face, or personality, of the individual to the world. This is rarely the real face, but rather a "compromise" reached by the ego between the id and superego. *Trying to have it both ways.*

Ego is closely related to what Jung called the **persona**. The persona differs slightly from the ego, as it negotiates with the outer world on behalf of the ego, or as the personal manager of the ego, directing the individual to adapt in order to accommodate both id and superego. The bruised ego is the one that forms the persona—and a non-self begins early in life once the child feels flawed.

D'Artagnan desperately wants that new job position of combing Justin Bieber's hair. But it goes to a person who doesn't deserve to even look at Justin's hair. Deep within—without his knowledge—he wants to scream and yell and hit or murder his boss for making the wrong decision. His now-stung ego looks at superego's moral imperative to never hurt anyone, and also at id's desire—the pleasure of sweet primal revenge for pleasure lost. But, his ego de-sides, and appeases superego against the wishes of id. He says nothing (enraging id) for fear of losing his current income and stature, and so a shadow forms to bury his unthinkable thoughts in the darkness. Artie remains silent—he doesn't even know these unconscious thoughts are taking place, his tension levels rise quickly as id goes un-promoted. His neck suddenly begins to lock-up and hurt. He thinks he has slept "wrong." The next day he holds in his expression; goes along with the decision, smiles, bides his time—waiting for his next opportunity for pleasure—surviving through his current environment using his neck pain as self-punishment against dark thoughts arising from deep within himself. What he is thinking is so heinous that it is hidden, even from him, by ego. It's hidden because the evil thoughts he is thinking would bring him great pleasure, but would also reveal the raging monster within him, and so must be suppressed by superego leading to a new body symptom.

Sigmund Freud called this an "ego thus educated" because it learns if it falls in line with others and accommodates them, that it may eventually get what the id wants even though the pleasure has been deferred and forever diminished. Here ego attempts to balance primal cravings (id) versus morals (superego) based on the realities at hand. Freud called this the **reality principle**, as ego tries to decide whether or not it should abandon a pleasurable impulse and antagonize id. The byproduct of deferring instant primal pleasure is always anxiety, and so in deferring these instincts, there is considerable increase in "drive tension."

Thus—what can be seen as **final representation** of an individual's personality to the world is nothing more than ego—and it comes at the cost of anxiety and tension if superego is extremely controlling. In the absence of a highly demanding superego there is dramatically lowered anger from conflict as the person can be more of himself resulting in less internal conflict—less caring of the opinions of outside observers.

> The ego can be THE primary obstacle to healing inner conflict—psychic conflict being the key component in the formation of physical symptoms.

Let's look at how this works: Jedediah's wife has suddenly died. His id wants to scream and kick and fall on the ground in a tantrum, or even worse, as in suicide. The pleasure, comfort, and love Jedediah has lost from his wife's separation are too threatening and powerful to express in an environment with outside observers. So his ego counsels his superego and they pull closer together to act as his family and his society would expect him to. Jed handles it "like a man." But he doesn't know that he is **not handling it at all** because his superego silently hides the magnitude of his fury from him, inside his body (his unconscious mind). Without his conscious knowledge, he simply casts his furious/deadly rage and panic into his body. His new acute back pain is a message of psychic conflict within. He feels as though he has slipped a disc, but he has only buried id.

Bartholomew's parents divorced when he was young. The pain of the abandonment that he remembers is so great that he vows never to do that to his own children, and so he sticks with his spouse through the bad times. However, his id, his selfish, his inner child, his greedy primal animalistic-side, sometimes wants to leave her and find instant pleasure with someone else. Id wants immediate pleasure elsewhere, but ego agrees with superego because of his past experience and so he pushes those unwanted desires deep down—never knowing they exist. He sees himself as "a good man." His tension rises and falls, his back pain occurs on and off his entire life. He believes he is at perfect peace inside and was simply born with a bad back. This occurs outside of his awareness, when ego stands between healing and suffering, as it leans too far toward superego (perfectionism) and away from id (pleasure). Often we become so identified with our public image—our superego, or persona—that we firmly believe we are what we are pretending to be. *Buying into our own press.*

When our truest desires rise in conflict with our public persona, rage begins to build as superego applies more and more guilt energy in order to allow the ego to maintain an image that the self knows is not really true, or even wanted. Whatever is unwanted and repressed always surfaces in the form of anxiety—as symptoms, that then surface to keep the individual from becoming aware he possesses a dark side, which is filled with socially unacceptable thoughts.

> *A symptom is a sign of, and a substitute for, an instinctual satisfaction which has remained in abeyance; it is a consequence of the process of repression…. The ego is able by means of repression to keep the idea which is the vehicle of the reprehensible impulse from becoming conscious.*

— Sigmund Freud, *Inhibitions, Symptoms, and Anxiety*[31]

So the ego as **referee** looks at your id's primal need for immediate satisfaction and also at the need to appear as you believe others wish you to be (superego). In a highly stimulating environment, every quiet and seemingly controlled individual, who thinks he has no anger or internal conflict, is being fooled by his beguiling ego. The need or desire of the individual to appear as he wants others to see him engenders perfectionism, and perfectionism just happens to be the primary personality trait behind mindbody symptoms. If ego coddles superego, less energy and attention is given to id—and psychic conflict rises quickly.

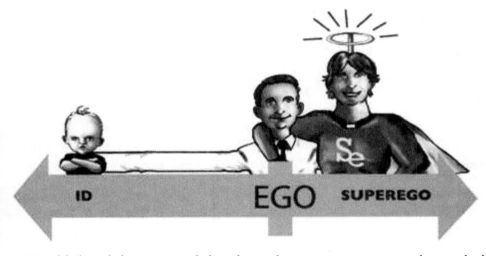

Freud believed that unwanted thoughts and emotions were repressed or pushed into the unconscious mind, which he considered to be a void—an immoral repository of energy that was not compatible with the conscious image of self. The problem with repression is that it's on automatic pilot. We don't consciously repress unwanted emotions, it just happens. The more the automatic pilot clicks on, the less the real pilot is needed, until suddenly the individual looks and sees that there is no pilot at all. He never sees that he is repressing his truest of needs, as he eventually becomes something other than his true self. As he attempts to please others, his ego buries his own wishes as they become subservient to his moral duties …*and the yin chases the yang… as this attempts to become that….*

This view is addressed in **humanistic psychology**, which emerged as an alternative to both behaviorism and psychoanalysis. One of its founders, Carl Rogers, PhD, put forth this concept in what he called **client centered therapy**. This therapeutic approach to healing utilizes **talk therapy** like psychoanalysis does, but in a more Socratic fashion in which the therapist allows the individual to resolve his own problems through his own personal insights. There is no advising the client or "interpreting or analyzing clients' statements."[32] Humanistic therapy refers to the "talking catharsis" as counseling rather than therapy. Carl Rogers wrote in, *On Becoming a Person*, "...it is the client who knows what hurts, what directions to go, what problems are crucial, what experiences have been deeply buried."[33]

> Humanistic psychology therefore asserts that individuals suffer from anxiety and depression because they are living a life that is not consistent with their true selves; that people in psychic conflict are living their lives as others want them to and not as they themselves wish.

A humanistic healing approach eases symptoms of pain, as it blends together introspective insight-oriented therapy with **self-discovery** as the sufferer moves toward self-actualization, which Carl Jung had stated was the most basic instinct of man.*

The problem for most of us, Rogers argued, is that we are often forced to choose between gaining the acceptance and approval of others or being ourselves.
— Kestner, et. al., *General Psychology*[34]

Each of these approaches to healing contains the same theme: The **Self**, and **ego**, in psychic conflict with each other for the outward expression of our inner truth— that is the mechanism behind TMS. *Normalcy vs. primal expression.*

Jung's ego-world:

Carl Jung came to understand that the unconscious mind was a much greater complex of thoughts, ideas, and emotions than Freud had earlier characterized. He expanded the unconscious and made it a more inclusionary and palatable part of self. He relabeled Freud's voids as the shadow—our undeveloped inferior self, which he contended contained not only unwanted immoral traits, but also great talents, good characteristics, and wealths of knowledge—**our inner gold**, repressed along with the bad.

Berlenetta longingly desires to be a singer, but her parents want her to teach school. Her parents will only pay for her to get a teaching certificate. They will not support her becoming a singer. Her ego, at the center, looks at her conscious and unconscious realities. Her unconscious id deeply desires to sing, but her moral superego says she

---

* Jung called self-actualization (Maslow's term), self-realization, a process that he thought of as **individuation** where the individual becomes Self, transcendent of ego.

should do what her parents want. Conflict! But she has only one choice, since there is no money for a singing career, and in wishing to please her parents, she casts her potentials, desires, and talents into her shadow. She chooses a life of unfilled desires, generating life-long anxiety—expressing skin problems, intestinal disorders, pain, and other symptoms—because her id-voice was silenced.

Whether Freudian or Jungian, ego remains the arbitrator. Every life-experience is first screened by the ego, and if the ego rejects aspects of that particular experience in order to preserve self-image, the emotion attached to that experience is then cast into our shadow. Both ego and shadow develop simultaneously from the existence of the other.[35] The more demanding the superego, the larger the shadow that is required to hide any unwanted truths. If a man hates his job, but also understands that others depend on him for the income, then his shadow must grow darker as he hides the truth of his disdain in order to please others. He never realizes any of this, as repression works outside of awareness—he suffers multiple physical problems that are then multiplied by faulty medical diagnoses.

How Do We Avoid Seeing A Side of Ourselves We Hate?

We innately know we are conflicted so we attempt to avoid admitting any conflict by casting our shadow, or undesirable qualities, onto others in what is called **projection**. We use projection to reduce our personal anxiety by slipping our own personal flaws past our egos—making us feel good about ourselves by judging and criticizing others—whose faults are simply our own faults that we deny. The other guy always has the problems, so if she can convince herself of this, she feels better about herself by "bringing down" others, assuaging her own guilt and low esteem.

While Freud saw the unconscious as a garbage dump for all the darkness that the ego had rejected, Jung brilliantly realized that the ego rejects not only negative unwanted emotions, but also undeveloped, unexpressed potentials. *Throwing out the baby with the bathwater.*

So from Jung we know that good things as well as bad get repressed. But why would one cast aside potential, or talent? Most often because our family or society deemed it as wrong, or irrelevant—not cool to our parents and friends, and so we may deny creative parts of ourselves in order to be accepted, to please—to belong.

Faylene's mother is highly critical of her hog-calling career. Faylene's squealing mad and wants to tell her mother off, but ego steps in and chooses superego's demand for value and respect over the revenge her id desires. The result is anxiety and tension as id is hogtied.

Now, we are in big trouble in understanding TMS, if you—the reader—can't see where this is all heading.

Let's recap. Whenever we intellectualize our emotions away at the behest of superego, we rob the self of the most instinctual pleasures of want or cravings. If the ego is not properly balancing the primal needs of the id with the demands of the superego, the id begins to feel persecuted—resulting in ego-induced tension. We also know from clinical proof that tension is the cause of most of our infirmities. This Freudian clash of unconscious desires with conscious behavior was characterized by British psychologist Donald Bannister as "a darkened cellar in which a struggle goes on between a sex-crazed chimpanzee [the id] and a Victorian spinster [the superego], with a nervous Swiss bank clerk [the ego] serving as referee."

> It is this superego-id clash that produces **rage-tension** that causes many physical symptoms.

Billy Bob had been physically abused as a young boy. As an adult he sees another young boy being physically abused. His id wants to kill the abuser for the instant pleasure it would bring it, but his ego looks at his superego and weighs the value of killing the abuser against a lifetime in jail—pouring energy into his shadow. Instinct is stifled by intellect. He chooses to say nothing, repressing the desire to kill, he internalizes the event, and his chest begins to hurt.

> Id Denied (pleasure deferred) = Tension
> ... and
> Tension = Mindbody Symptoms

Here is where psychoanalytical therapy was born and its successes unrivaled as early practitioners discovered a conflicted world within everyone. Healing catharsis, however, doesn't always need to come from psychoanalysis; however—knowledge, presence of being, self-expression, love and forgiveness must be present for healing to occur. In the deepest of healing, there needs to be a dialogue with the personal shadow as in humanistic or analytical therapy, a journey into the depths of the unconscious where psychic battles become physical realities. Behavioral changes by themselves can greatly ease symptoms, but only **true insight** can affect a permanent cure.

The Shadow Knows

The light shines in the darkness, but the darkness has not understood it.
— *John,* 1:5, NIV

In healing from tensionalgia pain, it is critical that she understands the power of her unconscious mind. The Jungian shadow is where emotional pain lives, and where emotional pain lives, physical pain is also a tenant. The shadow is the **alter-ego**, that part of self that has been repressed by the ego in order for relationships to meander and exist. The shadow contains both darkness and light, both the problems and the answers to relieving pain and suffering. Jung believed that the shadow-self contained "undeveloped, unexpressed potentials" that were "complementary to the ego"[36] and that tapping into that potential can make the individual whole again.* Healing is contingent upon opening lines of communication with the shadow self. A quick peek inward is sometimes enough for some people to heal. This is Dr. Sarno's knowledge therapy.

The unconscious mind is the source of all learning, behavior, corrupted memory, and change. Understanding the darker side of self is the king in healing. Long live the king who holds the keys to the kingdom of good health. People attempt to improve their lives by what they see, but what they **cannot see**, what they **fear** to see, underlies most of their psycho-physiological needs and provides motivation.

One does not become enlightened by imagining figures of light, but by making the darkness conscious.

— Carl Jung[37]

Change and healing ultimately occur at the unconscious level. If this were not true, a smoker who wished to quit would merely say "I am quitting." Clearly, this doesn't always work, and it is because his unconscious mind is the repository for old habits, conditioning, and motivations. Even when self desires change, the unconscious cannot be controlled, and reacts very cautiously and slowly to the conscious efforts toward change. Many psychiatrists and psychologists believe that self does not understand how to communicate with the unconscious side; or that the unconscious side gets mixed signals and therefore is confused as to how to change.

Some people unconsciously set themselves up to repeatedly fail. One method of making certain that failure occurs is to never try. This can be accomplished through repetitive obsessive behavior or more commonly to a lesser extent, by procrastination. Things such as cleaning and recleaning, thinking and rethinking, or doing and redoing or checking and rechecking, or practicing and repracticing are avoidance-flight mechanisms. Procrastination is merely the fear of trying **and succeeding!** But the ultimate question is why do we avoid and hide our light—our success—or true happiness? The reason isn't what you think. It is due to fear that we will become what we despise or were taught to consider morally wrong; what our superego most fears—that we may become ourselves reaping boundless glory and success, as the light threatens to cast out the shadow inside us for all to see.

---

* Freud's contemporary Josef Breuer had influenced Freud's understanding of how powerful merely talking out problems was, as Freud witnessed Breuer healing patients by enticing them to reveal hidden shadows. This is considered "the talking cure," or "chimney sweeping." This form of healing only comes through **insight-oriented healing** (analytical) and not through behavioral therapy. Behavioral therapy assumes that problems arise from a learning process that has gone awry; it contends that by treating the behavior you can then treat the cause by relearning what you had previously learned incorrectly. But as Dr. Sarno has written, behavioral therapy is "singularly ineffective" in stopping TMS.

Hiding Our Inner Gold from Ourselves and from Others

It's our light, not our darkness, that most frightens us.

— Marianne Williamson

Our deepest fear is not that we are inadequate, our deepest fear is that we are powerful beyond measure... we ask ourselves, who am I to be brilliant, gorgeous, talented, and fabulous? But actually, who are you not to be? You are a child of God. Your playing small doesn't serve the world. There's nothing enlightened about shrinking so that others won't feel insecure around you. We are all meant to shine as children do. We were born to make manifest the glory of God that is within us. And as we let our own light shine, we unconsciously give other people permission to do the same. As we are liberated from our own fear our presence automatically liberates others.

— Marianne Williamson, *A Return to Love*

As Debbie Ford describes in *The Shadow Effect*, the reason we engage in shadow-work, or try to pierce through our personas, is to forgive ourselves for everything we hate about ourselves. It allows us to forgive ourselves for our quitting, our parents' divorce, our talent, our stealing, our obsessing, our fearing, our child dying, our failing, and our succeeding. Most of us just don't feel deserving of success—to be happy or to feel good. As I mentioned earlier, part of the shadow's purpose is to hide our "gold"—our wealth of potential. Accepting the side of ourselves that we have hidden, allows us to forgive ourselves for having while others don't—being happy where others aren't—succeeding where others can't—doing what others won't—freeing us from all that guilty pleasure, and from mistakes that we have made and continue to hold ourselves accountable for. The recognition and acceptance of our darkness unites the divided self, making us whole again, and healing begins.

The greatest gift of forgiveness is that we free ourselves.

— Debbie Ford, *The Shadow Effect*

In conclusion, healing begins as we initiate communication with the personal shadow—digging for happiness. Now that we understand a little more of what is taking place psychologically, we can move forward to see how the interactions of these psychological forces affect physiological imbalance: that is, how the body reacts to the expansion of shadow energy. Later, we will peer into the more specific personality type that experiences greater pain and more tension equivalents. To heal, you must close your eyes to many things that you once thought to be true.

The Autonomic Nervous System—Behind the Seen

We unconsciously create a physical state to avoid an unwanted emotional state. Since the mind and the body are one, all psychological conflict alters the body's physiology in some manner.

To more deeply understand how pain is induced from unwanted and undetected conflict, it's imperative to have at least a cursory knowledge of the physiological role that the **autonomic nervous system (ANS)** plays in pain. We need to connect the previous psychological material to the body. The autonomic nervous system is the transducer by which thoughts are transformed into emotions, and emotions manifest into the experience of pleasure or of pain.

Early trauma—fear or separation anxiety—met with a freeze response due to helplessness—disrupts the ANS in a manner that causes it to dramatically malfunction throughout life by over-functioning or under-functioning—if the corrupted memories are never purged, or discharged. Infant separation trauma can lead to over-sensitization, to colitis, skin problems, allergies, mitral valve prolapse, irritable bladder, ulcers, asthma, immune problems, and of course pain. Anything the ANS controls can be overregulated (over-reactive) when it is disrupted. These disruptions are the TMS examples given throughout this book.

The autonomic system (auto, Greek, defined as "self;" nomos, Greek, defined as "rule") is autonomic, or automatic, because it regulates all involuntary body functions, usually outside of conscious awareness. Our minds unconsciously take care of certain functions for us as long as there is an unconscious will to do so. It's like your insides are sleepwalking 24 hours per day. The functions that the ANS oversees include: breathing rate, blood pressure, internal organ function, digestion, smooth muscle activity, body temperature, heartbeat, and the distribution of the blood supply within the musculoskeletal system. Most people recognize that one or more of these functions is altered under stress. But what if they aren't aware they are psychologically conflicted, or aware of the magnitude of any conflict? We know from those who have healed from TMS, that the ANS is functioning properly because pain leaves once the TMS process is understood and the changes are made that are required to heal. There is no external/physical manipulation of the autonomic system itself in TMS healing, so by deduction, there is nothing wrong with the system itself, but rather something influencing the system from within—that something is the shadow energy discussed in the last section. The thought process, or memory, is corrupted, not the "system" itself. When there is a change in any of the involuntary functions, the system is merely doing its job in reporting ego-shadow conflict. This autonomic system is truly amazing, in that it can increase or decrease the function of any of the systems it is responsible for in its attempt to hide or report unfaceable rage. Body functioning is automatically taken care of according to the workings of the unconscious mind, which just happens to be where emotions live.

The ANS (more specifically the hypothalamus) is responsible for **homeostasis** regardless of changes in the external environment. Homeostasis is the body's attempt to maintain uniformity and regularity: the attempt to keep involuntary functions going smoothly under ever-changing external stimuli. However—strong, repressed emotions can disrupt the process, by increasing or decreasing any one of the ANS' functions—which causes the TMS symptoms.

The ANS itself is further divided into three main subdivisions, **sympathetic**, **parasympathetic** and **enteric** systems. Only the first two are relevant to this discussion on TMS. It's okay to yawn here, I did when I read all this and more so again while I wrote it. I'll forgive you. Hang in there, just a couple more pages. You can do it! The fun stuff is coming up soon.

Under stress, that part of the autonomic nervous system called the **sympathetic** nervous system (SNS) is activated or engaged. Right now you may be holding your breath and tensing muscles as unconscious tension rises in the process of trying to understand complex material. Your sympathetic nervous system is now unconsciously and actively engaged. Our final concern is with these first two systems.

Boring System #1—The Sympathetic

The Sympathetic—From here is where TMS pain emanates. It is within the sympathetic system that the fight, flight, or freeze response for self-survival takes place. For example, you are a combat soldier and you come under hostile fire. The sympathetic system immediately activates to provide the energy needed in order to survive. It dilates the pupils of the eyes in order to increase vision. It increases heart rate in order to pump more blood to the musculoskeletal network, closes down the digestive process as well as urinary and bowel function in order to free up energy for one purpose—immediate survival. It will also raise blood pressure and opens bronchioles in order to increase oxygen to the system.

The sympathetic system **raises the acuity of the biological being** to align itself with the need for more acute perception. It **manufactures energy** when it is needed, and it burns that very same energy depending on the demands made of it. But a price will have to be paid later on for this demand.

Motivation is the mechanism that provides the energy for any task at hand, and motivation emanates from unconscious processes.* The larger questions are, where does the energy go if it is continually and needlessly manufactured by the SNS and there is no mechanism by which to purge all the overflow? And what psychological events keep the energy levels dangerously heightened?

---

* Motivation comes from the conflict in forces between **Eros** and **Thanatos**. Eros—the sexual instinct, or pleasure-force, drives us forward. But we have yet another—an opposing force within us called Thanatos, by neo-Freudians. Thanatos is the opposing force to Eros—it is a darker force, or destructive instinct. Where our Eros instincts drive us to sexual-propagation, creativity, harmony, and self-survival, Thanatos instincts drive us to self-destruction, OCD, compulsion, disharmony—TMS. This struggle between instincts of Eros (self-preservation) and Thanatos (self-destruction) creates the animating forces in our lives that we call—motivation.

Boring System #2—The Parasympathetic

The Parasympathetic—Contrary to the sympathetic system, the parasympathetic system restores and saves energy. It **reverses** the process activated by the sympathetic system. It constricts the pupils, decreases heart rate and heart-force, restores digestion, increases urinary output, lowers blood pressure and diverts blood back to the skin and the digestive tract. This system holds energy—storing it—saving it for future demands. The parasympathetic soothes the mindbody. It is the healer system we need to reengage to reduce anxiety and TMS. If this system never "restores," you will feel burned out, and experience any other of a host of mindbody ailments.

> These two autonomic nervous system components, the sympathetic and parasympathetic, work in an antagonistic manner for homeostasis. They work against each other to maintain balance within the body's system ...*and the yin chases the yang ...to balance this with that...* but the pursuit of perfection and the presence of fear, keep the sympathetic system actively engaged by demanding unneeded energy.

The following is a perfect example of how these systems work together with the ego for balance. You are hosting multiple engagements, such as weddings. Unknown to you, this is deeply enraging. Superego and id are now in psychic conflict because of these new heavy demands placed on you. Id wants to party big time, superego wants to make sure all RSVPs were sent out, all the food and drinks are okay, there is enough money to pay for the event, that the lamp in the corner won't offend anyone, everyone is happy, and that no one was left out of the invitation, etc., etc., and... the conflict parties on.

So ego unconsciously decides it's better (as in more socially acceptable) to experience pain, rather than to consciously experience the frustration and anger resulting from the demands placed on you, by you. Your sympathetic system obligingly engages in response to these conflicts and reduces the bloodflow to your back, or head, or neck, or knee, or shoulder. Your ego determines that an "internal freeze" is a better option than avoiding the weddings altogether, or fighting by saying "screw it, I'm not hosting anything."

All this has happened outside of your awareness. Suddenly, you have pain, and you erroneously think you have slept wrong or have thrown your back out.

When the parties are finally over, your parasympathetic system may once again allow the blood to flow to your lower back and your pain may leave, if you perceive the danger (demand) as being over. You should now be back in balance and happy. But what if your sympathetic side won't let go because your mind has fallen for a false proposition regarding pain and your body's structural integrity? If you've gone to a physician in the meantime, and he's told you that you need immediate surgery, then your parasympathetic system may never re-activate to bring you back down to rest and regroup—the physician has now prolonged your pain and symptoms.

With TMS, the sympathetic system appears to fail to drop out of survival mode. The anxious individual senses danger and outside observers at every turn, and so the sympathetic system appears to be "stuck" in the ON position. But a closer look may reveal that it is not stuck, but rather in a conditioned pattern. The brain may just be repeating false scenarios as the same false reality is repeatedly chosen to appear perfect in the eyes of those who observe you ...*as this always becomes that... over and over....*

In the case of symptom-chronicity and self-victimization some people will place themselves in the same situation in order to experience the same bad events, repeatedly. They are victims of biochemical reactions that are associated with certain emotions. Those very emotions begin with a single thought. If you think you don't deserve something, then you don't deserve it. If you think your body is failing then it will. If the thoughts become obsessive (through corrupted memory), the parasympathetic system will never calm the body, as self-imposed pain and depression are used to **victimize self** repeatedly.

Now here's another pretty amazing fact: the mindbody reacts to a stressful event from memory as if it was actually experiencing the event in real time. The pain resulting from TMS also has no useful physical function; that is, it isn't protecting anything except ego and others around you.

The autonomic nervous system is always engaged and at work. It cannot be easily controlled by conscious will but rather is indirectly influenced by our state of mind and mental imagery. Usually, we are only aware of the actions of the autonomic nervous system when it is malfunctioning as in the case of TMS. However, the ANS can be **influenced by new knowledge.** Highly advanced practitioners of Zen and yoga can directly influence the autonomic nervous system through visualization. Thus, the ANS is susceptible to conscious intent, but direct control of this nature is rare without special efforts such as bio-/neuro-feedback training.

Hypothalamus

The **hypothalamus** is the brain structure in charge of body temperature, emotions, hunger, thirst, and circadian rhythms. Its main function is homeostasis, or status quo for the body. Dr. Sarno has called the hypothalamus "an essential way station in the (TMS) process." It is the brain's "interpreter of" and the "reactor to" the information it receives. **The hypothalamus is the center of the mindbody connection.**

This begs the ultimate question, once again, as to whether tendencies toward pain are biological by nature or developmental through experience? It is both of course. But since healing can and does occur regularly through deepening awareness, the biology can be altered by the thought, with the ultimate reversal of biochemical events from new information, perceptions, and deep belief. The thought comes first since biology itself is a result of **consciousness.**

Our failing physical health is a reflection of our unresolved deeper emotional status through a disruption in the normal functioning of the autonomic nervous system.

> *Removal of the infant from the mother immediately after birth... to perform the usual rituals... does result in separation and actually traumatizes the infant in the process. Trauma is basically in its purest form dysregulation, (meaning) an interruption in the normal smooth regulatory patterns of autonomic cycling which we call homeostasis: optimal state of regulatory function within the brain and body, and that's what's disrupted because the part of the brain that develops and grows with attunement regulates that autonomic cycle and that brain does not develop as well if one doesn't have the early experience of attunement and bonding.**

— Robert Scaer, MD, *The Body Bears the Burden*

Attunement is a responsive, harmonious relationship. The lack of immediate connection, or attunement, especially with mother—beginning at birth—ignites a lifetime of longing to be reconnected, causing various sorts of autonomic irregularities, depression, and anxiety. Many TMS sufferers report they never bonded with their mother or father, leading to a lifetime of emptiness filled with continuous self-punishment. The father's role comes along a little later, but is just as critical in the emotional development process that feeds the child what it needs for harmony and balance. Without these connections comes a deep void that is often filled with drugs, depression, anxiety, violence, perfection, obsessive thinking—and of course TMS. That person who brings tears to your eyes when you reflect back in your life is the one you never made a connection with—and deeply longed to.

Early Separation = Fear = Anger = Energy

= Autonomic Dysregulation

ARISING SIMULTANEOUSLY

---

* From the work of Allan N. Schore, PhD, primarily from his book, *Affect Regulation and the Origin of the Self*, and Seymour A. Antleman, PhD, and colleagues—summarized by Robert Scaer, MD, *The Body Bears the Burden: Trauma, Dissociation, and Disease.*

Reading my old letters I notice a secret will.

It's as if another person had planned my life.

Even in the dark, someone is hitching the horses.

. . .

So many invisible angels work to keep

Us from drowning; so many hands reach

Down to pull the swimmer from the water.

— Robert Bly, "The Eel in the Cave"

3

Once Upon My Time....

Wisdom comes from great suffering.

— Aeschylus, *Prometheus Bound*, 478 BC

My battle with pain began in my lower back when I was 14 years old. It suddenly appeared and quickly knocked me off my feet. I had constant lower back pain, to varying degrees, for the next 27 years, that is, until I found Dr. Sarno's work.

I will never know why my pain began at that specific time in my life. Looking back now, with wisdom under my hat, the only thing I know for certain is that at that time my accumulated stress had increased to a point where it began to overflow and manifest itself as TMS tensionalgia. Today, I consider myself chronically free of pain.

Pain had been a part of who I was for 27 years, and I naïvely accepted it as a genetic defect. I had fallen for the many misperceptions regarding pain—costing me over half a lifetime of agony. Today I know that pain is a message of imbalance—self-inflicted distractions from unwanted thoughts and emotions. When these arising darker thoughts conflict with how we view ourselves, symptoms then become necessary to distract us. A brain attempting to distract you is a brain that is trying to deny something.

There was no accident or injury that initiated my pain, and the doctors were always visibly agitated when I told them that. In fact, one in particular was quite condescending in response to my not having an injury explanation. So, in wanting to please, I began creating an injury story to tell throughout the subsequent years. It appeared to make the physicians happy that they could fill in their records with a sensible cause. I did my job—avoiding confrontation. Idealized image of self (superego) remained protected, and as Karen Horney (pronounced "horn-eye"), MD, wrote in *Our Inner Conflicts*, the idealized image of self as a defensive function* "is to negate the existence of conflicts."[38] I would discover 27 years later that it was precisely that type of defensiveness, or avoidance, that ultimately creates chronic pain. Not being true to ourselves—knowing deep within that something is not right. When I first read Dr. Sarno's, *Mind Over Back Pain* in 2000, I reflected back to when I was 14 and how I had allowed the doctors to coerce me into creating a false scenario for

---

* The idealized image of self as described by Horney is considered to be a "defensive function" because it substituted the individual's true self-confidence, pride, and genuine ideals with perfectionistic traits so that he could avoid or "defend" his own shortcomings.

the onset of my pain. More recently, I read that in 1978, Dr. Sarno conducted a survey of 100 of his pain sufferers to determine how their pain first began. The results showed 60 percent had no physical incident, and the other 40 percent claimed a physical incident had triggered their pain.[39] And so three decades later I felt vindicated. Things were beginning to reconcile themselves, painfully slowly.

My pain had debilitated me at 14 years old. I was unable to raise my right leg more than a few inches off the ground while in the supine position, and I could no longer stride a normal length. My gait was more like a quarter step. I listened intensely while one chiropractor told my father, "He'll eventually have to go under the knife for this disc herniation. He's this far away from surgery (indicating a small distance between his thumb and index finger), but if you keep coming back here to s$$ me, I think we can avoid it." Those words, as untrue as they were, were insidious and added to the duration and intensity of my pain over the next few decades. He had set in motion a pattern of false beliefs that would eventually allow me to cripple myself. But this was only the genesis. My lower back pain was merely one symptom of a **mindbody process** that would manifest itself in me as my life unfolded.

For the next 12 years I suffered through varying degrees of pain, as well as numerous other mindbody manifestations. I would naïvely visit the chiropractor regularly, the therapists, the MDs, the gym, the bed, and the always welcoming floor. It was an on-again-off-again love affair with pain. That is until 1985, when I was 26 years old and the pain affair became a marriage.

The Shakespearean Flaw—Setting the Stage for the Play of My Life

One of several watershed years in my life was 1985. I was 26 and in the last couple of weeks of finishing my bachelor's degree in engineering science at Youngstown State University in Ohio. My wife, Susan, was pregnant with our first baby, and life, unknown to me, was becoming increasingly tense as a new birth of knowledge was about to spring forth. The accumulated stress of finals, graduation, career, physical training, and impending fatherhood were beginning to manifest within me as often subtle, but ever more powerful and nefarious, mindbody symptoms—working 40 hours a week while attending YSU full time.

My pain was increasing daily as Susan's due-date neared. Plus, my face was beginning to turn red, which I had never experienced before. This redness is called rosacea, and without exception, to this day, it only surfaces when I am under stress (i.e., hidden anger). For decades now I've explained to my dermatologist that there is a perfect (rho) correlation between the tension I'm under and the onset of any redness. Studies show that stress is the main reason for rosacea. A 2001 article published in Rosacea Review cited a survey conducted by the National Rosacea Society of over 700 rosacea sufferers. From the 700-plus surveyed, an overwhelming 91 percent reported that "emotional stress caused, or sometimes caused their rosacea to flare up."[40] My guess is the other 9 percent weren't aware enough to notice the correlation. In that same survey, the participants ranked the emotions behind their rosacea flare-ups in order as: anxiety, anger, frustration, and worry. The correlation between pain and rosacea is not known, but I believe it to be extremely high. The reason for the redness is the same reason for the various other skin manifestations like psoriasis and eczema: **chronically hidden tension—TMS.** These symptoms all result from psyche imbalance with accompanying autonomic nervous system imbalance, from chakra imbalance.

In *Deadly Emotions*, Don Colbert, MD, describes a conversation with one of his medical school professors regarding why the professor had switched from dermatology to psychiatry.

> *He told me that his work as a dermatologist had led him to conclude that many individuals who were suffering with psoriasis and eczema were actually "weeping through their skin." In other words, these people, for one reason or another, were unable to weep openly, even though they had experienced events that warranted a good cry.*
>
> — Don Colbert, MD, *Deadly Emotions*[41]

Windows of Opportunities... Closed

Two weeks before Susan's due-date, she began having ankle swelling, elevated blood pressure, and severe abdominal pains. On our primary care physician's directive, I took her to the local hospital's emergency room for further testing and observation. The testing showed she had become preeclampsic. This is a condition that occurs in the 2nd or 3rd trimester of pregnancy in approximately 5 to 8 percent of all pregnancies.[42] It is marked by potentially lethal, and stunningly rapid, increases in blood pressure and high levels of protein in the urine. The excruciating abdominal pain results from expanding blood vessels within the liver. Approximately 76,000 women in the world die each year from preeclampsia (a.k.a. pregnancy-induced hypertension), which is more deadly than eclampsia itself.[43] The danger lies not only from the deadly levels of blood pressure, but also from the rapid potential crossover into toxemia that often occurs and can quickly take the life of both mother and baby. So, Susan needed to be closely monitored for several days in the hospital. Over those few days, her abdominal pain dramatically increased and, with our baby's heart rate becoming more erratic, it was decided that our baby should be delivered by caesarean section.

The anesthesiologist concluded that she would require a spinal block since she had eaten too soon prior to when the caesarean operation was to take place—precluding general anesthesia. During the spinal block he punctured a blood vessel,[44] causing blood to pour into the spinal canal, gradually forming a blood clot that compressed her spinal cord, preventing precious oxygen from feeding the nerves of the cord.

After our baby boy was delivered, the anesthesiologist sent Susan back to her room before sensation and movement had returned to her legs because he was tired and wanted to go home. From that point, the nerves in her spinal cord began slowly dying from a lack of oxygen. When the cord is compressed there is a 24-hour "window of opportunity" to decompress it[45] for full motor function and sensation to be restored, or at least in large part. After 24 hours the window slams shut and irreversible paralysis quickly follows, due to the formation of scar tissue from the lack of oxygen to the delicate spinal nerves.

I spent the next few days trying to get the doctors back in to see why she hadn't regained any feeling or movement in her legs. I didn't have much success, and the nurses had no luck either. I was told that one doctor was gardening, another had a banquet to attend, and that there was probably just "residual anesthesia" in her spinal canal that would eventually wear off. But it turned out that this was the worst possible course of inaction. The negligence left Susan permanently paralyzed from her waist down. We were 26.

My own scars of personal guilt would be revealed painfully over time, but it was the doctors' ignorance and ego that crippled my wife. Her being handicapped was completely unnecessary and could have been easily averted. They could have stepped in at any time and helped her, but chose not to. They chose to follow doctors' "codes" and "honor," over their patient—fearful of stepping on each other's professional toes. They chose money and schedules over their patient. They chose everything at their disposal over their patient and she still struggles daily over the choices they made in 1985. People always pay a price for the poor choices of others, and this was no exception. Neglect is malpractice.

> Dr. Mel P. Ractiss [Susan's "doctor"] gets a call at ten minutes to twelve. He doesn't come in till 4:00, "because it's my day off, and I've got to come in anyway to talk to the nurses and give a speech," so he waits the whole day, wants to enjoy his day off, then he comes in and he doesn't go right to see the patient; he gives a speech first, then he comes down. When does the light bulb ever go on, and when should it go on?... We know from the speed of a spinal hematoma, it has to get worse every minute. It does not get better.
> — Robert V. Traci, Esq.[46]

It would have taken a simple CT scan of her spine (a CT machine was on the same floor) to see that a pool of blood was forming, and to evacuate it in a timely manner. But the lack of interest or action by all the physicians involved led to a complete and permanent paralysis at the T12, L1 level in her spine. Within approximately 24 hours of giving birth, at the age of 26, my wife was paraplegic due to the inactions of a handful of incompetent physicians. I was told a year later by a neurosurgeon that, after two hours, they should have been concerned, after four hours they should have had a neurosurgical team in there, after eight hours they should have been in utter panic, and after twelve hours she should have been back in surgery. But they never came back to do anything—nothing—for three days. A concerned nurse called the obstetrician who performed the cesarean section to inform him that the feeling hadn't returned to Susan's legs. He gave some general orders and then told the nurse, "If that doesn't take care of it, cut her legs off."[47] He laid the phone down and fell back asleep as she tried to reawaken him repeatedly. His job was over, he was going to receive his pay, and didn't want to be bothered anymore—as each physician felt the problem was the others' responsibility.

After 72 hours of paralysis, our attending physician decided it might be time to seek advice from someone else and finally called in a local neurosurgeon. After nearly three days of not sleeping—pacing the floor—worrying and not knowing what was wrong with Susan, within 15 minutes the neurosurgeon told me what he thought had happened—but—he "needed proof" from a CT scan. The CT was taken and he showed me the scan of her spine where the swelling from the pool of blood had permanently damaged her spinal cord. I will never forget that visual image as long as I live—her spinal cord ran down the CT about the size of my pinky finger, and abruptly toward the bottom it was swollen three times as large. On Friday, May 25, 1985, three days after becoming parents, standing there late at night in the darkened, cold, empty hallway of the hospital, I was told that my wife would never walk again. I was stunned beyond imagination—unable to speak—just staring at the neurosurgeon in dream-like disbelief. As I looked to my right I saw a nurse with tears streaming down her face—tears that let me know that it was not just a nightmare, it had actually happened. Life was about to change—forever.

Furious with the devastating news, and the lack of care or interest we received at the local hospital over the previous three days, I began to let the expletives fly and had Susan moved by ambulance to University Hospitals of Cleveland. I had contemplated moving her by Life-Flight helicopter but the surgeon told me the damage had already been done and that getting her there sooner wasn't necessary—what was done was done.

I was also advised by the neurosurgeon who had just diagnosed her spinal hematoma, that the director of neurosurgery in Cleveland, Robert A. Ratcheson, MD, was one of the most talented neurosurgeons in the world, and that he may be able to regain some of her motor function or sensation—if anyone could—by removing the clot. At that time Dr. Ratcheson was president of the US Congress of Neurological Surgeons and had never before seen a spinal hematoma as a result of a spinal anesthetic.[48] It was a long shot, but I was willing to try anything to help my wife. She was a part of me—we were one.

Upon arriving at University Hospitals, with Susan still in the ambulance, I was met at the emergency room doors by a startlingly large group of hospital personnel. After days of trauma and not sleeping I was in a state of dissociation* (a freeze

---

* The dissociation response is the opposite of presence (a healing mechanism for pain and other disorders). Presence is experiencing the moment—body and mind united—aware of your own feelings and thoughts in relationship to your surroundings—cognizant, conscious, and knowing. Dissociation

response), out of my body—in a mental fog as those emergency doors slid open in what looked like slow motion, with scattered lights and muffled voices. My mind's eye can still see that moment vividly. Standing there in the entryway were two rows of waiting hospital personnel lined up on both sides. The white-smocked assembled team members, clipboards in hand, were eager to see this extremely rare case coming to them from Warren, Ohio. University Hospitals of Cleveland is a teaching hospital—this had the potential to be a golden learning experience for them, plus, they actually cared.

As I began to wade through the two rows someone spoke up and asked if I was Mr. Ozanich. As I turned toward the voice, the chief resident stepped forward and made it quite clear to me then, that it was most likely "too late" for hope now, but that a laminectomy may bring about some small degree of feeling or function back to Susan. A laminectomy is a procedure where the surgeon chisels and saws the bone away surrounding the spinal cord in order to get to the subarachnoid space to decompress the cord by removing any obstruction. In our case, the obstruction was clotted blood that was approximately 72 hours old. It was a small and desperate chance and a highly dangerous operation that they told me could kill Susan. The physicians were now debating among themselves as to whether they should operate— unsure in their own minds—now wanting a decision from me as to how much I wanted them to take the gamble. Susan couldn't bring herself to make the difficult decision so she asked me to make it for her—she trusted my judgment but I had never faced anything like this situation.

It was the most difficult decision I had ever made because I would rather have had her alive and handicapped than not at all. I paced for about an hour and then decided to go for it because of Dr. Ratcheson's reputation. He had been waiting for an answer from me so I told him to go ahead and attempt the evacuation of the clot for that prayerful chance that she may regain some slightly increased quality in her life. Fifteen minutes later they came to get her—Susan and I held hands for a few minutes in silence—staring at each other, and as they began to take her gurney away she told me to tell our baby Matthew that she loved him if she didn't make it. I watched as a sea of green uniforms took her away—wondering if I would ever see her alive again. It was so overwhelming to Susan that she completely blocked it—shutting off her emotions and memory in order to cope through what must have been a nightmare within a nightmare for her. Her faith alone sustained her.

I then had to do yet another difficult thing—tell her parents and my parents what was going on. The four of them had been isolated in a room for a couple of hours, waiting impatiently while I spoke with the surgeons. As I entered their room all four

---

contrary to presence; severs the emotional impact of the moment from the individual to protect him from being overwhelmed. But a price will be paid later for the dis-connect.

parents stood up quickly and walked toward me looking absolutely exhausted—drained of life. The most beautiful event in life—a birth—had taken a turn that we could never have imagined. As I explained the situation to them I saw the despair in their faces—her father speechless and stunned—her mother in tears, my father and mother devastated. Now the gut-wrenching wait began—pacing back and forth for word of good news.

Susan and I had both sacrificed quite a bit while I was working on my bachelor's degree, but on the final day, we weren't celebrating at any graduation ceremony. On graduation day I was lying on the tiled floor in the surgical intensive care unit praying that she would walk again, and she was undergoing her second major surgery in three days. The 7½ hour microscopic operation to remove the clot went well, but it failed to bring back any motor function or sensation to her—too much time had passed and the window of opportunity had slammed shut.

Seven days after the surgery, Dr. Ratcheson and the director of anesthesiology came by our room to check for progress in Susan—after only a few seconds of inspection Dr. Ratcheson looked up at me soberly—hands in his smock pockets—he motioned with his head to follow him into the hallway where he proceeded to tell me that his prognosis "was not good" and that "this should never have happened." He told me in a rather stern tone, as he threw his clipboard across the nurses' desk, that it was inconceivable for physicians to have waited that long to come back in to see my wife and that, as her husband, I had an obligation to reconcile what had happened. Even though he told me he could not further advise me, he did tell me that all of his records, as well as those of his colleagues, were open to me when the time came that I would need them. The implication was crystal clear. The president of the 2600-member Congress of Neurological Surgeons was telling me the physicians in Warren had just committed an act of unconscionable malpractice—that I should be suing them—and that he was going to support me when I did. But at that time I was too devastated to even consider it. I was far too concerned about how we were going to even survive, let alone consider litigation. We had only been married four years and it all seemed over.

Dr. Ratcheson asked me near the end of our visits with him, "Where was the attending physician?" That was our doctor, or so we thought, but he magically disappeared when we needed him. Ratcheson told me that everything "hinged upon the attending physician," that he was the doctor in charge of all the other doctors; they were under his direction to take action. I told him the truth—I didn't know where the attending was. They had all disappeared when we needed them. Ratcheson just shook his head in disgust and said, "I think you know what you need to do now—you have an obligation—have your attorney contact me."

However, the Type T personality rises to the occasion, pushing aside any emotions that are subservient to duty. I was defiantly numb during this time. I felt nothing, in a zombie-like state—pushing onward—determined to make things right for us, somehow. I didn't know how, but I knew **I should** try to make a life for us, and so I pushed forward—dead inside.

> Coping requires that we repress emotions that might interfere with whatever we are trying to do and TMS exists in order to maintain repression of those emotions.
> — John E. Sarno, MD, *Healing Back Pain*[49]

To add salt to our open wounds, while Susan was still recovering from the C-section and spinal surgery at University Hospitals, one of the most devastating tornado events in American history began in our town. On that day, May 31, 1985, 43 tornadoes hit an area from Ohio to Pennsylvania to New York to Ontario—the third most costly tornado event in American history. The damage all began in our little town of Newton Falls beginning with F3s and F4s, increasing to F5 strength as they approached the Pennsylvania line—culminating in the only F5 to have ever hit Pennsylvania. The tornado destroyed much of our downtown and over 400 homes. It missed our apartment by about a half-mile, destroying all the homes on a nearby street. When the winds finally calmed, there was 88 dead and 450 million dollars in damages. It is the worst ever tornado outbreak in our region of the country. Life was literally becoming a whirlwind spinning out of control.

Life for us with our beautiful baby Matthew, and the new handicap, and the ensuing therapy was indescribably difficult. The only thing that got us through that time was our son, our parents, our friends, and our faith in God's unknowable plan. Only people who have gone through such an ordeal could possibly comprehend the magnitude of its difficulty. When enough time had gone by, and the bills had poured in (the anesthesiologist sent me a $90 bill), and I had my wife rehabilitated enough to take care of herself a little, I filed suit against the doctors who had senselessly handicapped her. I had the full support of the University Hospitals' neurosurgery group—an expert witness from George Washington University's anesthesia group, and was receiving a steady stream of phone calls from local doctors urging me to file suit against the negligent doctors.*

There are no easy lawsuits, no easy wins. Both sides go through hell in malpractice suits; however, I learned a great deal during those next 3½ years while involved in that suit. I learned that frivolous suits, although senseless, selfish, and self-indulgent, and even though they tie up the system needlessly, only add a small fraction to rising insurance premiums. Outrageous insurance premiums are primarily the result of bad doctors. Malpractice suits account for only about 1-2 percent of total health care costs. It is most often the same doctors repeatedly creating the same problems for the rest of the medical industry, but the good doctors are reluctant to speak up in what is called

---

* I've noted a distinct pattern over the past 25 years. The really good physicians were angry at the other physicians for paralyzing my wife, and the really bad physicians were angry at me for suing.

a "conspiracy of silence." Case in point, in 1997 the same anesthesiologist who performed the botched spinal block on Susan, permanently paralyzed another pregnant woman during her child's birth in Alliance, Ohio. The system had failed—once again.

This lead-in is not as much a vendetta against physicians (although I have certainly earned the right to complain), as it is a "setting of the stage" for the host of physical problems that I was about to encounter through my own suppression of anger and guilt in my personal id-superego conflict. Susan's problems are and were much worse, of course, than mine. But this book is an explanation of pain and of a syndrome called TMS and how I defeated a lifetime of pain and how anyone can achieve a level of happiness after adversity that they could never imagine possible. If they can find the strength of ability to open their minds to what is truly happening to them, anyone can heal if they desire—and **believe**.

With my wife now permanently handicapped, living in a tornado-devastated town, I had to go to the police station day by day to get permission to leave town to visit her an hour away in Cleveland because our entire city was in lockdown by the National Guard. For a month, at night, I sat in shock wondering what had just happened to us. It was a dream within a dream. I sat alone in our small apartment while Matthew was with my parents-in-law in their apartment upstairs, a single candle glowing since there was no television, electricity, phones, nothing—not a single luxury, like Robinson Crusoe, primitive as can be.

...and the vicious cycle BEGAN....

During the next 3½ years we were not only struggling for survival, but also deeply involved in high profile litigation. As I moved forward, I never stopped to deal with what had happened to us, never took time or effort to discharge the full impact of the trauma—and my tension level rose steadily. A tragedy such as this was much too painful for me to face in real time; the majority of it got repressed so that I was able to cope with the situation. I relegated it to my unconscious and naïvely forged ahead. This, I would find out later, was not only the worst thing that I could do; it was potentially deadly. But I was the **perfect** fool. I had no idea what was happening to me over that 3½-year period accompanying the lawsuit and in that new phase of our new lives. Looking back now I see so clearly why I had developed so many physical symptoms and pains, but darkness always precedes dawn.

I now know that I unconsciously felt responsible for what had happened to Susan. I felt (even at the conscious level) that maybe, had she not married me, she may have had a better life with someone else and would not have been handicapped. Every time I looked at her in that wheelchair I felt responsible. I also felt that maybe I could have done more during those first critical hours when the blood clot began forming. But realistically I never knew that a blood clot could even form, let alone damage a spinal cord. I'm not a doctor. The anesthesiologist that paralyzed her didn't even consider the possibility of a clot. How could I have known? The nurses' notes indicated my concern, to no avail.[50] I did my best to get her the proper care, but residual **guilt** was still buried deep. Child always blames self and I was no exception. After these many years it has become quite apparent that the physicians let us down, all by themselves.

Accountability has been well established and recorded into history, but it couldn't stop my ever-surfacing conflict. The degree of medical negligence that we were the "victims of" occurred to me one day in the rehab center when a handicapped veterinarian asked us what had happened to Susan. As we began to explain the anesthesia procedure, he suddenly cut us off and said, "It was a blood clot, wasn't it?" We were both shocked by his statement and asked him how he could have possibly known. He said it happened quite often with dogs during spinal anesthesia. I knew then that we hadn't received the care that a dog would have received. I became more angry and vengeful that day. However, true to my personality type, I turned the vengeance inward and my back pain increased. Off to the chiropractor....

At an unconscious level, I'm sure I wanted to do serious harm to those doctors because of their negligence. I(d) needed revenge, but ego sided with superego and said "no." And conflict was born. This is the cognitive level at which all psychic-stress occurs and my unconscious mind was in a furious state of **deadly tension**. In the years that followed in taking care of Susan, I wasn't letting go of my anger over what had happened to us because I couldn't feel or face its magnitude. I rarely talked about it to anyone, never dealt with it, and never looked back. I'm a recovering perfectionist—things like this were rejected by my psyche; cast into my shadow.

Symptoms Increase

While the malpractice trial was on-going in 1986, I began having constant sore throats and swollen glands, and my back was hurting more than it ever had—I was stuck in a trauma-freeze response—dissociating from the trauma. I became a regular patient in the chiropractors' office, and had even begun visiting them at their homes at night for adjustments. The back relief from the manipulations was always slight to none, and never long-lasting. My sore throats, however, lasted eight months. I had gone to an otolaryngologist but he could find no reason for the swelling in my glands. I had extensive blood profiles but they all came back normal.

I also began having a heart arrhythmia and my fingertips and face were becoming more numb each day while driving back and forth to Cleveland. I was becoming concerned that something was seriously wrong with my heart, so I made an appointment with a local heart specialist to have a series of extensive exams performed. After the EKG, echocardiogram, and a stress test on the treadmill, the cardiologist concluded that I was suffering from exhaustion and stress from what had just happened to Susan. After all, what had happened to us was big news in the local medical community. The cardiologist told me, "you have been through so much, Steve—you are hyperventilating which is causing excess oxygen to be pumped into your bloodstream, making your face and finger tips numb." He gave me a sedative and a clean bill of health.

During this time period Susan's father, Jack, was struggling with lymphocytic leukemia. Jack was doing fairly well, but after his daughter's needless tragedy, he succumbed to his own rage and disease and died two years later, after recently turning 47. We needed and loved him very much and depended on him being there for us, but he, too, was suddenly gone. Jack and my mother-in-law, Pat, lived in an apartment above our apartment and I couldn't have handpicked better in-laws. My parents and Pat were godsends, and Jack helped us with every last ounce of his life. I loved him so much, and when he died, he took a part of us all with him—he was truly one of a kind. Sadly, he never got to see the successful outcome of the malpractice suit, or watch his grandchildren grow up to become such beautiful people. After his death, I pushed on ahead, unknowingly setting myself up for more disasters. I felt I could make it all better by pushing even harder. Perfectionists don't feel in real time, they look forward in anticipation of heading off future disasters, by pushing aside current emotions. They brace for the worst through a high-speed mental scenario analysis that is called "what if" thinking—always on the defensive, waiting for the next shoe to fall, never really being thankful they have shoes, simply anticipating the next fall.

I have been through some terrible things in my life, some of which actually happened.
— Mark Twain

Soon after Jack's death in 1987, I developed a cough that started slowly but quickly worsened—lasting seven months. I went to several local pulmonary physicians, but all their medication and advice accomplished nothing. It was actually making me worse. My cough worsened to where it became a severe barking cough and I couldn't sleep because it would wake me. I was losing weight—its persistence eating up my appetite, consuming me like a raging fire. All I could think about was the coughing! It would be another 13 years before I would find out that the cough was due to tension from repressed rage, and it was serving its purpose in me like my pain had been doing. It was Mini-Me talking to me, and in my not listening to the message, it kept me distracted from my own wrath.

I decided I had better visit the Cleveland Clinic for a deeper look into my lungs, since I knew there must be something seriously wrong, of course. After extensive testing, the diagnosis was that nothing was wrong with my lungs. The Clinic physician gave me a big clean bill of health, along with another big bill, and told me that the coughing had become a "habit" and that I should "try to suppress the need" to cough. He gave me codeine to zap the urge and break the cycle of the echo (echo: as in my brain's loop of obsessive focus) that allowed my brain to erroneously feel the need for the cough. The need was not known to me then, but when I found Dr. Sarno's work 13 years later, I finally understood its purpose. The cough and pain and other symptoms were TMS equivalents; distractionary mechanisms—deceptions of my mind. I was experiencing the effects of a freeze-response due to the helpless state of trauma I had experienced over a period of years. If I couldn't **fight** (kill the malpractice physicians), and couldn't **flee** (leave my family) then for survival I went into **freeze** mode. The energy building up in me from the flight/fight response that was never utilized, got "stuck" or frozen in my neural network because it was never discharged through fight or flight. My autonomic system now was in a state of **dysregulation** (the manner in which the body handles energy). My pain, my coughing—all my symptoms—were the result of never having discharged the original energy from my system. The anger-energy was **stuck** in me, revealing its presence through all the body problems. It needed to be discharged but I didn't understand mindbody effects—yet.

Within two weeks of my visit to the Cleveland Clinic, my cough had disappeared. The Clinic doctor had given me back my confidence in myself and now the clean bill of health took my focus off the cough and into another unconscious arena for further battle... **and the vicious cycle continued....**

I soon developed a needle-like sharp pain in my bladder, along with a burning sensation. The human mind needs focus. Forcing attention away from fury and onto pain is the end result of TMS as described by Dr. Sarno. It is THE red herring. When stress and anger build to overwhelming levels, people cannot face the shameful, rage-filled emotions they want to act on because they alter the idealized image they have of themselves, and so the brain chooses to focus on the body instead of the underlying reason for the physical symptom. The rage is shifted from conscious to unconscious (body). Repression is a time transfer of energy... from now till then... and it is assisted by the presence of TMS to keep the unwanted from entering awareness.

My repressed fury was so overpowering that I began experiencing an assiduous series of mindbody manifestations—like falling dominoes. The systematic breakdown of my physical body began, as unwanted unconscious thoughts began reversing their flow back into my conscious mind; where they desire (id) to once again be confronted, and yet are denied (superego). **This is the classic battle for conscious thought.** The bladder pain would drop me to the floor when I needed the distraction from my surfacing rage. I would then crawl around until the needle-like stabs would cease. Bear in mind that my back pain never completely stopped with the appearance of these new disorders, but would sometimes lessen with a newer affliction. The random breakdowns in my system were becoming distractions from my original distraction, which was my severe pain. The mind prefers to hold one primary pain or symptom at a time, but in severe cases of chronic tension there is an overflow into other areas of the body. The focus then shifts from point to point, but the mind normally chooses one area to focus on at a time—but not always.

I was now hearing a loud gushing and thumping sound in my left ear near the carotid artery. The needle-like stabbing in my bladder increased as well, and I became increasingly concerned that it may indeed be bladder cancer. I was approaching the paramount of negative thinking, or so I had thought. Negativity is like a goldfish, the more space you give it, the larger it grows. Why would I not have a new major problem? The problem was that my negative vibrations were bringing on the problems, not vice-versa, since chronic pain is a self-fulfilling prophecy. It is also difficult to change that type of what-if thinking when it has been perfected. Conditioning to the negative can occur quite rapidly, but the longer it continues, the harder it is to break the cycle. *Time may heal all wounds but time also wounds all heels.*

I first went to see a urologist because my senses told me that the pain was coming from my bladder. I was later proven correct; however, when the urologist checked for bladder tumors and prostate problems, he found nothing wrong, and suggested that I may have pulled a muscle that "tied in and around" the bladder area. So I was off to see the gastroenterologist next, as the pain continued. He checked the sigmoid colon and tested the rectum for internal bleeding, but(t) could find nothing wrong. He suggested it was a spastic colon and gave me anti-spasm medication, which didn't work. All the tests that the two doctors performed had found nothing abnormal, and the medication did nothing as my pain continued. It wasn't for another decade that I would discover that my bladder pain was from an affliction often referred to as interstitial cystitis (IC). With IC, oxygen is reduced along the lining of the bladder— and is acutely painful. It was simply tension-related but I didn't have all the pieces of the pain-puzzle at that point in my life. My bladder pain was occurring due to the same process that created my lower back pain and cough.

I will NEVER forget the day my bladder pain vanished. I literally had not been able to move without that sharp stabbing sensation. But I was determined to get back to Perfectville, which was my residence in those days. So one day I just began some vigorous activity, giving my fool attention to that activity, and suddenly—the pain was gone. After months of pain, that particular pain was gone in a fleeting moment. But why?—because I ignored it. It had been kept alive by my feeding it the fear it needed. Just as in any relationship, if there is no attention paid to the partner in focus, that partner will leave the relationship. Without realizing it, I had pierced the veil by accident, and did the proper thing by shifting my attention away from the pain. I repudiated it through **activity** and shifted my focus elsewhere. We all need attention in life, and so does pain, because pain is a part of who we are. But my back pain increased to an unbearable level that very night. My focus was back-to-back.

Through ignoring what the body is doing and becoming active, the mind cannot focus on body or symptom anymore; it must focus on activity instead. This is **presence**.

The brain can hold multivariate scenarios in its decision-making, but can only make one decision at a time. We are binary creatures. For example, while sitting down, lift your right foot from the floor and begin making clockwise circles with it. While continuing, take your right hand and draw the number six in the air. Your foot will change direction to follow the latter decision (direction) of the hand. Conditioning plays a heavy role in healing, which guides the mind and the body follows.

I was taking care of my wife the best I could, and she was fighting bravely to try to live her new life from a wheelchair. I still admire her ability to move onward each day. She's a role model for people who feel sorry for themselves and don't know how to live a full life when things don't go as planned. She even later had the courage to try to have another baby, which thankfully we did, a 2-pound preemie girl we named Kelsey. The handicap experience was all new to us but we had tremendous support from my parents, Susan's mom Pat, and close friends. It took an entire team of family and friends many years around the clock through blood, sweat and tears, to get Susan back to the point that she could take care of herself like she does today. She was strong through it all. It was a tremendous group effort—and unparalleled success.

The Snowball Effect—When it Snows, it Actually Pours

During this period of chronic tension, it seemed as if problem after problem was becoming the status quo. My expanding symptoms fed into the negative thinking that brought on vibrations of even more problems. The symptoms I experienced in my late 20s and early 30s were not in isolation, nor were they mutually exclusive. The primary personality traits behind all these ailments were perfectionism and low self-esteem. The combination of these two traits generates tremendous amounts of conflict. The rage is then converted to a high energy state within the sympathetic system, as self struggles to hyper-cope.

It's very important to reiterate here that these symptoms are not merely psychogenic in nature, because additionally there were always physiologic changes within the tissues of the body. Although these processes all originate in the mind, the symptoms are not in the person's head.

My symptoms were real, and extremely painful—manifesting as emotional pain passing through my hypothalamus into my body. This communication between body and mind was made via neurotransmitters in the nervous system that act as both translators and couriers of emotion throughout the body, making mindbody one, with no distinction between the two. The neurotransmitters are merely doing their job in reporting the mind's status to the body, and vice versa. The body itself has the ability to think and to communicate with the mind, which is **embodied cognition**. But this was still the genesis for me. More truths were yet to be unveiled. My lesson was not yet over, as school was about to begin.

Over the next few years, life became increasingly more difficult for my wife and me as tensions mounted dramatically. Our relationship was strained from a lack of intimacy and frustration from her handicap, and also because we had little in common other than our tragedy and our children. Our relationship was falling apart, but I didn't consciously realize it at the time.

What We Don't Want to See Can Blind Us

I soon began having episodes where I was unable to see above a certain horizontal line. I couldn't see the tops of people's heads or read a book and see the lines. My field of vision was cut off halfway up. This was one of the more frightening TMS equivalents. I thought I might be going blind, of course.

At the edge of the cut-off in my eyesight, I could see what appeared to be a saw tooth or zigzag shaped waveform that looked like a rainbow. The zigzag is called fortification spectrum because of its resemblance to the walls of medieval forts. Not all the colors of the rainbow were always present; sometimes there was only a single band of red. The impairment of my vision would start as a small black dot, or tunnel, and would spread its way outward adding colors as it grew. The scintillation spreads out with a loss of visual field, or tunnel vision, leaving behind a scotoma (visual loss). The loss of visual field may not necessarily be scintillating either. A few former sufferers have told me that they merely saw a ball of light in the center of their visual field that obscured their vision.

It was another 13 years when I read in Dr. Sarno's book that he also experienced this symptom, and that it is called scintillating scotoma. How fitting a phrase, since the word scotoma refers to the notion that "the eye sees only what it wants to see"—turning the mind's eye away from the unwanted.

The colored spectrum in the eyes moves in a jagged oscillating manner, which is the scintillation part. The scotoma is the blocked/dark area within the visual field, often called "tunnel vision." Dr. Sarno had written that he also had the same symptom before his migraine headaches would begin, a precursor if you will, to pain; but after a colleague informed him that his migraines were from repressed anger, his migraines immediately disappeared, although the scintillating scotoma still appears to him without the pain of the migraine.[51] So it can be a prelude to migraine headaches, but it doesn't always follow through with the pain. This is called an acephalgic migraine, or silent headache. However, just like back pain, it results from a constriction of blood vessels that serve the eyes. Perhaps the magnitude of the fear of the loss of vision is enough to distract the individual without the need for pain? I have not experienced this vision problem since I healed after reading Dr. Sarno's books and acted on his advice. But it is further proof that he is correct, that hidden tension creates reduced bloodflow/oxygen-related symptoms. Thus, repression and scotoma are synonymous words, in that, we see what we want, and only that ...**and the vicious cycle continued....**

Ringing in the Steves,
We Shall Come Annoying, Ringing in the Steves

I soon developed severe tinnitus in my ears, which increased in proportion to my tension and attention levels. Tinnitus is a ringing in the ears or "the perception of sound where no external source is present." In Latin, it means "to tinkle; like a bell." Louise Haye has written in *You Can Heal Your Life* that tinnitus is born from an inner stubbornness through an unwillingness to relent in life.[52] There is no question that there is a stubborn component to TMS, a refusal to change direction. The American Tinnitus Association claims that the cause of tinnitus is not known, but does give possible reasons such as jaw misalignment, medications, wax buildup, ear and sinus infections, cardiovascular disease, or tumors. I had none of these. Although I still do get a ringing with certain types of medication, especially aspirin, the ringing at that point in my life proved to be from repressed rage, since it, too, left when all my other symptoms disappeared. No matter the cause, it becomes louder the more attention you give it, and the more tense you become with it. It can be quite maddening if you pay attention to it—or "listen" to it.

As with all TMS equivalents, it is the attention paid to it that keeps it in perpetuity. You must deny its existence by simply ignoring it. It sounds easy to just avoid symptoms and pain. But remember, it's the anger and anxiety never acknowledged that are the driving force behind the physical problems. If you knew which emotional attachments were present beneath conscious awareness, there would be no need for the symptoms to reveal themselves throughout the body. So ignoring the symptom, as in the case of tinnitus, is not as easy as it may first "sound."

Tinnitus is at the top of the list when it comes to ignoring symptoms for healing. Don't listen to it. Focus attention elsewhere! I remember reading about actor William Shatner saying that the ringing in his ears became so bad that he thought of shooting himself. But he went on to say that he just ignored it and it went away. Like pain, it's that simple, sometimes, depending on the depth of the need for the diversion.

My mind was still using my back as the primary source of distraction from my pleasure deferred. It held my attention stronger and longer for many reasons. One reason is that it was the most stable of the symptoms. A second reason was that it was the most painful symptom. A third reason was that it was suggested to me that it was a serious condition early on in my life, and doctors are always right, aren't they? They drive nice cars? The "white coat syndrome" not only temporarily increases blood pressure in patients but it can also have a permanent and damaging suggestive power to its presence, as we shall clearly see.

ZZGS: Zha Zha Gabor Syndrome, Dahling

My pain became more crippling in severity over the next decade into the mid-1990s. My doctor visits were more frequent, the dire medical prognoses more ominous. There were countless times where I was down flat on the floor in my family room with my knees propped up and pillows carefully placed under my legs and back and neck. I laughed when I saw Homer Simpson had hurt his back and he had a pillow with a rope tied around his waist to keep the pillow on. I call this the Zha Zha Gabor Syndrome (ZZGS) where there are pillows propped under feet, legs, around head, and neck and arms. All that was missing was the boa around my neck and the 25-carat diamond ring, dahling. In that same light, TMS specialist, Dr. Marc Sopher has written that many people erroneously feel that they cannot sleep on a soft bed or sit in a soft chair because it has insufficient support. He has referred to this as "Oh no, not the comfy chair!!" after the hilarious Monty Python "Spanish Inquisition" skit. The essence is the same; we are not at all fragile. We are stronger than we can possibly imagine, as strong as we believe we are—that is—until doctors convince us that we are fragile, and should sleep or sit on a certain type of surface. Softness does not cause discomfort, only erroneous beliefs do.

> *Everyone accepts it as gospel that a hard mattress is good for one's back. The idea has taken hold so firmly that a whole generation of people will never experience the joys of a soft, enveloping mattress.*

— John E. Sarno, MD, *Mind Over Back Pain*[53]

There were some days that my back was better than others, of course, since back pain is not from a structural problem. On those good days I would try to move around more, but then I would lose a range of motion in my knees. I wasn't able to bend them all the way, or only about halfway. Directly under my kneecaps would become painful and frozen. It's quite obvious now that the pain was moving because I was moving. The purpose of TMS is to keep the person down, to keep them from moving, and to keep their attention glued to the body and away from their problems. TMS (part of you) does not want you to become active. I was told that I had water on the knees, whatever that is. I now know that the statement was never true. I had a reduction in bloodflow to my knee because of high tension, that's all. The doctor that wanted to drain fluid from my knees was wrong, once again.

Neck-st, I began having off-and-on periods where my neck would freeze and I was unable to turn my head to the right or left in the morning. This would always follow a restless night of sleep where my unconscious mind would race with negative possibilities. I've heard people say they also had frozen and stiff necks but that it was due to sleeping wrong. This is not true, of course. You can sleep in any position you desire if your neck muscles are in a relaxed state. It's the persistent and unconscious squeezing of the neck muscles from night-tension that tightens and freezes it into a **TMS state**. This occurs because of increased unconscious activity—from relationship—finances/work—school. It would be more accurate to say that my unconscious mind slept wrong, and that the night was not filled with a relaxed sleep.

But night is often filled with the problems of today and tomorrow—and tension rises from the conflict. One can lie and sleep in any position he desires, when in a relaxed state of mind. The position of sleep, the hardness of the mattress, or surface is irrelevant to the physical condition of the neck and back in the morning. I now sleep in any position, for any length of time, with no neck or back problems. The only difference between then and now is that I integrated the concept of TMS and now sleep in a much healthier and more relaxed state of mindbody.

When I woke up this morning my girlfriend asked me, "Did you sleep good?" I said, "No, I made a few mistakes."
                                      — Steven Wright, comedian, not even close to ordinaire

I remember during the most stressful, tension-filled times that my arms and hands would fall asleep or become completely paralyzed. I found myself unconsciously squeezing my brain in the same unconscious manner that one holds the back or knee or shoulder in tension. It's difficult to realize this is happening, since it is an unconscious act, but the physical effects are consciously realized. I would catch myself squeezing my brain in a defensive manner, always on constant guard against the next thing that was going to go wrong. I saw nothing good around the corner, which I've referred to as a cognitive reuptake of negative default—never seeing any good, no light at the end of a long dark tunnel. No hope.

My poor wife had one problem after the other—she was strong, drawing from her deep faith—and I was there for her every step of the way. I became her legs—cutting, lifting, digging, driving—everything and anything to keep her going. She had the best support anyone in her condition could ever have and she was fighting as strongly as she could to get back to "normal"—to rebuild her life. We did the best we could with what we had—no doubt. But the demands on us both were taking a heavy toll. I loved her, but I did not recognize then that the entire situation was enraging because of the new demands that were thrust upon me—I was numb to the existence of tension in myself. Her problems were causing my problems. Therefore, as Dr. Sarno stated on ABC's *20/20*, "it (your brain) thinks it's doing you a favor" by diverting your attention to the pain and away from what you don't want to think about. By playing a shell game with the emotions, the pain sufferer automatically and continually represses, and relegates all potentially harmful emotions to the **shadow** in order to keep self-image intact.

Everyone automatically represses certain emotions. Some people necessarily repress more than others, especially if trauma strikes. Repression is a highly efficient tool and occurs in everyone, but this particular malady called TMS is more prevalent in people who harbor perfectionistic, driven, or obsessive personality traits.

Settlement—Unsettlement

Digressing back, 3½ years after my wife was paralyzed, we settled out-of-court with all the physicians involved in her handicapping. It was a large settlement, but a very hollow victory. What is the value of a person's legs? What is the monetary value of a person's life? The only consolation was that we could now buy better equipment and a nicer house for her. But there is no real victory in malpractice—only disability.

With the litigation finally and painstakingly over, I began to design and build a new home that was as handicap-accessible as possible for Susan, since there is no such thing as completely accessible. I once had a psychologist tell me that building a home is usually the most stressful event in a person's life. I would say he was correct, barring any tragedies. It was stressful, but I had now gotten myself back into graduate school and was trying to build a new house at the same time as studying. Push, push, push... don't look back.

I soon began having a tightening in my throat that is called globus pharynges. It was as if someone was squeezing my larynx with pliers. People remarked that they could even hear my voice changing pitch. Apparently, I sounded like Donald Duck on helium. For me, this was a repression of tears, and has the same feeling as the beginning of a cry—that never comes. To cry in public would be unacceptable to self, and so symptoms emerge instead of the healthier outcome.

Pop—Boing—Ouch!

Now in the spring of 1990, the stressful trial over, our new house was almost finished, only the driveway left to be paved. Life had calmed down dramatically since Susan's spinal cord damage and Jack's death—the medical visits were slowing. The eye of the storm was passing and I was feeling a little better. I decided to attempt to have some fun in life, so I took a golf lesson. During the lesson, as I swung the club, I heard a pop in my back and it knocked the wind out of me. By the time I got home, my left leg was partially paralyzed. I had lost all motor function in my left foot, calf, and most of my hamstring, as well as the deep tendon reflexes in my left ankle and left knee. The pain was so intense that I had to keep holding my breath on my way home because I had never experienced pain so deep. Ten years later I read this:

> *There is another interesting pattern that we see often. In these cases patients go through a highly stressful period that may last for weeks or months, such as an illness in the family or a financial crisis. They are physically fine as they live through the trouble, but one or two weeks after it's over they have an attack of back pain, either acute or slow onset. It seems as though they rise to the occasion and do whatever they have to do to deal with the trouble, but once it's over the accumulated anxiety threatens to overwhelm them, and so the pain begins.*

— John E. Sarno, MD, *Healing Back Pain*[54]

So like Forrest Gump would say, I went back to the doctor's office, uh-genn. This time the neurosurgeon sent me for an MRI which revealed multiple herniations, most predominantly at discs L4 and L5, and S1, of course. This generally correlated with the area my pain was emanating from and made perfect sense at the time. The neurosurgeon said I would never regain the deep tendon reflexes in my leg and that I needed to tell him when the pain was too unbearable for me to withstand, and then he would trim the discs around my spine. He was reluctant to operate on me and I didn't blame him. After all, he knew what had happened to my wife—he was the neurosurgeon that came in and within minutes had discovered the hematoma that had paralyzed her. Besides that, Susan and I had four legs between us, and only one worked now. The court trial was finally behind us and suddenly I, too, was handicapped. I had taken on part of her symptoms.

I was in bed for weeks and unable to stand on my toes or move my left foot and left calf for nine months. My left hamstring and calf were useless. If I had to walk, I would drag my left leg. Approximately six months later my deep tendon reflexes returned to normal despite the so-called herniated discs that were allegedly pressing the nerves. That fall, I began moving around again and was back in graduate school and returning to my normal level of chronic stress again.

My physical problems continued through the 1990s, as the relationship between my wife and I began falling apart. We had nothing in common but we also never properly dealt with our tragic situation. It was always, push, push, push on, and leave the past to history. We never sought counseling for what had happened to us, which was the worst possible move. TMS occurs because of unresolved conflict within interpersonal relationships, including and primarily the self. If the conflict in these relationships is too overwhelming for the mind, and if enough repression takes place, serious disorders may occur, and often do. But sadly, most people will never make the connection between their physical symptoms and their current environment because they never feel the magnitude of the conflict. Why is it repressed? The short answer is because of ego. Based on the pleasure principle, we constantly seek pleasure from unconscious instincts in order to avoid pain. When we defer the gratification of that pleasure for ego purposes, **tension rises** dramatically.

My symptoms multiplied in severity and magnitude into the late 1990s. Relationship wounds opened up and decades of minatory emotions attempted to flood back into awareness—dying to be recognized—held in check by superego. The worst was on the horizon. Conceptually, my anger bucket was overflowing.

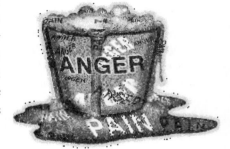

Itemizing Infirmities

My unfelt rage was always trying to surface, but superego resolutely held it in check with bodily symptoms. TMS remained my watchdog, always present to keep my emotions on a tight leash. I was taught as a child that it was wrong to do harm; that it was not right to hurt others, and that I should be... good. So I ended up as a "well-adjusted" individual who eventually clashed with overwhelming dynamic emotions. The end result is cognitive dissonance (an uncomfortable feeling caused by holding conflicting ideas simultaneously—knowing deep inside that something is wrong). Eventually, superego's steadfast determination to create distracting symptoms to hide id's revolt may result in the brain destroying the body. The mind will eat up the body to protect the persona. So by choosing a false self over authenticity, the brain creates an unlimited source of physical distractions—including deadly diseases.

Thus, the two main purposes of TMS are to keep the unconscious emotions from becoming conscious and also to send a message of energy or chakra imbalance. So there is an instinctual component to the mindbody process, a survival mechanism in play. But the medical industry has conditioned society to look the wrong direction when it comes to understanding health, and so there remains internal conflict and confusion. Modern medicine often does great injustice because it has convinced the collective thinking of society to believe that herniated discs, degenerating discs, stenosis, arthritis, spurs, etc., are the main sources of the pain. We now know that these structural changes almost never cause pain, but are merely the **source destination** of our rage.*

Back at the Urban Farmhouse

In 2000, I hit the bottom of the rocks on the bottom of the rock bottom. Years of repressing frustration and rage toward the physicians who had handicapped my wife and forever altered our lives was taking its final toll on me. I began separating from life. The dark side of my thinking began covering the light; my body began to fail rapidly. I knew somewhere deep down inside that there was nothing left for me to live for. It was as if the candle in my soul was flickering and ready to self-extinguish with the softest of breezes. Anxiety and depression set in heavily. Although I never had a conscious thought of doing harm to myself, I was allowing myself to simply fade away. This is depression.

My lower back pain was dominating my life and defining my daily activities. I was living my life as a slave to my back and so my life revolved around the pain. The irony was even painful. Slaves serve their masters with their backs, but my back was the

---

* Dr. Sarno claims in the *Mindbody Prescription* that it is very rare that an unconscious thought would break through to consciousness but had witnessed it once. So they can indeed shake hands quid pro quo, even if it is rare.

master I was now a slave to. I was now doing what has been called **bracing** for the next trauma to come along. I was tensing my body and brain for the next disaster, as TMS was working like a finely oiled machine in me. I thought, ate, and slept thinking about my back. Every event revolved around how my back would be today? On a scale of 1 to 10, with 10 being the highest pain I could possibly tolerate, my pain was at 11. I was now constantly soaked with sweat and had trouble walking anywhere or doing anything. It was too much.

How Much Can a Bucket Hold by Itself?

With my wife permanently handicapped, our marriage failing quickly, and my career floundering, there were more bad events that would come along for me to compartmentalize under the feeling of "negative" … **as the vicious cycle continued.…**

In the late 1990s, I attempted LASIK eye surgery to improve my sight, but in yet another act of medical negligence, the surgeon destroyed my left cornea and eyesight. I later found out that I was never a candidate for the procedure because I had an existing disease called keratoconus, which excluded me from candidacy for the surgery. The surgery resulted in iatrogenic keratectasia, a physician-induced, degenerative and progressive disease of the cornea that leads to loss of vision. My pain skyrocketed.

During this time I was unable to eat from the left side of my mouth because of a pain in my upper left mouth. The pain was deep and sharp as it shot through my head and down into my collarbone. After several x-rays, my dentist still couldn't see any problems on the imaging. When I told him I could no longer eat or tolerate the pain, he began a deeper physical probing of the gum line with his dental pick. There he found the root cause—a vertical tooth fracture below my gum, no doubt caused by the gnashing of my teeth. There is nothing that can be done to repair a severe vertical tooth fracture; the tooth needs to be extracted. I'll never forget the back pain I had when he told me the news. I don't think he'll ever forget it either, as he offered his sympathy as a back pain sufferer himself with an obvious Type T personality.

I couldn't sit down at all. I was on my hands and knees in his office waiting for the tooth to be pulled. But this was still only the beginning; the intensity of the pain in my lower back would continue increasing after the tooth and nerve were gone. The Novocain that numbed my upper jaw lasted 7½ hours. It was getting very late that night and I still hadn't gotten feeling back in my mouth in order to be able to eat. I almost went to the emergency room. But what could they do? My dentist was quite surprised when I told him how long sensation took to return. He later told me that sensation takes a little longer to return in the lower jaw, but two hours would be considered normal, and mine was in the upper jaw. Finally, at around 10 P.M. that night, the feeling began to come back into the area.

The teeth of this story is that there is something about chronic tension that also disrupts how people recover from injury, pain, or illness, as well as how they react to medications, food, and pollens. Tension creates mindbody imbalances to greater degrees than is currently understood, as it affects all systems involved in the mindbody process.

> *Ask a good neurobiologist, "What's the essential difference between the immune system and the nervous system?" They'll tell you that there isn't any—the immune system is a circulating nervous system.*
>
> — Deepak Chopra, MD, *Body, Mind & Soul*[55]

Swing Away, Merrell, Swing Away

During this short time span, I tried to stay active since I am by nature and nurture highly active. So I always attempted to push and make gains through the pain. No gain, no pain. So—one St. Patrick's Day evening I drove down to the local indoor golf dome to try to hit some golf balls through the intense pain. After several swings I felt a pop in my right elbow and the last two fingers lost sensation. I could no longer hold onto the golf club or close my hand. I left the hitting area and went to the bar to hunt some Wild Turkey for the pain. The agony must have been obvious, because a few minutes later the bartender brought me a bag of ice with pity in her eyes. But the ice didn't relieve much, as the pain spread from my collarbone to my hand. It became worse overnight, so a trip to the emergency room was necessary. The x-rays showed that I had broken the end of my elbow off, of course. The numbness in my fingers was from the piece of bone that grazed the bundle of nerves that run across the inside of the elbow—often called the funny bone nerves—it wasn't funny at the time. Like my friend Ricky says, "Golf is a funny game, but no-one's laughen."

The operation to remove the piece of bone was much more painful than the break itself. The tendon needed to be cut halfway across the elbow in order to extricate the broken bone from underneath. The convalescence was long and grueling and painful. I had to sleep sitting up, which was painful for my back, of course. After six weeks, I began physical therapy to get some semblance of range of motion back into the elbow. So I began therapy with elbow pain as well as back pain. I joked with the physical therapist that I would probably be returning for back therapy after my elbow therapy was over. Little did I know, before reading Sarno **...and the vicious cycle continued....**

During the fourth week of elbow rehabilitation, the therapist was bending my elbow backward against the bursa to continue regaining range of motion— straightening out my arm by bending it backwards over a rounded cylinder. I know I've used the word painful quite a bit, but pain seemed the only thing I had in my life. Only a person who has broken his elbow and had it rehabbed can understand the—let's say "uneasiness" of the therapy. As the therapist was bending my arm backwards over the cylinder, the dumbbell I was holding in that hand fell onto the therapy room floor. He picked it up and attempted to put it back into my right hand, but it fell out again. He said, "Can you grasp this?" I couldn't. In panic I stood up quickly. My right hand was completely paralyzed. I stared at my fingers in panicked amazement that I could not move them with all of my might. I immediately thought of my wife and her paralyzed legs, how awful it must be for her, and how spiritually tough she had been to endure it all.

For two hours they tried to understand what had just happened to me. They called in a supervisor who said that I might have had a stroke during therapy. I was told to go home and wait to see if motor function would return—if not, then I was to return for a brain scan to look for a possible brain tumor or stroke.

I drove home from therapy left-handed, extremely anxious to know whether I would ever be able to use my right hand again. After all, I was right-handed and it had always been like a right hand to me. When I returned home and told my wife that my hand was paralyzed, we got into an argument because I didn't stop at the grocery store for her on my way home. Our marriage was over—the worst symptoms on the horizon—relationship problems being the most common cause of severe symptoms.

I was concerned I may have had a stroke, or even have a brain tumor, but it didn't matter to her anymore. My increasing problems had become such a nuisance to both of us. I had taken good care of her but the time was nearing for our separation. It took years of deepening awareness to finally get past my resentment of her lack of support for me. My now ex-wife was merely grappling with her own shadow as resentment grew. There's a psychological phenomenon that occurs over time when people who are being taken care of begin to resent the caretaker. They hate needing people for even the smallest of things because they implicitly understand the drain they are taking on that person's life, especially if they are locked together in tight quarters. Familiarity breeds contempt. I was the one there and so I got the brunt of her deep frustration. Susan was a good woman—dealt a terrible hand in her life by modern medicine and many of the pretentious protocols that can drive the industry. She deserved better, we deserved better, but the situation brought our egos into conflict to a degree that no two people could manage—as our marriage dissolved and symptoms increased.

I had given her much of my life; I would now go it alone. The pain was about to increase in me to the greatest levels I had ever experienced, fired by the rage of separation. For relationship wounds to heal, the communication process must take place in real time; then and there.

Anger repressed, anger suppressed, anger inhibited, anger kept in the body is toxic.
— John Lee, *Facing the Fire*[56]

But continuing to be the perfect fool, I had no idea there were even emotions at play in me. I felt nothing, since I was accustomed to intellectualizing everything. Was I suffering from **secondary alexithymia** created by early conditioning and years of continuous trauma?

I'll Take Repression for $200, Alex

The intellectual escape is our first conscious refuge from anger.

— John Lee, *Facing the Fire*[57]

Etymologically, alexithymia, or **alex**, is Greek from "a lack of words for feelings," but this isn't precisely what alexithymia means. Alexithymia is "the inability to talk about feelings due to a lack of emotional awareness," but is not considered to be a disorder or disability.[58] It's simply a syndrome that manifests as a deficit in emotional cognition. Simply put, the individual is **unaware of any emotions**. They never discuss or communicate emotions because they don't understand that any are present. Alexithymic individuals suffer from many chronic psychosomatic mindbody ailments because they are unaware of the presence of strong emotions. Alex sufferers are often called human robots because they go through the motions of life, always rationalizing and intellectualizing their life away. There often has been a cycle of trauma and repression that eventually numbs the individual to all emotional experience. By repressing one emotion, or set of emotions, we can repress all our emotions. After repeated trauma and repression, emotions are eventually abandoned.

This would be a cogent explanation for the repressed emotions behind TMS and the clinical findings of Dr. Sarno regarding repression and psychosomatic disorder, but it may not be that simple. Alexithymia is not a simple repression of emotion; rather it is a void of the knowledge of the existence of emotion. With alexithymia, "There is just pain, nausea, and discomfort."[59] The alexithymic doesn't lack emotion; he simply doesn't recognize any emotions. It's the opinion of some alexithymia researchers that people become alexithymic because they never have a confidant, or safe person, in their life to express their emotions to, and so they learned to simply push emotions inside. Psychiatrists Peter E. Sifneos and John C. Nemiah, who coined the term alexithymia, are undecided on whether it is wholly biologic in nature (neurogenic) or if it's developmental (psychogenic). They have referred to its **biological** manifestation as **primary alex**, which would include being born that way (e.g., Dustin Hoffman's Rainman, Kim Peek in real life), or through head injury, disease, etc. The **psychological** alex is referred to as **secondary alex**; a defense mechanism against trauma, or a result of "parental conditioning" to "be good." Secondary alex is more often transient and the symptoms can often recede when the psychological trauma wanes. I was never diagnosed with secondary alex, but merely point out the strong possibility of it as a cause of TMS. Alexithymia should not be casually accepted as a cause of TMS, even though alex is prevalent in some form among most men in Western societies.

Handy Answers

Meanwhile, back at the urban ranch, I called my orthopedic surgeon immediately to look at my paralyzed hand. As soon as he saw me walk into his office, he knew that the rehab center had pinched the radial nerve in my right tricep. He had seen it before in people who wore casts on their arms, compressing the back of their triceps—causing the loss of use of the hand. A nerve impinged will cause paralysis in minutes, if not seconds. The notion of a nerve being impinged for years in a person's back or neck doesn't make sense. It took several weeks before I was able to begin using that hand, and months for it to be back to full strength. But my back pain increased as deeper anger settled in, as more repression took place and divorce neared.

Physically, I began to spiral downward—experiencing rapid bursts of vertigo. If I tilted my head slightly to the left, I would fall flat on the floor and my eyes would move back and forth quickly as my brain made a futile attempt to rebalance my body. This rapid back and forth jerky eye movement with visual field loss is called nystagmus. It looks like a robot acquiring a target. **This was the most frightening moment of all the TMS equivalents that I experienced.** I thought it could be a brain tumor or an acoustic neuroma, or autoimmune inner ear disease (AIED) or Meniere's disease, or any of a host of possible ear or brain disorders. I was certain my time had finally come, so I went to see a local ear specialist and had my ears examined thoroughly. Benign paroxysmal partial vertigo (BPPV) was initially diagnosed and then ruled out, as were all other serious disorders. My hearing and inner ear checked out **perfectly** as I heard all the test sounds in the booth. The doctor even commented to me, "Your hearing is phenomenal for a 40-year-old. Your thresholds are near those of a 12-year-old in their acuity." He then showed me a 12-year-old boy's chart he had in his office and held my chart up next to it. They appeared identical. I was beginning to slowly realize that I had a highly acute sensory system. Hmmm… another piece of the TMS puzzle in place.

The ear specialist eventually shrugged off my vertigo problem as a possible "earlier ear virus" and sent me home. It wasn't for a few more years that I would discover that the rapid bursts were due to TMS. There have been too many other TMS sufferers with whom I have spoken who have had this exact same problem (approximately 10 percent). All have been diagnosed as having BPPV, but I am confident that it is a tension-induced symptom. The symptoms were **suggested** to me by a friend at a very vulnerable time of high tension. Something occurs during high levels of tension to change the bloodflow either to the inner ear or to the brain itself, or both. A few pregnant women have also told me they have had similar bursts of vertigo, obviously from the tension of impending delivery.

I continued having rapid bursts for about seven months. It only began waning when I began moving around again, and ignoring it. This bloodflow alteration is another TMS equivalent and should be recognized as such, only after more serious conditions are ruled out. Serious symptoms should have serious examinations because they can have serious consequences, seriously.

I soon began hearing a very high pitch squealing in the same ear. It had the sound and cadence of those British police sirens. Eee-Aaaa, Eee-Aaaa…. It was so loud at times it kept me up all night. It was more tension needing more attention—yet another message being sent to me that I was deeply conflicted, deeply furious, deeply unhappy. It, too, left with TMS healing.

I desperately needed to get out of the house one night so I decided to accompany my wife, daughter, and a friend to a local restaurant. There I got food poisoning and threw up repeatedly throughout the night. I couldn't see well out of my left eye because of my damaged cornea and I couldn't lean on my right arm because of my elbow surgery and I had trouble chewing because of the recent tooth extraction. The poisoning, though, was a result of the state of my immune system at the time. My daughter, who also ate the same food, did not get ill. The immune system is dangerously susceptible when a person is in chronic tension. It cannot fight for you as it would when in a positive happy mindset with decreased tension levels. It also gives further credence to the Chopra statement (above) that good neurobiologists understand that the immune system is merely a circulating nervous system.

> *It is my impression that virtually any organ or system in the body can be used by the mind as a defense against repressed emotionality. These include disorders of the immune system....*
>
> — John E. Sarno, MD, *Healing Back Pain*[60]

I was now afraid to drive my car or leave my house because of the sudden bursts of vertigo. I began turning inward—more reclusive—edging toward agoraphobia for the first time in my life. I had always been a very social person, but the world no longer interested me. I saw it as merely another arena for more problems to invade my life. I felt that as long as I was alone, I could lower my risk of something else happening to me **...and the vicious cycle continued....**

The smell of food began to turn my stomach and I was nauseated at the thought of eating. I had broken my elbow, permanently damaged a cornea, fractured a tooth (the tooth was #13, of course), paralyzed a hand, had intense bladder pain, contracted food poisoning, and suffered severe bouts of falling down from verti-going into severe depression. The only time I was leaving my house was to see the back doctors, or to back therapy, but even that soon ended.

I had dropped 34 pounds and wasn't eating, was in a state of chronic tension but I didn't even know it. I was numb from the unconscious mind up, moving robotically through life's motions. I was experiencing the effects of deadly tension; in fact it was a textbook response for my personality and biography. But I hadn't yet read Dr. Sarno's books and so I was perfectly unaware—still thinking archaically that my herniated discs were causing me pain. Sometimes in life, we need to regroup. Pain and illness are messages from the inner self revealing that we have become out-of-touch with our inner self. The pain dramatically rises when we aren't listening—determined to hold our attention.

The interstitial cystitis (IC) soon returned with a vengeance. As usual, when it struck, it would have me crawling around on the floor on all fours (actually all threes because I still couldn't use my right arm) …**and the vicious cycle continued….**

The Patient Is Told He Has a Problem and the Problem Worsens

My back pain intensified to the point that, not only was it increasing in the lower right back, it also moved to my midback at the T12, L1 area (amazingly the same area of my wife's spinal damage). The two back pain areas were intense enough that I made an appointment to see a physician who sent me in for x-rays. The x-rays showed foraminal stenosis and arthritis, which is normal. It also revealed a strange malformation at T12. The doctor remarked, "When were you in the car accident?" I told him I had never been in an accident. He showed me the bony deformation and the severe narrowing between the discs at T-11 and T-12 and was surprised that I had never injured that area of my back. He also remarked that, since my back was such a "mess," he would prefer to never manipulate it again. It was a little disheartening at the time, but more important was what the x-rays had revealed. There was foraminal stenosis with osteophytes (spurs); a malformation at T12, L1 and my left hip joint was severely worn out, but I had no pain there—yet. However, through this new knowledge that my hip was now crumbling, this hip deformation would come back to haunt me later. After finding Sarno's work, I began getting more aggressive as per his recommendations regarding TMS healing, and voila, my left hip began locking up on me badly. I had been made aware of these physiological changes to my hip; my mind apparently wasn't clever enough to know they were there.

One by one, during my healing, the pain sought out the locations of wear and tear in me, desperately seeking a site that would convince me that I had somehow reinjured myself. Anything, give me anything, to not have to face these resentful, violent, guilt-ridden emotions! …**and the vicious cycle continued….**

I had twisted my right ankle playing sports at least seven times in my life and had been on crutches each of those times. I first tore the ligaments in my right ankle in our high school championship football game and had "rolled it" severely six times after that. The last time I rolled it my orthopedic physician called me in to show me the x-ray. Shaking his head, he pointed out that I had severe post-traumatic arthritis (PTA) in it. My ankle joint was largely gone; eaten away by arthritis. He put up another x-ray of a healthy ankle and the difference was dramatic. When I told him I normally didn't have any pain at all there, he was quite surprised—commenting, "You're a lucky guy; you should be in serious pain all the time." That thought now firmly planted in my mind, I was certain to feel pain there in the future from the Law of Attraction,* and I did, of course.

---

* The Law of Attraction, a.k.a. The Teachings of Abraham is the phrase introduced by Esther and Jerry Hicks. Its basic premise is that the solutions to life are always available to us from the infinite energy of the

Fast forward 18 years after he first showed me that ankle x-ray to the time period that I'm now describing in 2000, and the stage has been lit: the interstitial cystitis had returned, my lower back pain had intensified greatly and had spread to my middle-back where I was shown the strange malformation. I was still off-balance intermittently from the vertigo, my elbow still hurt from the surgery, I was losing the vision in my left eye, and I was now on crutches from the sudden onset of ankle pain, and had also developed piriformis syndrome (this is a cramping of the gluteus medial muscle near the hip as a result of reduced bloodflow to the sciatic nerve—from tension). The ankle pain was more debilitating than the back pain. With back pain, I could move if necessary, but not with TMS in the ankle. My final symptom came when my left knee began to swell with pain at the top of the knee cap. It was by far the most painful thing I have ever experienced—I simply could not physically move with it. Susan commented that I might have "a joint disease." I was beginning to think that same thought myself, but it was depressing to hear it from someone else. She had merely corroborated and exacerbated my own negative thoughts. All the emotions that I had pushed aside were now coming back to revisit me, as they chased my old injuries, as well as, defined new ones. But I kept pushing ahead ...**and the vicious cycle continued....**

Still Fighting for Answers—The Egoscue Method

By now, the only thing I could get out of bed for was to do my physical therapy program that was designed for me by a well-known therapist from California named Pete Egoscue. Pete had worked with golfer Jack Nicklaus and former president Gerald Ford. I also had worked with Pete a decade earlier and had gained some temporary results. So during this time, I contacted his company, The Egoscue Method, and had a therapy program tailored to suit my back pain. The therapy program arrived on videotape and I worked very hard on doing the exercises exactly as prescribed. I never missed a session and was extremely diligent. I did them perfectly. But it wasn't working this time. This time I was getting worse. My last resort was failing, and so was I.

As months passed, I remained indoors—lying on the floor as a fixed piece of furniture in front of the family room television, I worked on my therapy program.

---

universe; we just need to feel the matching "vibrations," for answers. Our feelings and emotions stemming from our thoughts are sent out into the universe and bring back a "match" to us. We bring what we are thinking to us whether they be good things or bad things. It is based in quantum mechanics in that we ourselves are given the power to create our own outer worlds from our inner self. The theory is that energy and matter are attracted to similar energy and matter by their vibrational frequencies—since everything living vibrates. If you hold firm to a problem or answer it becomes tangible by bringing it to you. We therefore bring people, scenarios and effects to ourselves as our vibrations created from our thoughts create matter and situations. It has been criticized as a "blaming the victim" theory but it has nothing to do with blaming and is often misrepresented as such.

But the harder I worked, the more the pain increased. The pain became so sharp that I could no longer do the therapy, or even think about it. Time was running out, so I emailed the Egoscue Clinic and the next day I received a call from Pete himself. We had a very good heart-to-heart talk about life and pain. He told me that he could tell I was in severe pain, and at the end of our discussion, he abruptly said, "as far as the back pain… we don't believe that it comes from there." That statement gave me **great pause**; I thanked him for calling and said goodbye. It was a beginning, a ray of hope in a very long dark period. I thank Pete for his candor and his advice. If it had not been for his honesty I may still be in serious pain today, still doing therapy, still struggling to survive like so many others who believe that back pain and neck pain and knee pain, are caused by physical or structural collapse. If not for his call to me and his final words, I would most likely have had multiple unnecessary surgeries. But within those succinct words of his, I sensed what Pete's implication was, and it gave me great pause to reflect, and so I did. I paused….

Pause—Reflection—Decision

I reflected, and reflected back again. Pausing is important in life, a pause is that short timespan in between the flight or fight responses where great ideas often emanate. Pauses can be great opportunities for constructive reflection, but also inroads for TMS to surface if there are unresolved issues. One must always be vigilant.

Pete's advice was a first step in my permanent healing. I can divide his therapy program into two parts. The first part is getting people to become much more active, to get off their lazy derrieres and to become physical, which is the most important element in healing. This is the exact manner in which to live life and also to heal from a lack of life. The second half of Pete's program is in retraining the musculoskeletal system into perfectly oriented 90-degree angles, or a returning of the body to its correct postural alignments. The former is a sine qua non for healing, and the latter is the death knell. Pete is correct on the first approach concerning activity and confidence, but the realigning of the body is absolutely unnecessary, as I found out in due time. The over-concern with proper body position and alignment allows the mind to be continually distracted from the emotional undertones by allowing the mind's eye to view the body as somehow flawed. This structural-deficit thinking feeds directly into the brain's clever strategy, which is the very reason for the existence of TMS. This is why the program wasn't working for me the second time around. I had severe tensionalgia, and that part of the program kept my pain ongoing by embedding in me a mental image that there was still a structural deficit in my spine, and that somehow I wasn't physically aligned properly.

> *As long as he (the sufferer) is in any way preoccupied with what his body is doing, the pain will continue.*
>
> — John E. Sarno, MD, *Healing Back Pain*[61]

The temporary fix I experienced with Pete the first time around is also common with epidural injections and surgeries, which have little or no effect after the initial placebo effects of the first round. So, I needed to stop therapy, but I didn't know it yet. The therapy was yet another culprit behind my continuing pain, but I didn't have any idea how important it was to stop at this time because I hadn't heard of a man named Sarno yet.

Patients are usually shocked when it is suggested that they stop the exercises and stretching they have been taught to do for their backs. But it is essential in order to establish firmly in the mind what is important.

— John E. Sarno, MD, *Healing Back Pain*[62]

Pete Egoscue is a well-meaning and honest person. I have only thanks for him, but I know now that when I was doing his therapy program eight years earlier, I merely had a temporary placebo reaction to his assertive writing and reputation. The more the patient or sufferer believes in the methodology, the more likely he is to gain confidence in self, to become more active and to be temporarily distracted from his pain. While this temporary distraction is helpful, unfortunately, the pain invariably returns with therapy or surgery. Surgery and therapy are rarely permanent cures, since the pain is not from a structural problem, and the body knows how to heal itself in a natural time frame. Chronic pain sufferers must stop all forms of physical, body-focused therapy. As Dr. Sarno has written, and I proved with my own experience, you can sit, walk, and lie any way you want, the back is the strongest part of the human body. One does not need to be aligned properly.

Humans are highly adaptive beings. They need to be active and confident, but they must also utilize their natural abilities as humans to discern what is true from what is not true. Today, people are finally beginning to question the efficacy of medicine, therapy, injections, acupuncture, manipulations, and surgery. More and more people are opening their minds to **mindbody healing** as greater successes are coming from healing the whole person instead of redesigning the body. Good health or bad health is contingent upon beliefs. But necessary changes don't always come easily, due to false conditioning and societal norms. Change often occurs slowly, and people who try to understand and believe in the mindbody process often pick and choose what they want regarding the needed changes, but belief is an all-or-nothing policy. It's like being kinda pregnant. Belief doesn't work unless you hand your entire self over to it. Yes, pain can reoccur after having been healed from TMS using Dr. Sarno's "cure." This only confirms as he indicated, that we all harbor anger as emotional beings.

Back (to) Therapy

After a short break, I decided to seek out a local physical therapist since I still hadn't heard of Sarno. I felt maybe a fresh start was warranted. I reluctantly got into my vehicle and ventured outside, which was a rare occurrence. The first day the therapist had me do a press-up (called the Cobra position), which is a therapeutic exercise that arches the spine backwards, when suddenly I felt a rush of tingling, as pins-and-needles climbed from my toes to my knees. I told the therapist that "something had just happened" and that my feet were "pinching and tingling." This sensation is called paresthesia and is described by physicians as part of the radiculopathy process. I've witnessed the manifestation of this sensation in TMS sufferers' arms, legs—even in their faces. It's the same feeling one gets when their leg falls asleep except paresthesia has no objective cause. However, we know from Dr. Sarno's work that this sensation of pins-and-needles comes from a lack of oxygen flow to the nerve, and is normally harmless. I was in high tension, the press-up had merely cut off the flow, and for an instant the nerves were not getting any oxygen at all. My brain was now immediately conditioned to expect the sensation of needles with movement.

The therapist's professional response to me was, "Really?...that's weird!" I thought it was weird too, his response that is. He was a therapist and didn't know what was happening. Right behind the pins-and-needles a twitching started in my calves. The twitching is known as fasciculitis. It was clear to me from the pins-and-needles and the fasciculitis that there was something much more serious going on than I would admit to. Soon after, my left foot began dropping when I walked, and I was unable to lift my foot or my toes upward, and the bottom of my feet began to hurt. The foot pain would move from day to day but the pain at the pad on the bottom of my left foot was now constant. On some days, my heels would hurt so badly that I needed to walk on my toes. On other days, my toes would hurt so badly that I needed to walk on my heels. I remember waking up daily and thinking, is this a toe day or a heel day? No wait, Tuesday was heel day, today is Wednesday isn't it? No, wait.... Focus was riveted to the body in fear. Fear is an elevator that never stops at the top floor.

Recapping Today's News: I had suffered from lower back pain since age 14. The catalyst that exacerbated my numerous physical manifestations caused by a perfectionistic personality was the traumatic experience of seeing my beautiful wife handicapped, accompanied by our subsequent failed relationship.

Years earlier I had a paralyzed left leg with loss of deep tendon reflex, failed laser eye surgery destroying my eyesight, a broken elbow and a temporarily paralyzed hand, fractured tooth, rapid bursts of vertigo with nystagmus, interstitial cystitis, scintillating scotoma, severe tinnitus, a thumping and screeching sound in my ear, sensations of pins-and-needles from my feet to my knees, bottom foot-pad pain and alternating heel pain in both feet, drop foot, rosacea, ankle pain, knee pain, neck pain, and food poisoning. My friends would often tell me that I had it made in life. Life it seems is always greener on the other side of dense.

The foot drop and lower back pain hit an all time high (pain high, foot low). I could no longer sit, walk, lie, or sleep. I crawled around in a constant pain and sweat. I had now dropped 45 lbs. and was beginning to have flashbacks of my life (man, I missed a lot of putts). While I still didn't have any conscious thought of harming myself, I was continuing to allow my life to fade. I often wondered what I had done to make God so angry with me. I would soon come to realize through a **great transformation** that I was instinctually doing these things to myself, self-punishing—without my knowledge. It had always been me, never Him. We suffer when we separate ourselves from the Truth—Truth never separates from us.

I was bedridden. The only sleep I could muster was when I was so tired from fighting pain that I would literally pass out. I physically couldn't move. Lying in bed, I began having cold shivers that would start on my right side and move across my body in a manner that felt like waves of ice. My central nervous system was collapsing. I no longer cared about living, although consciously I would not admit it to myself, thus my TMS—and its very purpose—to keep the unthinkable from entering consciousness.

I had gotten to where I knew that lower back surgery was inevitable. I was going to die from pain or risk surgery in which I had no confidence. After all, I had seen my wife become permanently paralyzed from a relatively routine anesthetic procedure, so I feared surgery with the best of them. I didn't want to risk being paralyzed, too. My family needed me healthy. They were my life. But the pain was so great that I was beginning to have trouble maintaining consciousness. I had lost the desire to eat or to move. But I had two children who needed a dad, so I reached down deep and once again gathered myself up and went to my orthopedic surgeon's office to ask for a recommendation for a surgeon at the University Hospitals in Cleveland. He recommended a surgeon, and I made an appointment to consult with him for the surgery... **however**...

When the student is finally ready, he will suddenly become aware that the teacher has been here all along.

In Vino Veritas!

Days before the surgery consult, for some unknown reason (to me at least), I once again gathered the will to push through the cutting pain and sluggishly pulled myself out of bed. I was having headaches from lying around and needed to get out. I still had within me that flicker of light burning to live. I pulled myself up, limped into my vehicle, and drove down the street a mile to my friend Mike's wine dealership to visit him and to buy a nice bottle of Chardonnay. I stumbled into the store, where he quickly commented on how bad I looked, "You look like you've been through hell." Little did he know that I had been vacationing there for months. I was unable to stand upright, but I exchanged some polite conversation and was on my way back to bed; but as I opened the door, he quickly picked up a book from behind his counter. He told me to hold on a minute and remarked that he had just read an article on back pain and it reminded him of me. I remember him leafing through the pages quickly searching for the article because he knew I was in pain. I shut the door and walked like Igor over to the counter where he showed me the article. It was an article in a book called *Boardroom Classics* by a Dr. John E. Sarno who worked at the Howard Rusk Institute at the New York University Medical Center. The article's description of back pain, and the personality traits that most often defined the pain, made a lot of sense. It sounded just like me; all that I was. The article's thesis was that back pain was emotionally induced and with the exception of extremely rare anomalies is never structural in origin. Mike wrote down the name of the doctor and the book for me and I went home and looked it up online, and bought *Healing Back Pain*. When the book arrived, I read the first few chapters, thought it was all bullshit, threw the book across my family room, and went straight back to ZZGS, after a glass of Chardonnay, or three …**and the vicious cycle continued….**

It would only be a short time more and I would return to that same Sarno book and begin reluctantly taking glimpses at it in a last ditch attempt to avoid the surgery that was rapidly approaching, as desperation breeds open minds.

> *One of the unfortunate realities about working with a disorder like TMS is that most people will reject the idea until they are desperate for a solution.*
> — John E. Sarno, MD, *Healing Back Pain*[63]

I had felt so bad for months now, that I wasn't able to spend time with my kids. I could see the helpless looks in their faces as they walked by me, unable to help me. Children are the greatest joy in life and they aren't little for very long. One day I was feeling bad enough that I couldn't play games any more with my littlest, so I decided to take her down to Borders Books and Music to find some type of intellectual game in a book that we could share together while I was lying down, ZZGS. While at Borders, my pain was out of control because my proxemic space was compressed—that space that people maintain between themselves when they interact. I decided to take advantage of this rare out-of-the house opportunity and force myself over to the back pain section of books. I couldn't stand up anymore, the pain was just too intense, and so I crawled around rifling through the books. Go figure, they had the back pain section on the very bottom where you had to bend all the way down to see them. I must have looked bad because as I was crawling around on the floor looking for the books a store clerk walked by and said, "You look like you really need to sit down, can I get you a chair?" I said, "No thanks," because I couldn't sit without screaming pain anyway. But what a kind thought from a stranger. So I crawled around until I saw a book by that very same crazy Dr. Sarno who I didn't believe before. This book, however, was entitled *Mind Over Back Pain*, which was his first book from 1982. I remembered the little that I had read from his later book *Healing Back Pain*, that I didn't believe then, but this time was much different. This time surgery was rapidly approaching, so I decided to read it; after all, it was short (not like this book you're reading now). I quickly read pieces of it right there, on my knees. I got the gist of it enough to know that this doctor had found something highly significant regarding back pain, and varying types of body and joint pain. I bought it.

I took *Mind Over Back Pain* home and devoured it—trying to avoid surgery like the plague. I read myself on every page of that book—as if he wrote it about me. It all seemed to make sense and it was well articulated and well researched. I slowly began to realize that he was correct in his observations. Pain is the resultant effect of a personality type that is exacerbated by periods of heightened anxiety/tension and unwarranted admonitions from the medical industry. Over the past several years I've also come to realize that it stems from a childhood separation anxiety/trauma, and unmet childhood needs, later triggered by unresolved conflict in relationships—or midlife crisis—manifesting as specific behavioral patterns, including TMS. I would also soon return to Dr. Sarno's second book, *Healing Back Pain*. The tears would finally begin flowing as I realized how much tragedy I had been inadvertently repressing. All of my unrecognized emotions began surfacing—the healing had begun. What had happened to my wife and between us was finally about to come pouring out of me. The vicious cycle was about to be broken and my healing was about to become complete and permanent. Dr. Sarno was about to save my life.

Whuh?—what is this salty discharge?

— Jerry Seinfeld, "The Serenity Now"

4

Chasing the Changes— A Time for Reflection

Uncle what ails thee? What is this suffering from?
— Parzival, *Quest for the Grail* (Wolfram's)

Had Parzival asked that question at the beginning of his search for the Grail (Truth), he wouldn't have had to suffer as he did, nor would the others around him have continued their suffering. But he also would have never learned (grown), and so there was higher purpose. So what is really happening here? Where does all this suffering come from? I was fortunate, I was blessed with the precious opportunity of time, to reflect on what had happened to me in my life, as well as what was happening to my friends and others throughout our shared world. People without the gift of time are at the mercy of those who have it. Looking back (pun fully intended), my pain was necessary so that I would have to deal with my unresolved biography. **The pain served as an enforcer.** During times of great tension my body was revealing to me through my past physical injuries and natural physical changes, that I wasn't happy. But, it becomes problematic when trying to connect the dots. For example, we feel that once we are injured, that we are never quite right there, where the injury occurred, but this is an error in thought— living in the past. When we heal, we heal all the way, but the mind remembers those past injury sites vividly and is reluctant to give up the fear that accompanies old injuries. We are conditioned by the medical industry to believe that there is an ongoing problem there, when in fact, there is not. The old injury site is simply a trigger for emotional outpouring, a perfect spot for tension to hide. People expect their knee or back or shoulder or neck to act up because they were once injured there, and so it becomes a haven for anger/energy/focus—once again, it is an error in belief. And so the individual erroneously feels that the pain came from the herniation or the post-traumatic arthritis, etc. But this assumption has been proven to be wrong in thousands, if not in tens of thousands of former sufferers. So chasing the changes is like the snake eating its own tail as new emotions present themselves to old injuries, which are a history of the entire person.

However, tensionalgia doesn't always follow this pattern of the mind chasing old memories. It can and does often occur where there is no structural damage (Phase 1 TMS). I was also surprised to see some TMS sufferers who actually took on the suffering of others. We share wounds in this world through empathic response in the great need to pull others to us, to be connected, and to belong. We pass on truths and also faulty information by which our mindbodies respond. If the information (experience) is perceived to be true, then it becomes a reality. I was beginning to see the larger picture of pain. I was growing, and the pain was my fertilizer.

The more empathic she is—**sensory-aware**—the more she shares others' pain. The more sentient she is, the greater her need for "the pull" in order to close any separation. She feels the others' pain. Is it through fear? Or is it through empathy? Is she living for herself or for others? One thing is for certain, during times of great tension and intra-psychic stress; there is greater susceptibility to **imitating** other people's disorders. She doesn't "catch colds and infections," she merely imitates them.

Old Wives' Tails

Quite commonly people will have surgery on a knee or shoulder or lumbar area, only to have the pain shift to the other knee or shoulder or lumbar disc. They then erroneously believe that they were somehow putting more pressure on the other side by trying to avoid the surgery side or that new scar tissue is causing new pain. This is not what is happening—not even close to the truth. It's merely unknown tension seeking out yet another area for attention because the individual has falsely believed that the area operated on is now "okay" as a result of the surgery. And so the mind seeks some other anger destination within the body. These pain sufferers aren't aware of the concept of TMS and so they head back to have the other disc trimmed or other knee or shoulder repaired. Here the tension isn't chasing changes, it's just desperate to hide and so it gets re-relegated to new areas of concern.

TMS also finds its way to people who have public conversations of new healing fads. To admit there is an emotional process is deemed a weakness in society, especially by men. Women are much more open to the truth but they also tend to harbor higher anxiety levels because they try to be nicer and tend to care more about more things—so it appears to be a wash.* The end result is that people suffer needlessly while others get rich off them.

So what is happening? People tell me their backs are bad because they "garden for a while" and their pain begins. Their pain is not due to a bad back; gardening merely triggers a conditioned response. At an unconscious level deep within them the child tires of the repetitive act. They often tell me that they love gardening and there is no way they would get angry from the act. But what they cannot sense is that it isn't the adult who is angered by the act. It's the id that is throwing the fit that is causing the pain. The id (the primary mind) is that part of them that is being denied its instant pleasure. *The squeaky kid gets the grease.* I see it all the time. Men and women running ragged coaching their kid's sports teams, running them to school, working two jobs,

---

* Approximately 95 percent of fibromyalgia sufferers are women.

hurry, added responsibility, rush, rush, rush… and then, sudden pain. They get imaging, and see arthritis or herniations, and naïvely believe their pain is due to these changes. When their lives finally calm down, their pain eases or goes away. So what happened? Did their back discs suddenly un-herniate? Their rotator cuffs un-tear? Their torn knee ligaments and arthritic hips magically reconstitute? The answer is that their hidden tension levels lowered.

The unconscious mind holds the center of emotion and sends messages to be interpreted by the conscious mind. In a fast-paced life there is no time to reflect, and so these messages go widely untranslated until there is stimulation overload whereby pain and illness form. Then follows a period of desperately needed understimulation (by missing work or being bedridden), due to that very same pain or illness, as the mindbody can no longer continue its balancing act. The individual, outside of his awareness, brings on his own pain or illness so that he CAN be acceptably removed from the stressful or unwanted situation.

A few people have told me that their surgery worked but they get tingling in their legs when they are tired. Well, their surgery didn't work. They believed it did at the time—the placebo sorta worked—the blood began to flow again because they felt "cured." When they become tired, they become angered within—both irritated and agitated—as the conditioned response kicks in. The structure of the human spine doesn't suddenly become less stable when the body becomes tired. The larger picture becomes clearer when the entire painting is unveiled. But life passes by too quickly to always grab the brass ring, and so they spin around on the pain-go-round in eternal circles—caught in the cycle of going along with the pack mentality. They aren't dumb, they just don't know yet because they're caught up in the frenzy of a modern society and blinded by tremendous misconceptions regarding health.

During this new era of the 21st century, the true knowledge of "what is going on here" is swiftly expanding. People are recognizing that surgery is not necessary most every time. A couple of people I know who have injured their knees have put off knee surgery against the wishes of their doctors. They ended up healing faster than other people I knew who had knee surgery, since the surgery itself is re-injuring the knee and making the convalescence lengthier. People are also increasingly recognizing that they have hidden emotions in play, and that those very same emotions often attack old injury sites. They are also beginning to recognize the timing of the onset of their symptoms. But the **pharmo-medical machine** keeps pushing them backward in order to keep them blinded by fear. All one needs is to watch a few TV commercials and he will begin having pains or heartburn or any host of suggested physical ailments—and right behind the ads are the class action lawsuit commercials for the damage the drugs and medical testing caused. Illness is big business and the sufferer is the client. After all, it is much easier to take a pill than to look within to find the cause of any dis-order, or dis-ease. Who are the drug manufacturers marketing to on television anyway? The Average Joe can't go out and buy most of those drugs. They do suggest at the end of the commercial however, to, "ask your physician about it!" But the physician shouldn't be giving you drugs because you saw them on TV and decided that you need them. So who are they targeting? They are directly targeting doubt and fear. Fear = money.

> *The various health disciplines interested in the back have succeeded in creating an army of the partially disabled in this country with their medieval concepts of structural damage and injury as the basis of back pain.*
>
> — John E. Sarno, MD, *Healing Back Pain*[64]

People often state that they were lifting or pulling on something when their pain began. But they rarely look at what was pulling on them at that time in their lives. There is always deeper causation and it is always from **cognitive dissonance**—acting in a manner that conflicts with how they truly feel inside.

During times of heightened tension, the body is already locked in fight or flight. The sympathetic nervous system is on high alert—the blood triaged to the organs most needed to survive. Then, all it takes is a simple lift or a pull or a twist for the blood to be suddenly cut off. When the blood gets cut off, there is a sudden and severe sharp pain. Now a domino effect begins. The brain begins protecting the affected area by further tensing. The individual, through repeated and unproven suggestion **believes** he has thrown his back out or herniated his discs. High tech imaging soon follows where the individual visually sees physical evidence of structural "damage," subsequently confirmed by the dire radiology report—further convincing him that his pain is due to a structural injury. Finally, the physician himself validates the person's skewed conclusion by advising that he "take it easy" or "have surgery" or "therapy" in order to become normal again. But the individual doesn't know the entire truth. The changes he saw on the images were most likely there before his pain began. One needs only to look at the 1994 Hoag Memorial Hospital/Cleveland Clinic study to see that many people have these changes and herniations and wears-and-tears but have no symptoms because the pain is not coming from these "normal abnormalities." Error upon error gets passed down through layer-after-layer, generation-after-generation, conscious-to-unconscious.

Pain does not come from having one leg longer than the other, or one hip higher than the other. Pain does not come from arthritis or herniated discs or bone warping. Pain comes from deep-seated unhappiness, monotony through lack of purpose, and fear, which in turn further angers the sufferer, increasing pain.

I remember watching Michael Jackson on TV during one of his child molestation trials. He came to court limping in pain (with snazzy pajamas on) being assisted by two bodyguards during one of the first days of the trial. He had claimed his pain was due to a fall he had from a stage years before (Phase 3 TMS). It was obvious that his anger had increased to **threshold levels** because he was forced to be in court and shamed. The area chosen was the result of an old injury site, but the pain was not from the injury itself, it was from his autonomic nervous system and that clever mind that never forgets, a posteriori. His mind's eye remembers the old injury, doubting it had ever healed—a place that can be used to run away from his thoughts whenever needed.

I once fell for the "needs a softer mattress" or "needs a firmer mattress" ruse propagated by the sleep industry. When I went to hotels, if the mattress was too soft I would wake up, invariably, in pain. I had myself convinced that the soft mattress was hurting my back, and so it did. Oh No, Not the Comfy Chair! Where the mind sleeps, the body does also. I was once told I had one leg longer than the other and that was the reason for my pain. How have we fallen this far in medicine? However— whenever I would forget my shoe lift, my pain would increase dramatically—snared by the trap—I created my own suffering. These days I sit, walk, run and lift any way I want to. The pharmo-medical complex has truly created an army of the partially disabled who constantly feel as though they are falling apart; and so they do. But this attitude can change, and is changing. Back pain will someday be "behind us," but a new, more beguiling problem, will certainly replace it as long as the body is looked toward for answers—as a focal point away from undesirable thoughts and emotions.

Fuh-Getuh-bout It!

Forget the shoe lifts, pills, mattresses, images, back braces, surgery, manipulations, therapy, creams, and advice. To be free of pain we must set ourselves free. Societal admonitions are enslaving to the human psyche because warnings are limiters. They imprison the mind, and the body becomes the cellmate. Also, to further propagate these misconceptions, people pass "the word" along concerning their own wounds and healing treatments. I've sat in public places many times listening to people share their woundology. People would say things like, "you should try this new elbow brace, it really works!" or, "my therapist has me doing this new exercise, it's really working!" or, "I tried this new over-the-counter medication to re-grow my joints and I feel much better!" "Try this new pillow I bought, I feel better already!" or, "this surgeon is really good, go see him." On and on, ad nauseum it goes, where it stops nobody really knows. The laymen and the physicians naïvely pass false information back and forth. It's not entirely anyone's fault, but some have more accountability than others. People are truly attempting to help others and themselves, like most physicians are trying to do. But what you don't know can sometimes hurt you. One of my favorites is Shaquille O'Neal's commercial. "I want a championship so bad it hurts." All you need to do is to rub this cream on the pain and kazaam, it's gone. There was another amusing advertisement regarding a talisman you wear around your neck to balance your energy. It made your balance better and your pains go away, and it even improved your golf score! I'm sure it works—if the believer believes it deeply enough. However, it is not a part of any solution—it is the problem. If you put your faith in the stone, it stays in the stone. We are defined by our beliefs—what we believe in, guides our lives.

Since I've been pain-free, I've slept on the floor, on soft mattresses, sat any way I wanted, lifted with just my back, and twisted and turned in any manner. I know what causes pain now—it cannot hold my attention anymore. When my tension level rises, my mind seeks my old injuries, sometimes. This is to say, during times of great tension I can feel my back tighten, or hip lose some range of motion, but no pain follows—I can stop pain by simply knowing what events are taking place in my life.

Sometimes pain seeks out the body area that is performing repetitious acts, like a job that is hated or just mundane. Understanding this is mandatory for healing—acquiring knowledge—the first pillar in healing. The second pillar is acting on this knowledge. These days I know when I get a stab of pain that I'm frustrated or angry inside and that my body is okay, and the pain never stays more than a few seconds. This has brought contentiousness, as several people have said to me, "I thought you were pain-free?" The idea that a human being will never have pain again is fantasy. When I say pain-free, I mean there is no chronicity or severity. I've gotten over-arrogant with the power and stability of my spine and tried to lift very heavy objects without using my legs. I get a twinge, but it dissipates rapidly. By pain-free living, I don't mean that you can shoot a bullet through your foot and have no pain. One must use common sense in discerning statements and false claims.

Don't Pull the Trigger—When the Gun Is Loaded

People often report that at that moment of [pain] onset, they hear some kind of noise, a crack, a snap or a pop… The noise is a mystery… One thing is clear—the noise indicates nothing harmful.

— John E. Sarno, MD, *Healing Back Pain*[65]

A trigger is an event, sensation, place, time, movement, substance, or inference that initiates a physical phenomenon, such as pain. It's the cork that is unplugged that enables the bubbling conflict to make itself known throughout the body. The trigger delivers the message of existing tension—reminds the brain of the past—recreating a conditioned response. It sets in motion the catastrophe of misinformation and allows the hidden anger a **specious focal point**.

The most well-known trigger is the **pop** that comes from lifting or moving or bending or pulling. The sound is from body parts moving against one another and joint fluid compressing or expanding. It usually means nothing. The vast majority of these frightening "pops" and "cracks" are routine sounds that the body makes in mechanical movement. It is rare, but also possible, that a cracking or popping sound indicates a serious occurrence like the structure being torn apart. So it's always imperative to get a physical exam to rule out the need for immediate medical treatment. These sounds do however open up a great opportunity to distract the individual—providing a physical decoy. We are mentally conditioned to believe that when our backs pop from twisting or turning that we have thrown our backs out or have slipped or herniated a disc. This is a physical impossibility, as I said, unless the structure is torn apart such as in an accident. There may be some sort of biophysical change occurring with these snaps and pops, but it is usually harmless and meaningless.

Discs are structures located between the bodies of spinal bones to take up the shock. They are firmly attached to the vertebral bodies above and below and in no way can they "slip."
— John E. Sarno, MD, *Healing Back Pain*[66]

The triggers' effects result from both conditioning and suggestion. That is, people are conditioned to believe something is wrong when they hear a popping sound. They also receive the suggestion through persistent warnings to be careful not to throw their backs out. The Law of Attraction now guarantees that they will experience the effects of those warnings at some point. But people need only to look at what is popping in their lives when their pain strikes hard.

Alleve-i-ating Triggers

Triggers take many forms. I communicated with an intelligent man who understood the pain process quite well, and understood it as an emotionally driven process. His symptoms were severe neck stiffness and rigidity that began after he got an Alleve tablet stuck in his throat. He was also working out hard in the gym during the week, and was stuck in a tense family situation wrought with tight financial constraints. His was an effect waiting to happen. The tablet merely pushed him over the edge of the tension threshold, and his symptoms began pouring out—Phase 2 TMS—resulting in severe neck tightness and dizziness, classic TMS symptoms. The tablet didn't alleviate anything, but rather triggered something much deeper. To his credit, he implicitly understood the process to be an emotional effect.

A common trigger is the **admonition**. Admonition ignites pain when the individual has been persistently warned to be careful of something that he was previously unaware of (The Law of Attraction in action, Jackson). I communicated with a man named Chris who had suffered from repetitive stress injury (RSI) and recovered rather rapidly after finding Dr. Sarno's work. Chris had written to me that his pain "went through the roof" soon after he attended a mandatory course on repetitive stress injuries and hand pain. Warning of pain... brings pain—because it gives the compulsive individual a legitimate and socially approved focal point to hide within when he needs a mental diversion. Chronic whiplash is a common example.

An odd, but interesting trigger I ran across while researching, was introduced by a man who had already recovered about 75 percent from RSI after reading Dr. Sarno's second book. Robert would have been nearly 100 percent recovered but he could not change the pattern of pain that occurred when using his right index finger to click the computer's mouse. In Robby's own words, "[T]he bizarre part is that my finger and hand doesn't [sic] hurt when I close my eyes and move/click the mouse. It's as if the screen (and software) is the trigger for the pain?!?" He reduces his visual acuity when he closes his eyes, one of his senses. So, closing his eyes allegorically opens them by removing the **sensory trigger.** If he unconsciously despises staring at his computer screen because staring at it is in conflict with his unconscious wants and needs, then closing his eyes "cuts out" the source of information that triggers his anger, i.e., his eyesight. Sight is one of the senses that blinds us (Lao Tzu).

Bad Luck Chuck

Then there is the human **compassion trigger.** I met a man, Chuck, in his late 30s who suffered from severe TMS with an extreme burning lung sensation as well as the common icy cold waves from head to toe, that are common with extreme tension. He described the cold sensation as feeling like someone had poured a bucket of cold water over his head. He was going through extreme relationship separation anxiety after his wife left him, and had experienced paralytic episodes and increasing tinnitus. I spoke with him on the phone after an episode that landed him in the emergency room, exasperated by tremendous anxiety, burning, weakness and vertigo sensations. He explained to me that a coworker had walked up to him that day and asked him "how he was doing" regarding his health problems? He described the following events, "...at that moment I felt a sudden weight on me, followed by a general weakness, which made me begin a controlled drop to my knees for fear of falling—then the burning began... the weakness, followed by burning, continued in waves while I remained on the floor." Two days later, after he had returned from the hospital, the same coworker called him at his home to see how he was doing. In his words, "...the second day when she called, I became increasingly anxious the more we spoke, burned more and more until I was forced to tell her it was happening again and asked her to hold on.... I sat the phone down to catch my breath but didn't want to keep her waiting, so I picked it back up before I'd really recovered at all, and as she continued, I had to end the conversation... the anxiety and burning had set upon me strongly... once it was out, I could not put it away... I deteriorated into, essentially, a full panic attack I guess you could say?...Vertigo, burning, panic, it began to pass when I began speaking with the ER staff."

This woman's show of concern, as he described was "genuine concern" and so it triggered his emotional description of "weight upon me." This was the tell-all in his open-hearted description of the circumstances that played out in his body, as it often does in mindbody **symbolism.** We ultimately get to a repressive limit, after stealthily "going it alone" in life—then suddenly comes a word or words of human caring and **compassion** that pulls the individual over the self-pity threshold. His coworker triggered a response waiting to happen by uttering the words he desperately needed to hear from loved ones, anyone, and yet had not—feeling alone and unconnected. We often desire to find vengeance against prior rejections by trying to become independent of others. When a sympathetic ear comes along, it opens the floodgates for self-pity and allows the previously repressed energy to surface. This can be healing and cathartic; however, if more repression and denial occur—things can worsen. A kind doctor's ear, or a friendly gesture, can heal wounds of isolation and disconnection. As this man wrote to me, it passed when he began speaking with the ER staff. I had previously communicated with Dr. Sopher about this same need to be heard, and as an MD skilled in the mindbody process, he agreed that the physician's caring ear can be a soothing and powerful healing mechanism. It can untrigger the triggered.

Third time's the charm, right? If we continue to try to be tough and independent, AND if the need to know if anyone cares remains, the subconscious battle rages on. Several weeks later, Chuck began speaking with the same "trigger girl" and began having waves of the same symptoms and then "suddenly collapsed." This is conditioning at its finest. The first time she, out of compassion, asked him how he was doing, the question triggered all the emotions he'd been holding in to come pouring to the forefront. Now each time she asks him about himself his brain reacts the same—like the gazelle escaping the lion. Besides telling him to stop talking with her, I explained the association process to him, which he fully understands. What he doesn't understand is that his symptoms are the result of repressing his emotions, holding back what he cannot face until he heats up to the point that a single trigger initiates a meltdown. So his symptoms arrive to save his day so that he can avoid facing his true feelings. His brain simply does him a favor.

Another man wrote that he had healed about "80 to 95 percent" with TMS healing—had become active with running and lifting. He was essentially fine, but someone made the mistake of asking him how his back was doing, to which he replied "good," that it "had never been better." Then in his words, "…next day, bam—I could hardly stand up straight!" The query regarding his back reminded his brain of the past—thoughts pushed aside now hit the front burner—bam! This is Phase 1 TMS.

We definitely need to get things off our chests. Who hasn't asked someone how they were doing, and the person suddenly began crying? What if they can't or won't cry under the superego's watch? They will then need to bury the need to cry in their bodies that will eventually fire when the right trigger is pulled. The **compassion trigger** can redirect the mind's eye back to all that has been thus far repressed. But the trigger won't fire anything unless the weapon is loaded.

Another common trigger is the **bump** or **twist**. Unconscious anger will rush to an area of the body that has hit something, or been bumped into. All the pent-up rage heads toward the banged-up area, like a dam breached. With an obsessive mind, the pain then will not leave for an extended period. This is Phase 2 TMS with autoimmune characteristics as the body overreacts to a sensation—turning red—swelling—seemingly attacking itself as in gout.

Other common triggers are **empathic triggers**. These result from great **sensitivity** to others during times of high tension and anxiety, such as when someone very close to us comes down with a serious or threatening disorder. My virtual friend, Scott Tovan, admits to being susceptible to others' symptoms. In his words, "I had experienced an onset of back/leg symptoms after a close friend had back surgery (a benign growth was found inside her spinal canal and was pressing on her leg nerves). I also developed vertigo a few months after she did." I, too, experienced this same vertigo-trigger as Mr. Tovan. During my severe TMS, a friend of mine told me of her bursts of vertigo. A few weeks later, when I entered critical TMS, I developed her symptoms, exactly as she had described them to me—literally spinning her details.

The King of Triggers may well be the **aging trigger**, a.k.a. the **Not So Happy Birthday Trigger**, including the perceived loss of health and loss of looks. My friend Allan's pain had crippled him when he turned 70. He freely understands and admits that it was the thought of aging badly that had debilitated him. In his book, *The Mindbody Prescription*, Dr. Sarno lists six basic needs that anger and frustrate us if they are not adequately met. Number six on that list is "to be immortal (we are unconsciously enraged by the inevitability of death)." Allan has a beautiful story concerning his crippling pain and his complete recovery after finding Dr. Sarno's books. He told me that he had witnessed friends and acquaintances turn for the worse after turning 70, and so this thought process triggered his own demise as he debilitated himself at the thought of following the same fate. He made the mistake of peeking into the future and not living in the moment. Not only does this prove that it is an **error in thought** alone that creates the imbalance in the mindbody process, but it also gives great credence to Satchel Paige's question, "How old would you be if you didn't know how old you were?" Allan was told he had severe spinal stenosis and needed immediate surgery, but he wisely refused. He eventually recovered completely through TMS healing.

Pain is, as Dr. Sarno has described, a "cradle to grave" phenomenon; however, TMS exists primarily during the years that we bear the heaviest responsibilities. When pain strikes beyond these responsibility years, it's almost entirely due to the anger of aging—of seeing friends and relatives passing away as separation rage increases. Pain is often a part of midlife crisis as people begin to look for answers beyond what they see—curious of a life beyond what they have. Swiss psychiatrist Carl Jung wrote, "Among all my patients in the second half of life—that is to say over 35 years of age—there has not been one whose problem, in the last resort, was not that of finding a religious outlook on life."[67] People need soothing answers. If they can't find it from knowledge therapy or counselors, then they need to look more deeply within themselves for a spiritual awakening.

Another common trigger is the injury, illness, or **death of a loved one**. A few weeks after my neighbor's wife died, he was in surgery having his back operated on (stenosis surgery). In *The Mindbody Prescription*, Dr. Sarno reproduced a list of stressors from psychiatrists Thomas Holmes and Richard Rahe, who studied "the role of stressful life events." The Holmes-Rahe Stress Scale is a list of events ordered from the most stressful (likely to cause internal rage) to the least stressful. The number one most stressful event likely to cause rage is "death of a spouse." Closely related triggers are those of the **ill loved ones**. Many of these pain sufferers' stories begin with, "my mother or father moved back in with me when they fell ill." Or, I had to "start taking care of my mother when..." The energy now demanded of them to care for their loved one, generates the unconscious rage that drives them over Dr. Sarno's anger threshold.

A very common trigger is **pregnancy**. Pain either starts during pregnancy, or more commonly postpartum—due to anticipation of new demands, fear of change, and from the prior emotional wounds of the mother's own birth/infancy. Since we know that chemical imbalances are a result of a mental process and not vice versa, we can surmise that it is the energy demanded of the new mother from the new responsibility of the baby (a new part of themselves)—creating great anxiety and in the process altering chemistry.

One of my favorite triggers I read about in *Healing Back Pain*, where one of Dr. Sarno's patients told him that she only got pain when she made herself a drink and tried to relax. This drink trigger is actually a **guilt** trigger. The conscientious individual doesn't feel she deserves to relax, and, she may have been in pain once when she had a drink, so conditioning pours another dose of pain on the rocks.

There are also **examination triggers**. The Type T often complains of ongoing pain after having been tested for urinary, bowel, eye, ear, and various other disorders—from procedures performed during medical testing. The pain and worry from the medical test now becomes their new focus—and TMS begins....

There are many other triggers, most of which can be taken directly from the stressor list that Dr. Sarno reproduced in *The Mindbody Prescription*. However, most can be combined into those triggers I've listed here, except for the food, chemical, and pollen triggers—substance triggers.

And it goes on and on.... The list of triggers is infinite.
         — Marc Sopher, MD, *To Be or Not To Be... Pain-Free*[68]

5

How I Became Pain-Free

The unexamined life is not worth living.

— Socrates, *Apology of Socrates* (469-399 BCE)

When I write that I am healed or cured, this means my back pain is gone after 27 years of continuous pain. People will always have various aches and pains because they are organic, thinking, sentient beings. I would consider myself back to normal, where I was when I was 12 or 13 years old. As humans who possess the curses of anticipation and ego, there will always be some type of symptom, but life is now fun and enjoyable. I can see clearly now, the pain has gone, I understand the obstacles in my way.

Through serendipity, I had found Dr. Sarno's work and thankfully, I have a curious and open mind. Did I believe he was correct in his assertions? No, not really; deep down inside I thought he was a bit whacky. Perhaps he had taken too many x-rays without his lead helmet on? But I was desperate to rid my pain and to avoid surgery because I had witnessed my wife being paralyzed by a much less invasive procedure than I was about to have. In addition, of the dozens of people I knew who had had back surgery, it hadn't worked for any of them. Yes, some will say that it did, but it clearly didn't. They still must be careful or sometimes have bad days. They were fooled by the beguiling and awesome power of the **placebo effect**, with most ending up returning for more surgery when the effect had worn off and hidden tension once again arose in their knees or chest, etc. Common statements from friends or acquaintances that have had back or neck or knee or shoulder surgery that had actually failed are:

> Yes, surgery worked, but I still have to be careful.
>
> Yes, surgery worked, but I have to have another surgery, and another, and another.
>
> Yes, surgery worked, but I need to "get down" quickly if I feel the pain coming on.
>
> Yes, surgery worked, but I cannot lift anything.
>
> Yes, surgery worked, but if I overdo it, it begins to "stab" a little.
>
> Yes, surgery worked, but I need to do many sit-ups each day or continue my therapy.
>
> Yes, surgery worked, but now my ankle, knee, or hip hurts, etc.

If the individual likes and trusts the surgeon, the placebo effect can be quite substantial. But this is rare. Most aren't able to discern that the surgery failed, and that they're still TMSing. With true healing, you can lift most anything you desire. There is no residual pain. There is no need to "get down" quickly. There is no more fear of lifting or bending, or even the **need** for fear, because healing comes from understanding that the pain was never structural in origin. For a lucky few, the surgery placebo may last a lifetime, depending on how deeply they believed it solved their problem. But with certainty, their pain will be triggered again when their tension levels are elevated because the surgery didn't remove the true cause of their pain. Real, integrative, mindbody healing is permanent, but also contingent upon dealing effectively with any emotional conflict. Any pain relief from surgery is due to the relief that the surgery is actually over, and to the confidence in the surgeon and the procedure.

I wanted to believe Dr. Sarno's findings; however, like most, I didn't at first. It takes time to integrate the fullness of truth with a little **desperation** thrown in as a motivational force by which to expand current awareness. Those who have patience, diminished egos, and open minds, heal nicely. I've witnessed it several hundred times—and more importantly I lived it. Those who refute the TMS concept remain in pain, or in constant fear of movement or activity. I was caught somewhere in the middle at first. But today I never fear the pain nor do I have any indications that I ever had pain. Some 18 years after I was in critical condition, I am still free. But I have aged since then and my back deteriorates further with age. So what happened?

Healing Stages

In our most private mirror we see ourselves as paragons of virtue or intelligence, even our most blatant faults and handicaps will disappear or acquire attractive coloration.
— Karen Horney, MD, *Our Inner Conflicts*[69]

I would have **never**, in a gazillion years, viewed myself as angry. I had always seen myself as serene and controlled—but this IS the problem. The outward appearance of control, serenity, and peace is fine and dandy—but when things like pain, skin, bowel, seizure, immune, asthma, and digestive problems arise—there is something deeper going on—you've hidden something from yourself and others. The apparent serenity that accompanies strong repression comes with a staggering price. Symptoms are the indicators that these emotions are indeed present, right beneath the surface, literally screaming to get out.

The Wobbly Beginning

In desperation, I began following Dr. Sarno's advice with less than a fervent attitude. It was the scales of justice with dangerous surgery in my left hand, and in my right hand, the concept that I could have repressive tendencies—enough tension to create physical symptoms of such hidden magnitude. However, in my right hand, I was now holding hope, and in the sinister hand—despair.

I started reading Dr. Sarno's first book, *Mind Over Back Pain* and also purchased his second book on audiotape, *Healing Back Pain*. I already owned *Healing Back Pain*, which I had thrown across the family room floor once I began to understand its implications. With 20/20 hindsight, it is clear that I threw that book in anger because I knew deep down that it was all true. The truth scorches the bitter darkness with burning light, and the object burned is—ego.

I lay in bed reading *Mind Over Back Pain* and how the autonomic nervous system is involved in pain. Reading was, and is, difficult for me because of my damaged left cornea but the book made a lot of sense and was backed up with solid statistical evidence and decades of experience. Toward the end of reading that little book, something strange began happening. My hands began to swell. It was one of the most amazing things I have ever witnessed. It had never happened before, nor has it happened since. As I was reading, I began understanding what Dr. Sarno was conveying regarding the autonomic nervous system and unrecognized anger, and suddenly both of my hands began swelling, full of blood as my bloodflow suddenly became erratic. My hands became so heavily gorged with blood that I couldn't close them or bend my fingers. Was my unconscious mind creating a distraction in order to keep me from fully understanding the real reason behind my pain? I believe this was the reason—to keep the hidden as hidden. But I still don't know why it happened in my hands. Perhaps it was because I was holding the truth in my hands, in that book. No matter the reason, my awareness had begun to expand along with my hands. The reality of the mindbody process was unfolding "write" before my eyes. **We all know the Truth within ourselves**; the conflict arises when our egos choose to separate us for reasons I described earlier. When we step into the truth our internal forces rebel—the shadow does not wish to have light shed upon it—that's the reason we hide aspects of ourselves within it.

I stopped reading and stared at my hands for about half an hour as the pressure in them mounted. I wondered if they might explode at some point. Would my health insurance cover exploding hands? Then suddenly, I began having deep chest pains as the swelling in my hands dissipated. I wasn't really worried because I knew something was beginning to change. My chest pain lasted for about 15 minutes and then disappeared. I had never had chest pains before and I have not had any since then. It was the first step in my long road to recovery. It was also my first awareness of the autonomic process in action. I felt hopeful. Change had just occurred and **change is what is needed** for recovery from chronic pain.

My days then consisted of lying in bed unable to move, reading Dr. Sarno's books and attempting to more fully understand his assertions. I tried many times to sit up or to walk but the pain was absolutely crippling. I feared it—which was just what my brain wanted. But I decided to try, and so I would sit up in bed and attempt to walk a few paces and to become more active and to challenge the pain as the good doctor was advising. But I paid a heavy price for my effort as the pain always increased—dramatically. In fact, I began having more pain and various other physical problems. These problems do magnify doubt in the TMS healing process, and people often quit here and shrug it all off as nonsense. But what the good doctor had written made too much sense to stop that soon—I couldn't give up—not yet. My stubbornness got me into this mess—my stubbornness would need to lead me out.

My doubts about TMS remained elevated along with my pain. However, there was something in the "way he wrote" that compelled me to keep pushing forward. There was confidence in his pen and it ALL made perfect sense to me—the testimonials from his patients appeared genuine and sincere, so I continued ...**and the vicious cycle also continued....**

Each day I would read—repeatedly—the sections on mild oxygen deprivation, and would try to walk. It was difficult to believe that something mild could cause such debilitating pain; it all felt so dangerously structural. After all, I had seen my medical images with stenosis, and herniated discs, and arthritis. Could this mild ischemia create such unbearably sharp pain? I wasn't sure.

The days blurred into months. I would read, and then attempt to move around as Sarno had suggested. But day after day, the setbacks were more frequent than the advances. Even though he had so elegantly explained that "you cannot hurt yourself," it was still difficult for me to fully believe, so I moved with caution. Caution, I would later prove, was the worst thing I could have adhered to. I should have cast doubt to the wind earlier on, but it was a natural course of action, as seen by so many others who have healed in the same manner because we have all been erroneously taught to believe we are physically flawed—by doctors.

The months blended into more months, following the same patterns of "one step forward" and "five steps backward." But I had nothing to lose, and more importantly, I wasn't getting continually worse. By that, I mean, as I increased my activity, the pain did increase on many days but there were also days in which the pain was not as sharp. So, logically, if there were structural problems the pain should have worsened with increasing movement. The only explanation could be that Dr. Sarno might be correct, but I still wasn't convinced. I could not walk, I could not sit. I could not enjoy my kids, I had a handicapped wife; all three needed my help. Dr. Sarno had at the very least given me hope. I could at least make a half-assed attempt at healing. So I continued, receiving half-assed results. As living beings, we get out of life what we put into it, or what we believe of it. We vibrate at various frequencies and we receive vibrational matching back (The Law of Attraction).

My doubt in the early stages of healing was not singular. People I have met and who have all healed, tell me they, too, doubted greatly in the beginning. David

Schechter, MD, a TMS physician in Beverly Hills (California that is, swimmin' pools, movie stars) who met Dr. Sarno while attending NYU has said, "Doubt is part of the (TMS) process." It is indeed. If there were no structural doubts planted by physicians, there would be no continuing pain. Therefore, doubt regarding TMS gives pain leverage for continuance, as the irrational fear feeds into the brain's strategy.

Half a year or more had gone by and it seemed as if I was pinned down in a vicious cycle that could not be broken. I began to wonder if I was being overly naïve in following this Sarno's advice. After all, I was desperate, and desperate people often take desperate measures. I implicitly knew that I needed to take things up a notch in order to prove TMS as the correct diagnosis (self-diagnosis) or to prove TMS as a witch-doctor's ruse.

To strengthen my belief I began listening to an abridged audiotape set of *Healing Back Pain*. This was a priceless step on my healing journey. When the audiotapes arrived, I put my headphones on in anticipation of hearing Sarno's voice. It was not the sine qua non in my healing but it was the biggest step forward I could have taken. I found hearing to be a more powerful sense than seeing (reading). In my case, hearing was believing.

When one is depressed and debilitated from prolonged periods of torturous pain, confidence is either nonexistent or very low. Confidence is necessary in order to heal from pain—**confidence in the diagnosis**. It is crucial to find something to build up confidence, step by step, no matter how small those steps may be. Hearing the good doctor's voice explaining the TMS process catapulted me forward.

When Helen Keller was asked which of her senses she would choose if she had her choice, she replied, "I am just as deaf as I am blind.... Deafness is a much worse misfortune. For it means the loss of the most vital stimulus—the sound of the voice that brings language, sets thoughts astir and keeps us in the intellectual company of man." Helen knew the connection power of sound.

Tracordification—The Connecting of Hearts

Sound is awesome in its power because we feel the vibrations of connection where we cannot feel (at least consciously) the vibrations of sight (light). I believe this begins in the womb as the baby hears the vibrations of mother's heartbeat and voice. We need to hear that we are safe—connected and doing okay. I needed to hear it from Dr. Sarno directly. However, as a **visual spatial learner** with a marked weakness in auditory learning, I had to listen to those tapes non-stop. After hearing his voice, I began visualizing the entire process he had written about—in symbols and images. Reading alone wasn't moving me forward rapidly enough because of the type of learner I happen to be. Hearing Dr. Sarno's voice somehow connected him with me and enabled me to visually imagine the process better than reading his books had done so far. On the audiotape he was telling me I would be okay—much like I would expect to feel during a personal visit to his office.

Finally—hearing the words that I had been reading and memorizing vaulted me ahead. He was confident in his findings—neither arrogant nor dogmatic, but professional and matter-of-fact in what he had witnessed and knew to be true. He knew that tension-rage caused the vast majority of the pains that doctors attributed to structural wear and tear all over the body. He was asserting that structural degradations were merely normal aging of the body and that the new high-tech images, like MRIs, were showing the body changing normally through life. The scientific community had erroneously linked pain to these normal structural changes. Even though pain was only sometimes located near the sites of degeneration—the consensus had transformed the common error into a **spurious correlation, or apophenia—a pattern or connection that doesn't exist.** This was proven in a study on intervertebral and nonintervertebral disc abnormalities as seen on MRIs, performed at the Hoag Memorial Hospital in Newport Beach, California (see Chapter 4), which concluded: "The discovery of bulges or protrusions in people with lower back pain may frequently be coincidental." The key words here are frequently, followed by the word coincidental.

I once sat down and estimated how many times I listened to pieces of the abridged audiotapes of *Healing Back Pain*. It was well over a thousand times. Many people can merely read the book and heal through the understanding of each page, line-by-line, but, as a visual spatial learner, I needed to conceptualize the bigger picture by listening and by imagining symbols and images.

During this entire healing phase, I was also thinking psychologically as he had advised. I was mentally perusing all the possibilities for my symptoms, looking for any and every possible source of the pain and other symptoms. My list was shockingly long and it began with the phrase, paralyzed wife. But I still didn't feel any anger about anything. I knew I **should** be angry at what had happened to Susan, Matthew, and me, but I wasn't. This was the problem—superego had stealthily buried all rage in my body ...**and the vicious cycle continued...** however, all my years of playing sports were about to pay off. A sport teaches you discipline. When you are banged up and knocked down, you get back up on your feet no matter how bad it hurts, you pull yourself up by your bootstraps (or jock straps) and get right back in—to continue the goal.

One must confront TMS, fight it, or the symptoms will continue.
                                        — John E. Sarno, MD, *Healing Back Pain*[70]

I had been keeping a boombox ten feet from my bed so that as I rolled out of bed I could crawl over to the tape machine and hit play and listen to the audio of *Healing Back Pain*. Day by day I pushed on, increasing activity, reading, listening, and visualizing. I fully understood that I needed to move, to visually imagine a healthier body, and to integrate full belief in the process.

Yes, I Would NOT Like a Wake-Up Call for 6:24 A.M. Please

For several weeks, every morning at precisely 6:24 A.M. a very sharp back stab would awaken me like a lightning bolt. It was like the movie *Groundhog Day*. The pain would strike and knock the wind out of me. I would sit up quickly, look at the clock and fall back onto the pillow to start yet another day of the same old thing (no Sonny Bono playing). It was a classic example of a conditioned response and of the preciseness with which the unconscious operates. Right after that first wake-up call, my back would initially feel über-good in a drowsy state of somnolence. AAhhhhh—if I could only bottle that feeling of drowsiness. This brainwave-activity state is called theta wave time—just after waking. After theta, I jumped directly into high-gear beta—where the brainwaves begin to rapidly oscillate following the deep delta sleep of 0.1–4 cycles per second toward theta activity of 4–7 cycles per second. During theta, my back felt flexible

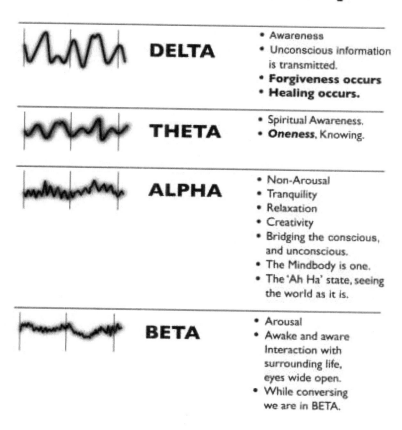

Brain Wave Activity

DELTA
- Awareness
- Unconscious information is transmitted.
- **Forgiveness occurs**
- **Healing occurs.**

THETA
- Spiritual Awareness.
- **Oneness,** Knowing.

ALPHA
- Non-Arousal
- Tranquility
- Relaxation
- Creativity
- Bridging the conscious, and unconscious.
- The Mindbody is one.
- The 'Ah Ha' state, seeing the world as it is.

BETA
- Arousal
- Awake and aware Interaction with surrounding life, eyes wide open.
- While conversing we are in BETA.

and pain-free. Sleep specialists often call theta drowsiness **second gear** and it would only last about a minute at most before I would awaken and shift into a beta state of increased brainwave activity and extreme pain. **Beta is a state of stress and anxiety**…. Hmmm?—another piece of the healing puzzle… I was missing a state of mind.

Between the relaxing theta and the anxiety-ridden beta is the highly desirable—**alpha activity.** Alpha is a beautiful state of gentle relaxation between theta and beta—peace and harmony—yet not quite meditative. Alpha alertness is the state of deep relaxation that is paramount for well-being and overall good health. Alpha is the goal in life, but much like breakfast, I skipped it every day.

> Healing takes place in delta, the deep sleep state. A restful night's sleep is critical to fighting doubt and dealing with the new day's stress. However, some people sleep well and still have TMS symptoms while others have chronic sleep issues and no symptoms. Sleep is not THE answer, but a lack of sleep can exacerbate the pain—preventing the individual from recharging to face the new day.

After being awakened from a restless night, I would lie for that heavenly minute before the pain began increasing rapidly and conditioning kicked in. I would then drop one leg at a time over the edge of the bed and crawl over to the tape machine to listen to Dr. Sarno's voice in order to renew my confidence to have the strength to fight the pain again—Groundhog Day-after-Groundhog Day. The recovery was slow, neither steady nor consistent. **TMS recovery is nonlinear.** In healing, it's best to integrate this concept of nonlinearity or the recovery time is prolonged due to increased frustration that accompanies each setback.

What the (Expletive Deleted)—I'm Getting Worse!!!

One day I had a major setback. I couldn't move my legs or stand. I even had trouble crawling without excruciating (Latin, defined as "out of the cross") pain. My structural doubts quickly began flooding back over Sarno's dam(n) idea. Was I doing the right thing by becoming active? After all, I had seen my x-rays where the stenosis was so evident—nerves looking pinched. I saw the arthritis on my x-ray and the herniations on my MRI, at the exact level of my pain. So what was I doing becoming so physical with a crumbling back? How naïve was I? Everything had fallen apart in one day as my pain level flew off the painometer. I remember slowly crawling across the floor as wave after wave cut through me—soaked in sweat—losing the ability to discern conscious awareness from reality. The room was looking distorted and I couldn't focus. That day was the pinnacle of TMS in me. I will never forget it; to this day it continues to motivate me to always move forward and never give in to doubt—a fortification of my faith.

I continued fading in and out of consciousness as the room was distorting and oscillating. Often when people are in prolonged periods of pain and depression they have flashbacks to happier times, but I didn't. I began having flashbacks to all the bad times in my life. I began a mental slideshow of the worst days of my life. My first flashback was to when I was seven years old and had rheumatic fever and had to lie motionless in a coma-like state for months. My second slide was of my wife being handicapped, the third was of the day my father-in-law died… and on and on. It was all the fun of a horror movie, but with no popcorn …**and the vicious cycle continued….**

This is a good time to talk about pain. I've had people tell me, "oh, I have aches and pains, too, but it doesn't bother me"—"I just stretch a little and keep going" (LOL—laugh out loud). Fortunately, most of these extremely naïve people may never understand the intensity of severe TMS pain. If you took a dull spoon and cut your leg off, and poured gasoline into the wound, it might come close to the pain of critical TMS—but I doubt it. There are indeed your run-of-the-mill aches and pains with TMS, as they are also a part of its mysterious nature, but with critical TMS people have committed suicide. What I'm describing here isn't your mama's nagging lumbago.

… it (TMS) could produce more severe pain than anything else I knew of in clinical medicine.

— John E. Sarno, MD, *Healing Back Pain*[71]

Everything had suddenly fallen apart. Why had the pain become so intense? Perhaps my unconscious mind did not like the fact that I was attempting to become more active? Maybe darker thoughts were resurfacing? I suspect that it was a combination of things, including prolonged and disrupted sleep patterns and poor physical conditioning. For certain—I was afraid to make the changes necessary to heal, and so I suffered greatly as I approached the threshold of transformation.

I was in dire straits that day (no, not the band)—as I literally crawled and limped to my computer. I wrote to my friend Graham Tuffee in Adelaide, Australia, telling him what was happening with me. He was also healing at that same time with Dr. Sarno's information and he gave me much-needed confidence. Fortunately, he emailed back immediately telling me to "hang in there" and to soothe myself and "not to worry." I remember printing out his email and reading it on all fours with sweat dripping from my face onto the page. At the time, I envisioned the sweat as blood, as though I was being sacrificed for something that I could not yet understand. I also remember that as I lay the email down to read it—it was upside down. It brought a brief smile to my face as I realized it had been sent to me from Australia and was probably intended to be read that way. Thank God for good friends in times of need—Graham later told me that when I finally healed, my healing pulled him along to finally heal as well—together we won.

I read and reread Graham's email and all the while Dr. Sarno's voice was playing in the background, "You cannot hurt yourself... TMS is harmless... mild oxygen deprivation." I was now stuck between the structural and the emotional—the medical industry and Dr. Sarno, illusion and reality. The images of my crumbling spine were flashing before my mind's eye. I could hear all the doctors' voices over the years telling me to be careful and to rest and that surgery was necessary due to structural decay and herniation. But Dr. Sarno on the audiotape was "telling me" to become more physical and to not worry. What should I do? Quit or go on? This is one of the toughest decisions in healing from pain because the "not wanting to go on" is one reason behind the pain. I didn't know whether to give up trying, or to keep believing. I was in a stalemate, at a crossroad, near a fork in the road without a GPS to tell me what to do—paralyzed with indecision.

The Watershed Event

During this time of intense indecision, I heard a Nike commercial on the bedroom television—**Just do it!** It was an epiphany—a true light bulb moment. Those words resonated in my mind over and over and over that day—sending a shockwave of sudden determination through me. What did I really have to lose by trying Sarno? Was I really living now? I began to stand up. Agonizing pain ran down the front, back, and sides of my legs, but I didn't care anymore. I had nothing to lose. I decided then—it was all or nothing. The Nike commercial, and my Ozzie friend, and my own will to persevere—all contributed to the move forward with the belief that my emotions were causing such intense pain and that those damn disc bulges, and stenosis, and arthritis, and the plethora of medical labels, were not causing my pain.

Although my unfelt rage had taken me further down than any time in 27 years, I could now see a road leading toward Recovery Highway. What a great slogan from Nike! "Just do it" has many connotations (Nike is the Greek goddess of victory). It reeks with the concept of jumping into life, of taking chances and pushing past doubt for life's sake. If I ever run into the person who came up with that slogan I will buy him or her dinner. I will—I'll just do it.

I decided to take that slogan to heart and not lie there and die, wallowing in self-pity. I was going to follow Dr. Sarno's advice to become more vigorous in my activity. I pulled myself up by the bootstraps (actually Nike shoe laces) once again and got dressed to run. I could hardly walk, but I was going to run around the neighborhood. I had trouble getting my running shoes on through the pain—but I did it. I hadn't jogged for 10 years—was weak—45 pounds underweight, out of shape and in the worst pain of my life. However, it's often desperation that is the motivation needed to prompt individuals to react and change. I knew I needed to begin, and that the time was now. In *The Republic*, Plato had written, "The beginning is the most important part of the work." Recovery from TMS begins with confidence in self and confidence in diagnosis.

Confidence is also freedom and freedom generates positive energy, the seeds of which grow from a single beginning.

Running On Empty

I dragged myself to the front door and with great courage, opened the door and looked out and saw a new world. With my portable tape machine playing Dr. Sarno's voice in my headset, I made up my mind that I was going the entire mile around my neighborhood. It was "2-a-days" all over again, just like the old football days. It was time to get tough again.

I started down my driveway and into the street in an attempt to make it around the entire neighborhood. It was one mile exactly around the hood. Given the fact that I hadn't even walked properly in months, I didn't know whether I could make it, but, I was determined. As I began to run, it was difficult, not only because my pain was so intense, but because I had trouble raising my foot because of drop-foot. It must have been quite a sight to watch, too, but when a person is in deep suffering, he tends to care a little less about appearance, as ego pulls back from superego. It was a start in the proper direction. The road that I began to run on that day was the road to recovery.

Thank Heaven for Harvey Kennedy

I lumbered to the first corner of the block before I had to go down on all fours in pain, pretending to tie my shoe. With TMS, when the bloodflow is cut off, it can feel like a bolt of lightning zigzagging down the leg and into the ankle or calf. It's no wonder that millions of people confuse the sensation of back pain with a nerve being pinched. After all—we have been erroneously inundated by the notion that herniated discs and stenosis are impinging nerves. If you combine that with the feeling of the blood withdrawing, it's no wonder we are caught in a confusing dilemma. I kept rewinding the tape to the statement below—listening to Dr. Sarno as I ran:

> ...the idea that they (nerves) are being pinched is usually fantasy and, once again, there is much ado about nothing.
>
> — John E. Sarno, MD, *Healing Back Pain*[72]

I kept rewinding because it was the part I doubted the most. I also kept rewinding the tape to the story he told of the now famous "30-year-old attorney" from *Healing Back Pain*. The attorney ran through his pain and that same night he was awakened as his pain attempted a tactical "break out" in another area of his middle back, and then disappeared forever. I was hoping during the entire jog that the same thing would happen to me that night. It did not; in fact it was another year or so before I eventually reeducated my brain and autonomic nervous system to react differently to movement. But I had begun....

Full of It

There was something very important about to occur in my recovery following that painful jog (probably painful to watch, too). As I ran, my focus on the pain was necessarily reduced. One must watch their step when running, one foot up, one foot down. Cars going by, wind blowing, dogs biting, bees stinging (these are a few of my favorite things). This is **presence**. It must have been a 20-minute mile but as I was coming down the home stretch I noticed that my pain was not as sharp as when I had started. I was striding normally, even though my foot was weak. My back seemed fairly loose and there was only a dull sensation of pain. I made it around the block and into my driveway and through the front door of my house, when It happened.

I closed the front door behind me and felt a sense of endorphic euphoria from the jog and the noticeably lowered level of pain. Then as I walked into my family room—It hit me. I was fine one moment and in a New York Second, the blood began withdrawing so fast that I had to get on the floor as waves of intense spasms washed over me. I could actually feel the blood withdrawing in my low back. It withdrew so hard that it almost pulled my legs back behind me, in severe cramping. The intensity was absolutely fantastic to experience. There was no reason for the pain to be that suddenly intense since seconds before I was standing tall and feeling relatively well. It was at that very moment that I knew Dr. Sarno was correct—it had been a distraction all along because it had **overreacted**. It was the watershed moment for me in my recovery. I was thrilled beyond explanation. I never looked back after that point. Thinking there were structural reasons for my pain was a thing of the past. In overplaying its hand, I realized that it was doing exactly what the good doctor had described. I had experienced a fundamental shift in consciousness. What I had been led to believe as true—I now knew—was false.

> *I now believe that the physical restrictions imposed by TMS are much more important than the pain, thus making it imperative that the patients gradually overcome them. If patients cannot do this, they are doomed to have recurrences of pain.*
> — John E. Sarno, MD, *Healing Back Pain*[73]

My unconscious self didn't like the fact that I was attempting to become active! I smiled through the agony. I knew that I had TMS now and that I was going to win the war. But would I win the peace by releasing my pain for good? It would still be a long road to recovery, but I now knew **how to attack pain**. I needed to become much more physical. There would be no more resting my back, or babying it, or therapy, or comfy pillows, or back braces, or special mattresses, or acupuncture, or manipulations, or anti-inflammatory drugs. As I said—I had hoped that I would be awakened that night like the 30-year-old attorney had been, and it would all be over. But it wasn't to be with me. It was still a long and bumpy road ahead, but that jog was THE turning point. TMS had overplayed its hand. It did a dumb thing for its own self-survival. The jig was up. I was onto it. I had had an epiphany.

My entire attitude shifted. I thanked God that night for turning me toward a truer path—a deeper level of consciousness. Now I had both hope AND direction. Hope without direction is like a Ferrari without fuel. It sure looks nice, but you can't go anywhere with it. I was now armed with the truth about pain and ready to begin attacking it and healing.

I increased my activity 10-fold, but day-after-day seemed like setback-after-setback. I was doing what Dr. Sarno had advised—attacking my pain through movement. But wild patterns became the norm instead of slow and steady healing. One day I would feel great, the next three days I would be worse. It's an awesome sight to witness how quickly one's confidence can collapse at the first onset of pain. It's embarrassing. One day I would be standing on Mount Olympus and the next day I was flailing in a Marianas Trench of doubt. Confidence falls like a house of cards when pain comes knocking at the back door. Nevertheless, I continued jogging and using my Total Trainer workout station. I first set small goals for myself when doing leg presses. I could only do about 10 reps at first but I eventually got up into the hundreds of reps. I would work out, always listening to Dr. Sarno's voice on my tape player, for confidence. Each day became the day before; work out hard, roll off the training station, run... and the pain would increase ...**and the vicious cycle continued....**

I continued with the same routine through the winter, but the setbacks were beginning to frustrate me. However, what I hadn't been paying attention to was how far I had come in my recovery process. Six months earlier I could barely get out of bed. Now I was lifting and running, but still couldn't sit down. This was a biggee for me. I wanted to be able to sit without the pain burying me in spasms. My brain was conditioned to withdraw blood whenever I would sit down. I needed to change this Pavlovian response.

Milty

One day my golfing partner-in-crime, Milty, stopped by to see me. I was lying on my stomach over a big exercise ball watching TV, since I still couldn't sit after these many months. I told him that after all these decades I had discovered what was happening to my back and that I needed to become more physical in the treatment, so he suggested we go golfing the next day. Golfing is the most fun you can have with your clothes on, but I had long since given up on the notion of ever playing again. The thought of me swinging that club and twisting hard gave me the willies. However, if I was to truly believe in the TMS process, and that there was nothing wrong with my spine, I needed to put up or shut up. I decided to putt up. We set a time to golf the next day.

I was tense that night—wary that I was going to injure myself the next day. But I understood Dr. Sarno's contention that, "the fear of becoming active is a **more powerful force** of distraction than the pain itself." We teed off the next day and, par for the course, the pain hit me hard. I was so fearful that I was going to further injure myself that I was inviting it back to me RSVP (Return, SteveO, Very, Painful). On the way to the golf course, just the thought of swinging a club generated spasms. At the first tee, I was afraid to swing the club but I managed to roll the ball around the ground. After each hole, I grimaced in pain, lifted my golf bag and started to the next hole. I remember walking and thinking to myself, "this Sarno guy had better be right" because this really hurts, and also "I suck at golf." A golf swing exerts tremendous torque on the spinal column and I could not get the mental images of my stenosis out of my mind's eye, and so my pain increased dramatically as we played. I even swung and missed the ball a few times, which brought a pitiful laugh from good ole Milty. It was his idea to get me out and moving around. I made it through the course though, and my "turkey brother" and I went into the clubhouse to hunt some wild ones. I had done it—faced a fear—piecing yet another part of my healing puzzle together that day, as the next day I was not in increased pain. But why wasn't I?

Paying Too Much At-tension

I can look back now and see why I wasn't moving along as fast as I had wanted. TMS feeds off your constant attention to the body. Each day I would run and exercise vigorously and then try to assign percentages to how good I felt that day. Was it a good day? Was this a better day than yesterday? Today was a 6.42 and yesterday was 5.87. If tomorrow is a 7.16, will I be happier? I was giving myself daily report cards. This was a critical error in recovery. Even though I was becoming much more active, I was still paying attention to how my body was healing.

> As long as he is in any way preoccupied with what his body is doing, the pain will continue.
>
> — John E. Sarno, MD, *Healing Back Pain*[74]

I mistakenly graded my progress—fighting—and delaying—my recovery. On one hand, I was pushing my physical envelope, and on the other hand, I was keeping my mind riveted to my body by giving myself minute-by-minute mental updates on my progression. It was like trying to applaud with one hand—there's lots of movement but no actual noise. I knew after nearly a year of trying to recover from TMS that one of two things was going to occur. First, I may be one of the two percent Dr. Sarno had reported who don't heal and needed intense psychoanalytical counseling. I understood that having a loved one handicapped could be something that would anger me forever because it was so senseless—so easily averted—stealing so much pleasure from our lives. This doubt haunted me and further slowed my progress. Second, I felt just maybe that I needed to step up my attack on TMS. I may need to confront it at the highest level. I may have been crazy not to see a psychiatrist, but I chose this second option. I had adopted a new mantra (mantra, defined as "a vehicle of the mind"). **...but the vicious cycle continued....**

Part A: Getting the Balls to Step Up My Activity

I altered my strategy and began a new, more intense, twofold attack. First, how could I pick up my physical activity? I knew that I loved golf and that it hurt very much to twist and turn when I swung the club. So, I decided to begin hitting 500 golf balls each day. I didn't care how much it was going to hurt, I would "just do it." Besides, it might just improve my golf swing. Second, I needed some type of mental soothing to disengage my sympathetic nervous system. I was obviously still in a state of chronic gridlock: chronically hidden tension. Little Stevie needed to let more go.

I will never forget that first bucket of golf balls. I could not transfer my weight. I could not move the club back. I could not swing all the way through. I hit the ball sideways and into the dirt. It must have looked like Arnold Palmer's golf swing, but I had fully committed myself now. I would hit a ball, and then drop down and pretend to tie my spikes because I was embarrassed by my own suffering. Now when I reflect back, when I had full-blown TMS, my shoes were always well tied. Ball after ball, I would swing the club and go down to the ground. The first day that I tried my new approach, I hit about 25 of the 75 balls and had to drag my legs back to my vehicle and lie across the hood before I could get in. This, too, became routine. Each day I would hit a few balls and then drag my legs to my vehicle and lie face down on the hood and hold on.

Daily, I was punishing the (k)id within me for throwing such a fit by giving me such pain. I did this by running, lifting, and going to the driving range and pounding golf balls. Day by day, Little Stevie fought back harder. Some days I would hit just a few golf balls and go into full spasm. I would try to walk back to the parking lot with some semblance of dignity, but my gait was disrupted because of the pain. So I dragged one foot or the other back to the safety of my welcoming, yet burning hot, vehicle (spikes always neatly tied). When I got there, I would hold onto its side and wait for the waves to subside. After a few weeks, it's possible the other golfers began to think that I really loved my vehicle a little too much. After a few minutes of spasms, I would attempt to get in. Getting in and out of a vehicle is a difficult task when your back is in spasm. But I stubbornly continued. It was becoming personal for me—a battle of me against me, and I was determined to defeat me.

This all-out attack went on for months into summer. I was absolutely, "kind of" positive that Dr. Sarno was correct in his clinical findings, sort of. I was fairly certain I needed to aggressively attack TMS if I was to ever become pain-free. I knew I had to continue to raise the bar to the ultimate level to succeed because I felt stuck and worn-out and frustrated. Confidence was slowly slipping.

I remember exactly where I was standing the day I decided to give up. I was drained of trying, feeling I was the exception to the rule and would never heal. As I stood there I heard a tiny little voice say, "Just keep trying!" I spun around quickly as the words stunned me. I looked down and there was a cute little boy about five years old looking directly at me, his arms crossed—smiling at me. I stared at him in astonishment. Were these words coming from him? Or through him? Little things can be big things when you're discovering what sustains you as a person. His words and angelic voice sustained me for a little longer. I couldn't give up.

Sic Vis Pacem Para Bellum
Latin: *If you want peace, prepare for war*

Something very subtle was happening during this time. I had become so invested in my daily routine that I hadn't noticed that I was hitting more golf balls and getting stronger. This is an important aspect of recovery. My focus had now shifted from one obsession to another. My mind's eye was no longer primarily staring at my body or my recovery pace. It was now about 75 percent on my body and 25 percent on my activities. My attention and focus were being shifted away from my pain, and reeducation was occurring. My recovery was progressing, but more importantly, it was progressing in the correct manner—by shifting focus.

Part B—Soothing My System

During these months of increased activity, I continued the mental scavenger hunt. Part B of my recovery plan was to **soothe my sympathetic nervous system** by making the narcissistic child in me happier. I began reading books and listening to audiotapes by a few very enlightened mindbody physicians. I knew that in conjunction with my ever-increasing physical activity, I also needed an equal dose of soothing relaxation— I had no pleasure in my life.

> The rage-energy has pulled your health out-of-balance, and you cannot sense it. So think deeper, open your mind—peel away the layers of your persona. Take a good inventory of your life and note how happy you currently are. Be really truthful with yourself as you consider this question. Since rage and fear and unhappiness are rooted in early separation anxiety, they're deeply buried, repressed and difficult to exhume. Therefore, as the sufferer, you need to take yourself "out of yourself" and look back at yourself in a highly objective manner. This can be thought of as disassociative self-analysis. Everyone holds anger, but most people don't internalize it at such high levels. Chronic symptom sufferers normally have much better capabilities to quickly recall past traumas or memories. In speaking with people who have few symptoms, it's quite clear that they simply don't remember little things. This is why it appears that Type T individuals have more detailed memories since they don't let go as easily.

It's Miller Time, When It's Time To Relax—Miller Comes Through

I began regularly listening to recordings by mindbody master, Emmett E. Miller, MD, and integrative medicine pioneer, Andrew Weil, MD. Each day I would aggressively move—and pay a price for it. As in any free market (I chose to believe in TMS freely), some days the price was higher than other days, depending on demand. Nevertheless, I paid my bills when they came due. So, each evening I would try to relax myself and to soothe my sympathetic system from the invisible knot it was tied into. Carl Jung often referred to these unconscious muddles as **snags**.

Nighttime relaxation was all new to me. Normally in the evenings, I would begin working on projects, reading and studying. I was a freight train out of control at night when I should have been parked in the station. I had fought relaxation by planning and working and goal-setting my entire life, like the "Little Engine that Should"— pushing ahead of the light.

It seems to me that it's erroneous to think that one can accomplish all his dreams in life. It is a tremendous error to believe that you can make people like you more by driving yourself into the ground and toward perfection. I needed to stop calculating the consequences and outcomes of all my actions. I needed to learn to live in real time through **presence**, to forget the past (let go) and to stop thinking about the future (let go). I needed to begin to **flow** and to *feel* once again—stop preparing so much, and just live.

To think is to say no.

— Alain, Emile Auguste Chartier (1868-1951)

I strongly recommend the healing material that I listened to during my recovery process—Dr. Miller's *Deep Healing, Healing Journey, The 10-Minute Stress Manager,* and *Easing Into Sleep,* and Dr. Andrew Weil's *Spontaneous Healing.* I also read Dr. Weil's *Spontaneous Healing* book and it is a fantastic source for understanding the nexus between mind and body. Dr. Weil balances emotion, nutrition, thoughts, imagery, and beliefs. I also bought his *Breathing: The Master Key to Life* CD set. I was gathering more and more tools, where really only one tool was necessary for the job. All I really needed was stronger belief—not more information—but we learn as we grow. Some people need more information to overcome fear.

During this period of intense relaxation came a new symptom—severe restless leg syndrome. The id-child within me was reluctant to relax because id didn't understand the concept. This is similar to beginning new breathing techniques for the first time. Individuals often report that they get very dizzy when they first attempt the new breathing rhythms.

I hammered my body by day and soothed my sympathetic nervous system at night. Day by day, beguiling pain would show its face and run. But month by month, very slowly and progressively, I was moving around more freely. I had now been on my recovery program for an unknown number of months (I stopped keeping track, which helped). My confidence in myself and in the TMS diagnosis was growing, as years of misleading information were slowly fading from memory.

I was now hitting a thousand golf balls each day—at 4½ hours a session. That may sound like a lot of golf balls to Mr. Joe E. Normal, but as a compulsive personality, I would have loved to hit more. This was real progress from golfing with Milty that first day in the spring, just a few months back, and being in so much pain that I could barely swing.

I often listened to the late Zen philosopher, Allan Watts, while meditating. I also began watching more comedies after reading the miraculous recovery of Norman Cousins in *Anatomy of an Illness* (who essentially cured himself through laughter). Daily I twisted and turned as hard as I could stand it. Evening I relaxed and soothed my being. Gradually, and I mean very, very gradually, I found myself not thinking about pain. I had moved to yet another plateau.

I Read Fred in Bed to Get Ahead—Nuff Said

Sometime during this period I found another TMS help-book by former pain sufferer, Fred Amir. Fred is a mindbody health specialist who authored the TMS book, *Rapid Recovery from Back and Neck Pain*. I wasn't thrilled with the progress that I was making thus far—I felt I needed more proof. This is characteristic of the Type T personality, the need for more information. Deeply ingrained patterns tend to make them cynical and doubtful. Reading Fred's book vanquished a little more doubt about the process, as I read about myself once again on every page of his book (I am featured in more books than I had realized). Fred had suffered from a classic battle with TMS. I was astounded because he had suffered from many of the same problems—initiated in the same manner as mine and in the same order. There was also a section that made me laugh hard for the first time in many months. While talking with his physiatrist about how many physical problems he had on his checklist, they both began to laugh at the length of his list. For some reason it made me laugh at my own long list of ailments. It is the absurdity in life that can make it hilarious. But more importantly, we all share life together. It's very comforting to know that others are going through similar scary events in life as you are. Fred humanized his own story and this gave it life. I've teased Fred that his pain made me laugh. He's replied to me that he was glad his pain was my pleasure.

Here Boy, Sit Boy—Good Boy....

Now that I was physically moving with greater ease and strength, I wanted to be able to sit down without squirming in pain and feeling that my back was spasming, which it still was. I could sit for about 5 to 10 seconds before the pain came searing through me. It would send me into full spasm and then begin to "refer" (sciatica) down its leg of choice. My social life was nonexistent since I couldn't sit and talk with my friends. Seldom do friends want to come into the bedroom or converse with you while you lie on the family room floor (except that time Zsa Zsa Gabor came by to visit).

So I decided one day to stand against this sitting problem. I wanted to be full of "sit." I was 99.999 percent certain that I had TMS, and that I needed to push forward. So one night I told Susan that I was going to sit down in my office chair, and that I wasn't going to stand up no matter how excruciating the pain became—I wanted the sitting problem to be gone that night.

We went into my office, where I was mentally preparing for some serious pain because I hadn't been able to sit for quite a long time. There are many ironies in the acquisition of knowledge and in the healing of TMS, and this was no exception. When one expects pain, one gets pain. But I hadn't quite integrated the bigger picture of TMS recovery yet. Recovery is a solid black puzzle at first, with no corner pieces, that must be pieced together one piece at a time through the light of personal revelations.

Dr. Sarno had clearly indicated that sitting was "such a benign activity,"[75] that it could not cause pain. The only reason pain reoccurs when an individual sits down is due to **conditioning**. If a person holds tension in his lower back, and he sits down and pain strikes, his brain is conditioned to withdraw blood each and every time he sits. When the cheeks hit the chair there's nothing butt despair. So the brain expects pain, and so it gets pain. I was unwittingly about to do the same thing—by bracing for it. This type of conditioning can occur anywhere in the body and it is instantaneous. If a person picks up a rock and a back stab or pain occurs, that person will be instantly conditioned to have a back pain when picking anything up, especially rocks.

I sat down in my office chair and asked my wife to hit me on the legs when I signaled. My intention was to break the focus by creating an alternative distracting pain. Within a few seconds of sitting, the spasms began. I held out for about a minute, holding my breath because the pain was so intense. I told her to hit me on the leg and she happily complied because our marriage was in trouble (but she didn't have to have that cigarette after). I then told her to hit me harder because my pain was so overwhelming that I was beginning to swoon. Soon the waves began to cease for about a minute. I began breathing full breaths again, but I could sense the spasms beginning again—each increasingly more intense. My unconscious mind did not want me to sit normally (just as the first time I ran around the block). This pattern continued, waves of spasms increasing and then ceasing, and then starting over, for about a half hour. Each wave was intensely more painful than the previous one. I eventually began to break down from the pain. It was bad, but I wasn't going to yield—I refused to stand up. If I wanted to sit again, I would need to break the conditioned response... **Now!** I could see in my wife's face that she could sense the agony that I was going through, but she was helpless to help me. Healing comes from within.

Toward the end of the half hour I was exhausted. The waves were ceasing to be as strong, their duration was shorter and their intensity less. Thirty minutes later the pain had ceased altogether. I sat silently; tears of joy replaced tears of pain. My breathing regulated and I began to relax. I had won. Thereafter I could sit any way, in any shape or form, for any time period I wanted with no onset of conditioned pain. It has been 10 years since that night, and I have had no hint of pain when sitting. I successfully reeducated my autonomic nervous system. I taught id that it had no more reason to fear sitting, using the same technique that bronc busters use to break wild horses, by riding out the pain that bucking night.

What I did that night was comparable to letting a bull loose and pointing it toward the good china, but it worked. "Not crying" is a control mechanism. As an adult I almost never felt the need to cry, because I had repression down like a finely tuned, well-oiled, invisible machine. My superego mindset was ingrained so deeply that I never even felt as if I warranted a cry. I merely never felt the need, and so the pain was always with me, to keep me from sensing the need.

Once again my main man, Dr. Sarno, was correct—we were best buddies by now and he didn't even know who I was. My confidence in his clinical findings had again increased, now to 99.9999 percent. My heart was again filling with hope that one day I would be free from pain's prison with no surgery or therapy or medications. Day by day I came closer to that realization.

Standing Pain-Free in Public

My next goal was to stand pain-free in the supermarket with my feet together. I've been amazed at how many sufferers I have met who have complained of the same problem. It's common in TMS that pain or dizziness increases dramatically when standing in crowded store lines waiting to be checked out. I can always tell when someone is in pain in the stores because they are either standing with their feet very wide apart, or they are squatting down. This is because the blood is withdrawing more strongly, because public places create anxiety and impatience; therefore, greater distraction is needed. And so I would squat down and pretend to tie my shoes. This was especially embarrassing when I was wearing sandals that didn't have laces.

There are multiple reasons for this effect and they all have to do with the inner self not wanting to be there—due to intrusion into our **proxemic space**—that degree of spatial separation that people maintain in social and interpersonal relationships. Self would rather be receiving **id-soothing*** than impatiently waiting in public and spending money.

---

* It isn't always the individual's stress or anger being "too high" that is causing their TMS, but a lack of soothing their id-self to counter their stress and pent-up anger, given their personalities and demands of current environments or self-imposed lifestyles.

I healed from this conditioned response by reeducating my reaction to the situation. I stood tall in line when the spasms began and I became more present. I held my feet together and focused on the nice people around me and began talking with them and asking them how they were doing. I began noting that most people are good, kind, and caring. It is amazing to see the reactions from people when they are offered a kind word or a simple hello. Those that are too grumpy to say hello are probably in their own pain from wounded relationship.

After each store visit, I would go for a relaxing walk in my neighborhood or watch something funny or listen to some relaxing music or eat something unhealthy. Slowly, very slowly, my pain lessened during the store visits as I repatterned my mind. Today, there is no pain at all when I stand in line or in life. I decided that I would no longer think of the glass as half full or half empty, I would be thankful to simply have water. However, there was still reeducation to occur, the child still feared …**and the vicious cycle continued….**

I was still running each day; it didn't matter to me if it was pouring rain or suffocatingly hot. I ran, and thought about reasons for pain. I was 42 years old at the time but I never missed one day of running during healing—plus 101 degrees or minus 20 degrees, I ran and thought. I didn't know it at that time, but I was performing a power therapy by redirecting the trauma accompanied by movement—running through all of my past events—literally and figuratively (more later on these therapies).

Never Fear Sopherman Is Here—TMS—Trust Marc Sopher

It was during this timeframe that I got a much needed confidence boost from Dr. Marc Sopher. Marc is a TMS mindbody-experienced physician who worked in Exeter, New Hampshire and had trained with Dr. Sarno. I will forever be grateful to him for helping with my recovery by responding to my email questions to him. After advising me that he could not ethically treat me over the Internet, he did give me confidence by writing that, "if you have TMS" (adding that "it certainly sounds as though you do"), I should drop all the timeframes I had "preset" for healing. He also told me that "any doubt" at all that I have TMS must be abolished—any "shadow of doubt" and the pain would continue. So with regard to monitoring my progress and in speeding my recovery, I had to cease and desist and to let those memories all fade. I needed to focus elsewhere—to forcefully guide my thoughts to someplace other than the painful areas.

I felt the best way to do this was to visualize and force my thoughts to areas on my body that felt great. So each time I would move, I would think of the upper-middle of my back instead of the painful lower area. I imagined that this area of my back was how my back should actually feel. I also visualized a perfect spine like an anatomical skeleton with perfect floating discs, wide foramina, and no arthritis.

After a few weeks of this technique, something truly astonishing happened. I dressed to run one day and was walking toward the front door while forcefully thinking about my mid-back, and suddenly a sharp scintillating pain hit me right in the spot I was focusing on! I was thrilled because I had memorized Dr. Sarno's books and tapes and anticipated the part where he said, "...when it moves—you got it beat." I had it!! I actually enticed the pain to move for a brief moment by visualizing it. This movement in my pain only lasted about two seconds, but it was a very welcome change of venue after thirty years of pain in the same location. So chronic pain can be healed no matter how long you have suffered from it. The pain quickly returned to my lower back after the scintillating sensation. My mind could not yet hold the focus away from my lower back, since I hadn't the mental discipline—yet—but I soon would.

I describe the new short-lived pain as scintillating because it was a sparkling sensation like one of those Fourth of July sparklers that kids play with on **Independence Day**. Those two seconds will always remain in my mind as a symbol of freedom. I had a sudden realization—and had just proven—that the mindbody connection was not only real, but that we as free and discerning people do indeed have control over our lives by the manner in which we visualize ourselves. I am a co-author of my own life. We have great control by how we see ourselves, and in what we believe to be true. Our persistent thoughts become our current reality.

Your experience is a product built from your attention. Be a wise investor of your attention particles... Unity is the truth; separation is the illusion. We are all one!
— Victor Daniel, Mindbody-Soul.com

My energy levels were sky high. I reflected on how much I had recovered in over ten months and I felt great—just as you can, too! My pain was much longer and more severe than in most cases, so you probably won't take as long to heal as I did. I was prostrate months earlier and now had just run a 6-minute mile. I was lifting heavy weights and sitting as long as I wanted. But the pain lingered like a politician at a fundraiser. I still had some lower back tension and pain, albeit much less, when I ran, and in doing certain movements. My emotional basement still needed cleaning. There were still spider webs in the shadows ...**and the cycle continued**....

It was now turning toward winter. I had healed about 90 percent. But why wouldn't it disappear completely? Why did it return at random times? My final goal was to be able to sleep on my stomach. I don't like sleeping on my back or sides. But I was still tight in my lower back and couldn't quite stand upright without my back pushing me forward. I emailed Dr. Sopher again and he told me again to be more patient.

Despite him telling me to chill a little, and telling me that impatience was incongruous with healing, I wanted my pain to be gone, now—so I modified my strategy. Each time I would move and get hit by pain, or run and "get hit" with pain, or get up in the morning and be in pain, I would punish my inner self severely by running longer and lifting more weights. I can now see that this punishment I was putting myself through was my way of letting out my frustration and guilt slowly. It was psychologically safer than letting all that repressed energy out at once—for me, and for those around me. I now realize I was discharging a freeze-survival response from my system, finishing a last act of survival, by running from a situation where I previously felt powerless. Running became, metaphorically, running. When we feel helpless we can flee, fight, or freeze to survive the situation. I chose to freeze instead of fighting or fleeing, which is a dangerous thing to do because freezing never allows for the resolution of the trauma—it freezes the trauma in your system, encoding a very dangerous state of existence, disrupting autonomic function. If you don't fight or flee under trauma, you lock the memory of the event into your system because you never "escaped" the situation in your mind.

I was so tired of the pain returning after I thought it was gone. Nevertheless, it relentlessly returned. I began to wonder if this would be my fate. Would I live my life with intermittent pain? Would I be on a roller coaster of pain for the rest of my life? After all, how could Howard Stern or John Stossel heal so quickly after seeing Dr. Sarno only a couple of times? Even though I knew TMS was true, and that I had been suffering from it most of my life, I remember Dr. Sarno stating that a small percentage of people don't heal. I appeared stuck at 90 percent, so I once again hit up Dr. Sopher for some more confidence and explained my concerns to him. He wrote back, "Steve, 90 percent is still very good!" It isn't good to a perfectionist—and it would be failure in my eyes if it were a necessity to manage my pain for the rest of my life. I needed complete healing for my own inner peace of mind—which only served to slow my healing. I continued pushing ahead of my own light, returning back into my own shadow.

I decided to turn my frustration of the possibility of pain-in-perpetuity into a healing mechanism for the final stage of healing. I would turn this pain against itself. Archaic anger is negative energy without a purpose. I decided to direct this frustration-energy toward movement and activity. From now on, when I woke up in pain, I was going to run twice as long, lift twice as long, and punish my inner brat twice as much. Surely, this would be the panacea? No, not quite.

However, I began to notice that each time I had a day of increased pain, the next time that I had a better day, the pain was less. So with each fall, came a higher high—the old dark before dawn platitude. Change was indeed occurring in a nonlinear fashion but I was also moving ever upward, toward the pinnacle of healing. TMS was holding on, but slowly losing its grip on me, or my grip on it.

The Final Stretch Home—Pain's Last Desperation

One morning out of the blue clear sky I woke up in so much pain that it was as if I had not healed at all. I was disgusted—furious with anger—but this time I could actually feel the frustration, which was new ground for me. I got dressed to run. It was pouring rain sideways. I pulled open the front door and took off running down my driveway and out into the street at a faster pace. I didn't have a distance in mind; I was going to run until…. I was both depressed and furious—I was defurious. I felt as if I was being used by my brain, and that particular feeling has always enraged me. I felt a hostage—I wanted to be free. So like Forrest Gump, "I just felt like ruh-ningg." I didn't run until my beard grew long, but I ran quite a distance. After mile four, my knee began hurting so much that I had to go down and embrace the ground. My back pain was completely gone but I couldn't walk or move my leg. I got up and continued limping down the street and after a half mile or so my knee pain disappeared and my back pain came back strong—I had it on the run. There is sweet victory in turning the tables on hostage-takers. I continued to run until my right ankle locked up on me, and I had to go back to the ground for about a minute to regroup. I got back up and started to slowly run again. My ankle pain disappeared and my lower back pain came back. I felt I had made my point to myself that day; I was kinda tired, I thought I would go home, and I did. It was almost over.

The periods between pains were lengthening. I was healing. My wife and I had been through much in our relationship. We were only married four years when our lives suddenly went in a direction that neither of us could have imagined. My pain also started at age 14, which is a very young age—and a very long time to be focused away from a side of me that I never knew existed. So I knew healing would take time. The million-dollar question was, how much longer? Once again, it is this type of thinking that perpetuates TMS symptoms. One must forget about TMS altogether. Live as though pain never existed—in real time—do what you love, and never keep tabs on it …**and it continued through winter**….

When springtime came, I began to hit golf balls again and twist my back as hard as I could with each swing. On worse pain days, I would hit a thousand golf balls in order to try to gain control over the inner-child that I felt was throwing a temper tantrum. On days with little pain, I would hit 75 as a reward. There were days when I would walk off the driving range, thinking about my golf swing-plane, and not even notice that I was once again walking properly. I didn't need to drag my legs or kiss the hood of my Blazer until the back spasms settled. I just got into my vehicle and drove home. Some days I made love to my hood and other days I went straight home to the wife. One day while driving home, a new pattern began emerging. My left hip socket began to lock up on me. It became so painful that I could not get out of my vehicle once I got home. I would pull into the garage, lift my left leg out with my arms and then kneel down on the garage floor. Then I would struggle to get back up after a few minutes and drag that leg and hip into the house. The pain was on the move and it was seeking every old injury site. Like a checklist, it was shifting to every point where I had once injured myself, or where there was considerable acceleration of the aging process. But I was healing. I changed my way of interpreting the messages by merely **allowing it to happen**, feeling the pain as a momentary wave of anger flowing over me that needed to express itself because I had never learned how. "Ok, you've said what you wanted—be gone with you now, Pain!"

A day came in **healing summer** on which I got up to run and the bottom of my right foot hurt so intensely that I couldn't stand on it. It was on the bottom right pad. Doctors call this neuroma or neuropathy, but it clearly is not. I laughed at this point, almost feeling sorry for the TMS in me. **I no longer feared the pain.** I can only describe the pain on the bottom of my foot as a golf ball on the right pad of my foot (no, I know what you're thinking, I checked the shoe, it wasn't a golf ball). I dressed to run. As I started down my driveway I slammed that foot into the cement as hard as I could slam it. The first few hits were excruciating and sent a tingling through my face, but by the end of my driveway, the foot pain was gone. I focused my attention on a part of my back that felt great and continued running. Some mornings the pain would be in my heels so I began slamming my heels on the ground as hard as I possibly could without breaking my foot. Too many people whose feet hurt begin to placate their pain, they let their foot pain hold their attention by babying their feet, needlessly controlling their lives because doctors erroneously diagnose them as having foot neuropathy (there are over 100 types of so-called neuropathies). I have helped many people get rid of their foot pain and know another individual who has gone from trouble walking, to jogging, through TMS healing. Never yield to pain—if you do, then you give in to your unconscious motivation for it.

There is a hierarchy of order to the universe—in hidden dimensions. The body follows the energy directed from the mind, and the mind follows the orders of the spirit. In this life we are spiritual beings with physical bodies, we are not physical beings trying to live spiritually. The body follows the mind—fueled by the energy of the spirit. How bad backs and bad necks and pain are viewed today, in an era of modern medicine, is a disaster. When an individual is in pain, the orders are bed rest and/or surgery and/or stabilization of the area through bracing and/or fusion and/or muscle strengthening. These are the very opposite approaches to take regarding healing. The appropriate therapy is to defeat fear and to become happier, more involved, and more productive. This isn't easy—but it's well worth the effort.

The truth be told, people feel sorry for themselves, and so they often unknowingly place themselves in pain and dis-ease for attention or self-pity. Their anger then seeks out any previously abused area of the body or any newly recommended center of focus and attention as new modern diseases multiply as needed. People who are aware and fearing of their aging, naturally begin to feel sorrier for themselves. People losing their looks or status (retirement) are depressed—greatly enraged by the anticipation of their own fate (aging, death); through self-sorrow, self-pity, and anger, they take their fear and frustration out on their own bodies. We live as our very will directs us.

The 18th Hole—The Final Shot

Golf season was now in full swing. I began actually golfing (yes, on a real golf course). I was once again busy and active around the house and in life. My pain was disappearing in a most erratic fashion. It had moved around my body in almost every area except my head. I was about to experience the final level of healing, but no one knows the hour when it will occur—it just suddenly—happens. My final goal was still to sleep on my stomach. At this point, if I lay on my stomach, my feet would still begin the tingling sensation as a conditioned response to the Cobra position that triggered the response earlier. I increased my **progressive relaxation** sessions and a few weeks later I was relaxed enough to sleep in any position except on my head—although I never really tried.

After 27 years, I was free. It was a life I had never known. I've since then had one deep back pain. A year after I healed, I got the flu and had a 103.5° temperature for three days. Lying in bed tossing around, my back sent me two or three very deep stabs of pain. I smiled through the fever because I knew the inner child did not like being sick because id only wants pleasure.

I had read and watched Allan Watts. I had read Andrew Weil and Emmett Miller and Edmund Bourne. I was finally calm and at peace. I had faced all that had happened to me and to Susan and now understood how I reacted to life. I was moving in real time, few emotions held in my body, no more pushing ahead of the light for tomorrow—no more living ahead of today. I had stopped my obsessive thinking and was now allowing life to evolve right in front of me as it happened. Presence had saved my day... and my life. I had healed, paradoxically, because I stopped trying to heal by reading books about healing and had stopped all rituals like journaling and structured healing programs which were continually creating and perpetuating the problem by focusing awareness on the problem.

...and the vicious cycle was BROKEN....
(Insert canned applause here)

Walking off the golf range one day, I was awakened to the sudden realization that I wasn't in any pain, nothing. Peace....

I stopped and looked up at the blue clear sky and felt a **unity connection** with life. I had experienced a spiritual expansion—life would never be the same. I had tripped over, stumbled through, and survived the rugged journey that allopathic medicine had sent me on, and returned with a deeper understanding of the awesome power of the mindbody. I had been through the belly of the whale and had been spit out on the other side, a more centered man. I am thankful for all that I have been shown in my life. The truth, once seen, is impossible to deny.

The mindbody reveals itself in the form of itself. Pain is a message that isn't understood by the self, and with the understanding of its purpose, comes healing. I had healed because I had pulled away from the herd of sheep that believe that structural changes cause pain. However, when a sheep breaks away from the herd, it opens itself up for attack by ego-hungry wolves, and so I have.

[Reality]…is a socially programmed hypnosis, an induced fiction in which we have collectively agreed to participate. And once in a while, somebody breaks out of that hypnosis of social conditioning—it's an interesting and motley group of sages, psychotics, and geniuses.

— Deepak Chopra, MD, *Body Mind & Soul*

Anchors Aweigh, My Boys—Anchors Aweigh

Last week for me was one of the worst I've had in months, if not years, between the pain and the anxiety—oh, and by the way, when the pain level jacked up, I couldn't think about the anxiety.

— Susan M. Canes, personal correspondence

After my pain was gone, extreme anxiety bursts began surfacing. I began having violent swings into heights of anxiety I had never experienced before. The pain I had endured my entire life was gone—my emotional anchor gone. Now there was nothing for my mind to focus on when it needed distraction. My mindbody attempted to substitute anxiety for physical pain. **Anxiety is an equivalent to pain and pain is an anchor for anxiety.** Pain, as we know, comes from the repression of emotion. *If he doesn't deal, he'll ultimately feel.*

At the very end of my pain, my back would hurt one second, and the next second it would be gone, and I would be spinning with dizziness. The next second the anxiety would be gone and the pain would return. The two were swinging wildly back and forth; anxiety and pain battling for consciousness. It was like being in a three-ring circus. I fully understand why the brain chooses pain instead of facing emotions. Anxiety resembles your nerves scraping their fingernails on a blackboard. Pain anchors such emotional energy to the body—when the anchor is raised, anxiety sails freely. So the pain syndrome serves its purpose as Dr. Sarno wrote, to "keep from tending to emotional things."[76] The wild swings lasted only a week or so and then abruptly ended.

I was back in balance—symptom-free for the first time in my life. However, I was about to be astonished—amazed—by unfounded arguments and denials against the very successful process that I had just experienced. The truth was about to be violently rejected.

6

Opposition to TMS: JSBS

John Stossel's Brother Syndrome

You can tell when you are getting close to the truth, by the vehement protests of those desperately clinging to positions that are growing weaker all the time. You can tell when you are getting close, by the number of bullets zipping by. The incredulous accusations and attitudes not just on your theory, but on your very character itself, by those who know nothing about you, have never met you, and have never evaluated your work... People shoot at pioneers.

— Clancy D. McKenzie, MD

My pain of 27 years was completely gone. Everything every MD, every chiropractor, and every therapist had ever told me about back pain was absolutely wrong. My back was very strong and healthy despite all the "problems" the high-tech imaging had been revealing. That initial misdiagnosis of the cause of my back pain when I was 14 years old, had initiated a cumulative process that propelled me into nearly 30 more years of unnecessary pain.

Three decades later, I found the truth, and it had set me free, as it has many others. However, despite the massive successes, there remains strong opposition to the reality of TMS. In denying that TMS is true, people often use, The Argument from Ignorance, also known as **The Argument from Personal Incredulity**. These tactics are used whenever the arguer decides that something is not possible because he personally can't understand the premise. It's incredible to him, "not believable," and so—untrue. He then asserts his own inability to understand as "proof" that the premise or proposition can't possibly be true and that there must be some other reason for certain causes and effects—because the answers aren't immediately obvious to him. Simply put, if he can't understand it, that's his proof that it's not true. People have gotten red in the face mad at me when I explain what is happening to them because they either know that it is true, or they just aren't in enough pain yet to open up to the truth. When anything comes along that conflicts with their idealized self-image, anger quickly spreads.

This is precisely why I threw Dr. Sarno's book across my family room after I began to understand its implications. I had the wrong image of myself.

I once asked my then 16-year-old son, Matthew, shortly after I became pain-free, "Why don't people merely call TMS false, instead of getting red-in-the-face angry?" He answered, "I guess it's because deep down inside, they know it's true." He had gotten to a point of awareness, at age 16, that many older people simply can't reach (he must have a good father).

In denying the process of TMS, the distraction is still working, as Dr. Sarno, among many others, has proven to be true. **The more vociferous the rejection that TMS is the reason behind symptoms, the more likely that it is indeed the cause of their symptoms—the overreaction reveals the shadow's threatened response.**

Marc Sopher, MD, co-author of *The Divided Mind—The Epidemic of Mindbody Disorders*, described a patient who stormed out of his office when told that his pain was most likely emotionally induced. The patient insisted that his pain was "real pain." The patient came back two days later and apologized, telling Dr. Sopher that, because Dr. Sopher had stuck with him and his family through tough times over the years, he was willing to listen to what he had to say. The man read Dr. Sarno's *Healing Back Pain*, along with some other TMS information, and his "pain simply vanished."[77] The TMS diagnosis can be seen as deeply offensive because it threatens an undeveloped-self that the persona has spent a lifetime concealing. Once the man pushed his ego aside, he healed. You will not heal if you think you know it all—or if your ego is threatened by what it doesn't want to hear; at this point—your pride is more important to you than your very life. Everything you think you know prevents healing.

There are many reasons people do not want to believe their symptoms are from an unconscious process. They have trouble believing that pain from a reduction in bloodflow can be so deep and sharp—it must be from skeletal or nerve damage. I felt the same way—so I, too, summarily rejected it.

Another reason people refute TMS is the stigma of emotional problems. Many people don't like the fact that the word psychosomatic starts with the word "psycho;" and they should forever be referred to as mindbody disorders, avoiding the pejorative. Another reason for rejection of TMS is that in Western culture we want to see things with our eyes, proof on imaging, something concrete to blame.

I once jokingly coined a term for people who refuse to believe the truth of **The Mindbody Syndrome** after I watched John Stossel's brother disputing TMS on ABC's *20/20*. I called it John Stossel's Brother Syndrome, or JSBS. John Stossel was an ABC news reporter at the time who suffered at least two decades with severe back pain. After one visit with Dr. Sarno, John was essentially pain-free. His brother, Tom Stossel, MD, however, is a classic example of someone who opposes TMS as the basis for pain—as being too simplistic an answer.

Tom is the Director of the Translational Medicine Division, at Brigham and Women's Hospital, and suffers on and off from chronic neck and back pain. Both brothers appeared in a 1999 ABC News *20/20* episode entitled "Dr. Sarno's Cure." Tom was not yet open to the concept of tension-induced pain and stated, "If anyone told me this was all in my head, my rage would not be repressed." Yet the week ABC taped the show on Dr. Sarno with the brothers, Dr. Tom Stossel's neck pain resurfaced. The timing of his pain is further proof of the efficacy of TMS and its often direct correlation to pain in Phase 1 TMS. John's report attempted to reveal the truth behind TMS, and so pain must resurface to biologically bury any unwanted emotions. My intention is not to pick on Tom; he appears to be a good man, but I make a point by using him as an example of a process that includes doubt. I initially reacted the same way Tom did.

The unconscious does not want the truth revealed and can put up an epic battle—hence the pain. These opposing forces create even further hidden conflict as belief confronts behavior and **rage approaches consciousness**. When we can gain the strength to face who we are, and how we react to life, openly and honestly, pain and illness have few places to hide in the body.

Similarly, I read a woman's post about how her pain was resurfacing. Her husband had insightfully pointed out that her pain was probably TMS that had moved from her back to her shoulders, as it often does, and that she should **reread** Dr. Sarno's book. She wrote: "As my husband pushed me to read the book again, my symptoms got worse." Many have reported that as they began to open-mindedly look into TMS, their pain skyrocketed—much like an exorcism—just as when my hands swelled while reading *Mind Over Back Pain*. Any attempt to uproot deeply buried issues with insight and awareness threatens the nature of darkness, which is to shadow the light. The following exchange occurred between the Stossel brothers on the ABC *20/20* show regarding TMS and Dr. Sarno's clinical findings:

Tom: There are a lot of [other] ridiculous things that I could do that probably don't work, that I'm not doing.

John: But it [TMS healing] worked for me, your brother.

Tom: Well, as a scientist, I have to say, anything's possible, but I'm not convinced.

Dr. Sarno's response to Tom's reaction and the TMS diagnosis was, "If they can't demonstrate it in the laboratory, [they think] it doesn't exist." According to Aristotle, "It is the mark of an educated mind to be able to entertain a thought without accepting it." Tom was arguing from The Argument from Personal Incredulity and rejecting clear evidence.

Why is there so much opposition to the clinical findings of TMS healing—when it works virtually every time? Few physicians or scientists want to admit that their years of training and hard work have been looking at pain from the wrong direction. The most absurd rejection I've heard from other physicians regarding Dr. Sarno and TMS is that he screens his patients—looking for "easy cures"— so that his success rate will be higher. There are few things in this world that could be further from the truth than that argument. On the ABC show, "Dr. Sarno's Cure," Janette Barber said her doctor told her, "It looks like you've tried everything." He had nothing more to offer to heal her pain, and yet she went to Dr. Sarno and healed quickly. These TMS physicians are seeing the hardest, most difficult cases—the ones other physicians cannot help. Sufferers only go to see TMS practitioners when they have tried everything—and are at the end of their hopes. This was also the only reason that I read Dr. Sarno's work—I had tried everything else. Dr. Sopher confirmed this for me—they (TMS physicians) mainly see "the worst cases, the ones who have failed all other treatment." These patients are ones that doctors have often abandoned, telling them there was nothing more that could be done for them—the situation was so frustrating to their physicians, that the doctors cringed when they saw these patients' names on their schedules. The TMS physicians—led by Dr. Sarno—do not pick winners to boost their healing rates. They accept the lost ones who have open minds— and they heal them at extraordinarily high rates of success.

TMS healing works, but it no doubt will be refuted by people who cannot look outside their medical experiences. I know many people who have healed from their pain just by understanding and believing that their emotions were causing their pain—yet some physicians still say it is not possible.

But what is a scientist? Aren't scientists open-minded and seeking the truth— following chains of evidence? A major source of controversy and opposition to TMS, as seen in the Stossel brothers' conversation, is that scientists want to be the ones spreading the word about cures. It is a decisive blow to ego for experts to be told by laymen the causes of body ailments, and so ego's first reaction is resistance.

> *This is why my work has been so studiously ignored. I have demonstrated conclusively that a truly physical-pathological process is the result of emotional phenomena, and can be halted by a mental one. That is, first of all, rank heresy, and secondly, beyond the comprehension of most physicians.... Paradoxically, thoughtful laymen are much more able to accept such an idea because they are not burdened with a medical education and all the philosophical biases that go along with it.*
>
> — John E. Sarno, MD, *Healing Back Pain*[78]

Ego has no place in science. Ego stands as an antithesis to science because it determines outcomes before results are established. Plato has been quoted as saying: "We can easily forgive a child who is afraid of the dark; the real tragedy of life is when men are afraid of the light."

John Stossel is a 19-time Emmy winner. He is an open-minded and astute individual, and now basically pain-free thanks to Dr. Sarno. John writes in his book, *Give Me a Break*, "… I notice Tom, too, now mostly ignores his back pain rather than nursing it and focusing on it—and it goes away."[79] Tom, just as I did, at a deeper level probably already knew the truth, but it was more difficult to accept and admit because of the burden of his medical education. The definition of burden is an oppressive responsibility. An education can be so oppressive that it may lead to ego over science—hubris over service.

The wrong view of science betrays itself in the craving to be right; for it is not his possession of knowledge, of irrefutable truth, that makes the man of science, but his persistent and recklessly critical quest for truth.

— Karl Popper[80]

Scientists clinging to slipped and herniated discs as the basis for back pain are not only failing to help their patients, but are also turning a blind eye to Karl Popper and his groundbreaking body of work regarding **Falsification Theory**. Falsification, as Popper argued, is what separates science from nonscience.

Falsifiability, as defined by Popper, says that a scientific theory is not scientific if it will not admit to the possibility of being false. This is good science because it delves more deeply into what is true and what is not true through contradiction. Succinctly, Popper said that scientific theories should be questioned, and that through this questioning, we uncover even more truths. Back surgery, steroid injections and traction therapy have proven to not work, and yet many still cling to these methods because they believe the majority must be right. As Popper stated, it is the "quest for truth" that makes the man of science, not his possession of knowledge.

Often doctors' medical certifications blind them to the obvious. They may claim: "Hey, I went to medical school, I will tell you what is wrong with you, you won't tell me." As we know from well-documented evidence regarding back and joint pain, this often makes symptoms worse. Physicians need to stop telling patients they are physically flawed, and begin asking them what changes or stress they've been experiencing.

If a physician can shut up for long enough, the patient will tell him what is wrong.... The chronically ill have an intuitive-visceral sense of what is wrong with them.
— Majid Ali, MD, Capital University of Integrative Medicine[81]

Dr. Sarno admits that it was when he began talking with chronic pain sufferers that he saw the personality tendencies that commonly accompany pain. The days of doctors' house calls are over, as doctors have moved from friend/healer to medical care providers. This is bad science.

Hopefully, someday all physicians will adhere to the methodology that Don Colbert, MD, utilizes with his patients. In *Deadly Emotions,* Colbert writes, "In my practice, my staff and I take the time to sit down with patients such as Karl to see if there is an emotional event that might be triggering a particular illness or condition. Again and again, we've found that emotional upheaval appears to be linked directly to disease."[82] Dr. Colbert is a scientist because of his critical quest for the truth.

If falsifiability were applied to TMS we would find that it is not merely oxygen deprivation (see Chapter 1) at work, but also alterations in fluid levels. The autonomic system also maintains thermoregulation by controlling sweating. Most pain sufferers have chronic dry skin with psoriasis or seborrheic dermatitis, severe dandruff, pseudo-gout, etc., as well as popping and clicking joints. So when rage becomes hot enough and the autonomic system can't maintain homeostasis—all and any of its functions can become erratic, not just the function of bloodflow as described in Chapter One.

Egos and Eye-Rollers

But this is only the tip of the iceberg. A man I communicated with who was suffering from chronic psychosomatic mid-back and neck-tension stiffness went to a neurologist at the UCLA Migraine Institute to get some relief. When he mentioned Dr. Sarno and TMS to the doctor, he said she "just rolled her eyes and waived off the issue...." She wanted, expected, and needed, a physical cause because she was educated to look for one—misguided and burdened by her medical training.

> *Science, based on the materialistic model, has attempted to understand the mechanisms of disease in the hope that if you could understand the mechanisms of disease and interfere with those mechanisms of disease, you should be able to get rid of the disease... unfortunately, that hasn't worked, because mechanisms of disease are not the origins of disease.*
>
> — Deepak Chopra, MD, *Body Mind & Soul*

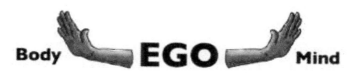

Ego is currently fighting any attempt at merging mind and body. There are many with a vested interest in suffering. Their livelihoods—or lifestyles—depend on the scientific engineering of pain, and this would be threatened if TMS was generally accepted by society. There is also the sufferer himself whose ego often clashes with his own beliefs as he brings pain upon himself for reasons that even he doesn't understand.

Caveat: We need doctors—we need good healers. In 2003, my dad had to have his heart pacemaker's J-lead removed at the Cleveland Clinic after a local surgeon broke it while putting it in. As I sat in the SICU at the Cleveland Clinic, I saw that it was packed with families. So I began asking people where they were from. Some were from the Far East, one couple was from Israel, another from England, and others from Canada. These people had loved ones who were very ill, and guess where they brought them? To the United States of America. I asked a couple of people why they had brought their family members here, to the Cleveland Clinic. They told me, "Because it's the best." This is not an anti-doctor book. Symptoms sometimes need to be relieved by professionals. People in need are being saved by the hundreds of thousands in places like the Cleveland Clinic, Mayo Clinic, and

Johns Hopkins through transplants, and reconstructions, grafts, etc. Modern medicine is good—but often overzealous.

The question is, however, how did these sufferers get to this point that they needed such interventions? What brought the 20-year-old boy to the point that he needed a heart stent already? Why has the 30-year-old banker had two bypass surgeries? Why is the 17-year-old athlete in chronic pain before every game? Once the individual gets too far out of balance, he will need to get good medical intervention. Be very careful; however, it is of course possible to have a physical/structural anomaly outside the psychosomatic realm such as a congenital disorder (being such by nature or birth). This book is about reasons, and questions in the attempt to shift erroneous perceptions and attitudes. So the larger question is—when does the doctor stop caring about why the patient is in his office? The medical industry, as necessary as it is, has become the **ouroboros** in fighting itself on one end, and keeping itself going on the other as the snake eats its own tail. Dr. Chopra points out that today there are more people making a living off cancer than are currently dying from it. The reason is that it has become too similar to an assembly line in its attitude toward the patient's needs; needs which are manifest in the form of his illness.

Two-Trauma Mechanism

Psychiatrist Clancy McKenzie revolutionized the understanding of schizophrenia and depression as well as post-traumatic stress disorders that produce depression and anxiety. He discovered a **Two-Trauma Mechanism** in the 1980s by "identifying the mechanism by which emotional trauma produces change in brain chemistry and structure." Early separations in life cause later problems, depending on **when** the first major separation occurred; that is, the stage of brain development at the time of the first trauma/separation.

McKenzie's findings are nothing short of brilliant. He identified one of the main mechanisms of these mental disorders in a detailed study that he conceptualized as *child-mother separation and trauma from the birth of a sibling*. Understandably, he was excited to bring his clinical findings to the entire psychiatric community, but they were soundly rejected by the majority—so he took a hiatus and waited for the psychiatric community "to catch up." To his amazement, they continued heading in the wrong direction. He states, "they were making important findings, but looking only at the biological results of the disease process, or genetic predispositions, and missing the cause altogether." This is precisely the same stage Dr. Sarno is at right now with TMS. The medical community must now catch up to his findings.

Today, Dr. McKenzie's work is more widely accepted and being disseminated by the psychiatric community. The brightest psychiatrists and brain specialists, such as

Paul MacLean, MD, understood his groundbreaking work immediately, as they saw the brilliance in its simplicity and accuracy.

> *Only the truly great scholars are able to entertain new concepts that differ from widely held views… too often persons do not trust their own minds to evaluate simple things; and they await the opinions of others before casting their lot. This holds true even for professionals in high places.*
>
> — Clancy D. McKenzie, MD

It takes scientists who think outside the medical box to discover and develop deeper understanding. But as Dr. McKenzie wrote, "They shoot at pioneers." Scientists such as McKenzie, Sarno, Sopher, Chopra, Colbert, Weil, Northrup, and Miller follow wherever the truth leads them. They don't live inside the medical box since their desire is to heal, not simply to treat patients. They help people based upon observation and re-observation and they won't hesitate to stray from the norm when the truth takes them elsewhere, since only dead fish swim with the stream.

> *Conventional medicine has become very narrow in its focus on the physical body…. Conventional medicine is now seen as being reckless, dangerous, forcing on people things that are toxic. It has become out of balance in its enthusiasm for external technological solutions to problems.*
>
> — Andrew Weil, MD, *Pros and Cons of Integrative Medicine*, PBS

In the early 1990s, pre-Sarno, my brother and I were seeing a neurosurgeon for our back pain. When the surgeon suddenly retired, a new neurosurgeon took over his practice. The first thing this new surgeon did was to go through each of his new files and get rid of each patient that he couldn't immediately operate on. If he couldn't operate on you he didn't want you as a patient. I spoke with many former TMS sufferers who said their neurosurgeons were absolutely irate at them when they wouldn't allow surgery, immediately. Is this medicine? Or business? The ultimate Truth always hangs somewhere in the middle. There are no absolutes.

Excuse Me, but Can Eye Borrow Your Rose-Colored Glasses?

It is so much easier to say, "I have inherited a bad back, or injured my back and neck," than it is to admit there may be some hidden emotions that I can't face right now." Or that, "I need some downtime; I just can't take all that is being thrust upon me right now—I need to be released from my responsibilities, even if for a short time." As a child, psychiatrist Carl Jung was picked on by other children to the point that he began using sickness as an excuse to avoid them. He even mastered the art of being able to make himself faint at will in order to avoid the taunting from others. Sometimes we just need an acceptable way out.

People who feel they have pain from injury to their backs and necks and knees or shoulders or feet just cannot admit that their lives have not gone as they had planned— that they fear aging—and that some of their primary needs have gone unfilled. They are stupefied by the fact that their bodies could be strongly reacting to emotions that they cannot feel. The smoldering and destructive thoughts just beneath conscious awareness often reveal themselves through multiple physiological problems. If these symptoms allow the individual to change his life in a manner that enables him to slow down, seek a hiding place, or less commonly, to complain (to be heard), then that's all the better because that's often what he needs in his life at the time.

Many are relieved by the idea that there is a herniated disc or torn rotator cuff, or the appearance of some structural damage on the imaging, because we all possess a **self-destructive instinct**—a hidden guilt—which many feel will be relieved through cutting part of their body away. Twentieth century psychiatrist, Karl Menninger, MD, recognized the phenomenon in his clinic in Topeka, Kansas.

> *Sometimes an operation seems to be necessary for a sick person's emotional comfort, and sometimes we emerge from the hospital with some serious problem solved or some needed adjustment made.... Menninger interprets this repeated submission to the surgeon's knife as an expression of unconscious guilt.... After the operation, Menninger points out, there is a marked period of relief and wellbeing... the almost aggressive demand for surgery is a symptom of the self-destructive force on the rampage.*
> — Arnold A. Hutschnecker, MD, *The Will to Live*[83]

The guilty appendage can be operated on and their unconscious guilt physically severed from them on what Dr. Hutschnecker called "the altar of the operating table." The patients' destructive thoughts, the frustration and anger from their overly demanding responsibilities and guilt, can remain hidden from others. At a deeper level of consciousness, they sacrifice a part of their body to atone for their sinful thoughts or desires. The destructive side that all people possess momentarily overshadows their loving and creative side.*

People look for answers with their eyes and ignore their heart's message. Illness, pain, and suffering are a result of imbalance from persistently being unaware of, or ignoring, personal needs. When an individual states that life is good, both to himself and to others, but he is also suffering from pain and/or paralysis, he is looking in the mirror and seeing a wishful reflection of his life. When an individual says life is good and he is not suffering, then life is probably good; he is in balance—seeing himself in the mirror with all of his senses as he truly is.

To admit that things have not gone as planned in life, yet also to be thankful, reveals a great sense of maturity and spiritual growth. It is seeing true self in real time, which is the power point in life. Now is where power reigns. The time to be happy is

---

* The argument continues over how many instincts we actually possess but Freud had come to the conclusion that at the base of all instincts stood only the two I mentioned earlier: the loving creative instinct, **Eros**, and the opposing self-destructive force that neo-Freudians call **Thanatos**.

now, not tomorrow. Life is living in the moment; it is not preparing for the potential of the future, or clinging to wounded relationships from the past.

Thus, there are two opposing ego-sets in play in TMS.

> The ego of the individual sufferer is refusing to consider that hidden emotions may be causing his symptoms. He can't believe that his mother-in-law (or father-in-law or wife or kids or job) is so internally enraging that it could cause his intense pain. He will never understand the concept of repression unless he seeks higher planes of truth within himself.
>
> ...AND....
>
> The egos within the medical industry will not allow for the notion that aging spines and deteriorating bodies are not the actual cause of most pain. Herniated discs rarely cause pain, but the notion that they are the standard cause of pain is so deeply integrated into the collective unconscious of society, that even open-minded people have trouble imagining a different picture. It's nothing short of a medical disaster.*

This point must be made so that there is no doubt in the reader's mind. It is the individual's ego that will not allow him to believe that TMS is true. The formation of the superego is designed just for this purpose—to appear to be above the human processes of anger, fear, anxiety, and humanity.

I have come to understand TMS tensionalgia as the key culprit behind all of my physical symptoms. I have helped people overcome their fear and ease their pain by increasing their understanding of what is happening. But, these people were open-minded and observant of self. They, in essence, healed themselves. Of those people whom I have not been able to help: each and everyone agreed with the truth of Dr. Sarno's TMS concept, until it came to their own pain—believing it is true for everyone but them. When people are screaming angry, pointing their finger in my face and sweating from my telling them that their pain is not due to partial ligament tears or spinal damage, I can see that what I am telling them is stinging their egos. Their anger and pain are emanating from their furious denial of any internal conflict—knowing in their heart-of-hearts that what I am telling them is true.

The lady doth protest too much, methinks.

— *Hamlet*, Act 3, scene 2

It was clearly evident in Richard Nixon's face as he stood at that podium vigorously maintaining his innocence in the Watergate scandal and vehemently stating, "...people have got to know whether or not their President's a crook. Well, I am not

---

* A herniated disc may indeed impinge on a nerve causing immediate paralysis, but as the nerve dies it will no longer send pain signals to the brain, and so a nerve impinged will not cause pain for long.

a crook." It could be seen in Bill Clinton's rosacea-red face as he pointed his finger and angrily stated, "I did not have sexual relations with that woman...." Both were lying, and it was evident by their **over-reaction** to the truth as it threatens ego. Many chronic pain sufferers are relieved to be finally rid of their repressed anger, and buried emotional pain. Deep down inside, people need the healing truth of light. Those who have vested energy in their own images may not desire change, even though it requires more energy from them to reject new ideas. Belief takes so little energy. The bulk of the energy is consumed in the fighting of any truths that may desire to surface.

Death, divorce, adoption, injury, criticism, abuse, indifference, midlife crisis, deep-seated marital strife, and various other forms of **perceived** rejection are the primary directors of pain—generators of psychic conflict. The ultimate fear is in becoming disconnected or experiencing further rejection and so self-punishment provides a reprieve from unconscious guilt.

Societies around the world have stigmatized people with emotional pain as somehow being failures, yet some of the greatest of people experience emotional pain. Edgar Allan Poe's brilliant body of work originated from extreme separation anxiety. Western society teaches that we are not normal if we have emotional conflict and yet all people invariably experience it. Since rejection forces emotional experiences that would never have been realized without the clash of opposites within, emotional pain can give rise to great talent, creativity, and insight.

Denial Aint Just a River in Egypt, It Flows Through Eight Other Countries

Sufferers are primarily (but not always) outwardly calm and quiet, obsessive, phobic perfectionists; slightly, to deeply, anxious, overly responsible, and highly conscientious individuals. From them, I often hear, "Oh yeah, there is no doubt, Steve, that emotions can affect the body and create pain—but not in me—mine is structural." The greatest stumbling block in my own recovery was seeing my MRI with the herniated discs and seeing my x-rays with the stenosis, bone spurs (osteophytes), and the arthritis.

> People often say, "Hey, I know a person who is not at all responsible, and yet he suffers from TMS." This seemingly "irresponsible" person may be caught up in a complex of such deep personal responsibility, that he ends up appearing irresponsible or lazy due to negative chatter gridlock. He is so afraid of failing or succeeding that he unconsciously brings failure upon himself and appears irresponsible when he doesn't truly want to be. So irresponsibility can also be seen as TMSing... and the yin chases the yang... as this becomes that.

Watching as the neurosurgeon hit my knee with the rubber hammer—my deep tendon reflex absent—was a tough memory for me to erase. As my feet began to drop in paralysis, and as numbness and tingling set in, it was very difficult to accept that what I was seeing was purely an emotional effect. Yet even seeing this, I chose not to believe a structural defect was causing it all. It was the best, and yet most difficult, decision I have ever made regarding my health, and it has paid off a thousand times over. My life is pain-free for the first time that I can ever remember, because I chose to open my mind.

The brilliant German scientist, Max Plank, felt that it took one generation to accept and to integrate new scientific ideas. Once upon a time, researchers believed ulcers were from defective stomachs. Through a single generation, society came to understand that ulcers were born from stress—they began to recede as the reason behind them became "accepted." Still today, scientists continue to seek the ulcer bacterium and once in a while they find one, too. But the bacterium is already present in most people—whether they have an ulcer or not. Dr. Sopher informs me that he has seen people take antibiotics that get rid of a bacterium, but they don't get any better. So the bacteria are often an **incidental finding** such as the herniated discs and stenosis and arthritis as seen on the x-rays and MRIs. Dr. Sopher's point is reinforced by Henry Bieler, MD, who studied the causes and cures of diseases for over 50 years, penning a book on the subject. Bieler's first conclusion was that the primary cause of most diseases was not germs. His second conclusion was that treating patients with drugs was almost always dangerous.

However—the scientific industry, in its fervent desire to head forward, often takes us backward by seeking a magic cure through the body. In the early 1980s, Australian scientists finally discovered "the ulcer bacteria"—finally finding a target at which they could aim a magic bullet. Robert Sapolsky, PhD, winner of the MacArthur Foundation's Genius Fellowship Award, stated regarding the Australian discovery, "I'm willing to bet half the gastroenterologists on Earth went out and celebrated that night—no more need to sit down to work out their patients' personal lives, it could now be cured with a pill."[84]

However, only a few years later it was discovered that just about everyone on planet Earth (at least two thirds) carries this same stomach bacteria, but only those under stress got ulcers. When stressed, the immune system is inhibited, preventing the repair of stomach tissue, allowing the stomach bacteria to run rampant. Most of us have these stomach ulcer bacteria, and herniated discs, and arthritis; all are similar normal physical abnormalities, and as in the case of herniated discs, the bacteria are almost always incidental to the physical problem.

Now, as people began to understand and believe that ulcers were caused by "stension," there was no longer the ruse of physicality in the stomach—the unconscious process had to find new hiding places such as the back, hands, and feet.

The brain continually scans to find a symptom we will fear—and there it stays. Viruses and bacteria can be extremely dangerous but are not the cause of most disease.* They only slither into the body when the individual becomes susceptible, depending on their state of physical and emotional health. Pneumonia, for example, normally kills only the very old, the very young, and the very weak—targets of disease.

> Not everyone exposed to the parasite gets sick with malaria.... Not everyone who meets up with flu virus gets flu.... Agents of disease do not cause us to get sick. They are merely potential vectors of illness waiting for chances to do their mischief. Given a chance, they will do it.... Agents of disease are all around us.... A person solidly equilibrated in a phase of relative health can often interact with these agents and not get sick. Since internal factors determine the nature of our relationships with them, the true causes of disease are internal.... Forgive me if I repeat myself; this point must be stressed: external, material objects are never causes of disease, merely agents waiting to cause specific symptoms in susceptible hosts.
>
> — Andrew Weil, MD, Health and Healing:
> The Philosophy of Integrative Medicine and Optimum Health[85]

Two people I knew many years ago were in terrible pain. They told me that they did indeed believe Sarno was correct, but that their back pain was "real." Both are still in pain today. They have given up many activities they love in order to avoid accepting the truth. They fear lifting, bending, and living normal active lives. As the title of Dr. Sopher's book suggests, To Be... or Not to Be Pain-Free, being pain-free is a choice (also a good "play" on Shakespeare). Sometimes the best way to prove someone wrong is to let him have his way.

I met a 40-year-old man who was having neck spasms, and as a result his hands and arms were becoming numb. His life was going badly, he was depressed and anxious, and riveted to his body symptoms. He obviously had TMS. His doctor recommended surgery, of course. I begged him not to have it. I told him that it would not work and when it didn't work, they would then find a medical excuse as to why it hadn't. He had the surgery, they placed a titanium plate in his neck, and it didn't stop his problems. Months later they told him that they had "missed the spot" and wanted to operate again. The same scenario plays out every day, but people are afraid, and so they want to believe what the doctor tells them is correct. But they are not correct regarding pain. I have seen opposition in many forms, from medical to therapeutic to psychiatric; however, they are all clinging to positions that grow ever weaker.

In the past, I contributed to worldwide pain forums in order to help ease needless suffering. These forums are organized to help people understand and to heal from tensionalgia and other mindbody disorders through the sharing of success and wounds

---

* These would include Biosafety level 1 and 2 viruses, and possibly BSL 3. Biosafety level 4 viruses are always deadly and are causative agents for disease and death.

(spread the pain, diffuse the fear). I felt strongly obligated to spread the truth because I had been blessed by having the truth revealed to me. In one such group was a man I will call Bernabe because his name is Bernabe. He used to email me from time to time, asking me questions about how I healed from my lifetime of pain. He appeared to be a very mild-mannered and intelligent man whose belief in tension-induced pain vacillated back and forth, as happens with most everyone at first. Pain has a way of distorting and skewing the truth. Pain is darkness—that wears people down into a bundle of bitterness and doubt. Part of the function of TMS is to create doubt—to doubt the conversion of emotional to physical and to lay the problem at the doorstep of the physical. This is called **somaticizing**—psychic events that convert emotional upheaval to physical events—leading the individual to wrongly believe that she has a physical problem when she actually has an emotional one.

At the time, Bernabe was a 37-year-old man (most likely is still a man, but not 37 anymore) who suffered from the normal misdiagnosis of pain due to disc protrusions at L4/L5 and S1. These levels are the disc number gold standards for back pain—we all have some degree of herniation there. Bernabe could no longer work because of his pain and was spending most of his time in bed. One day in frustration and despair, he posted the following message to a pain forum. The grammatical mistakes included are the result of his being from a foreign country and not having a full grasp of English syntax and spelling; nonetheless, he was a highly intelligent man who simply referred to himself as "a sufferer":

Date: Mon, 18 Feb 2002
From: Bernabe————
Subject: My 'provisional' Conclusions

After having read all TMS related books and tried to figure out what do them mean and reading tmsers opinions I have concluded the following thoughts: (I challenge anyone to discuss every point one by one).

1. tms has not basis to hold itself. The conclusion one can draw of it is that no one knows exactly about many back pain conditions. TMS is another poor and contradictory explanation of chronic back pain.

2. Dr. Sarno has found a nearly closed theory of back pain.

3. etc. [my words]

4. etc.

5. etc.

6. ad naseum, etc. [my words]

Bernabe went on to list nine points on how TMS was a false proposition (he would have made Karl Popper proud). I could tell through his words that he was in quite a bit of emotional pain, which was making his back pain more severe. When this occurs, people are less patient and more prone to observing the dark only. My friend Debbie responded to Bernabe with the only words she should have, "I feel very sad for you after reading your post... because if you believe what you wrote, you will not recover."

Another posting quickly followed Bernabe's from a person who identified herself as a Nerve Signal Interference (NSI) Specialist, which is obviously a field that doesn't promote the notion that emotions and mild oxygen deprivation are causes behind pain. *Where interest lies, honor dies.*

The posting reads:

DATE: Mon, 18 Feb 2002
From: Ms. Guided———
Subject: Options
Hey Bernabe:
You've given me new hope in reaching this group [it appears we were not intelligent enough to understand something (my words in brackets)]. So here goes.

Back problems are DEFINITELY caused by a structural aberration. And yes, mindset also plays a part, as does biochemistry. The most logical methodology, I feel, is to correct the physical element first if it is possible :) Then, what many perceive as massage therapy, is freed to truly work its magic. And of course any depression or psychological problems will soon dissipate with the new life granted in true freedom from pain :) However, if an individual's mind doesn't allow them the opportunity to benefit from the plan that I have described above, then... well, you know... nothing can be done to set that person free at the level that IS possible.
Sincerely,
Ms. Guided
Nerve Signal Interference (NSI) Specialist

Besides being an obvious plug for something called nerve signal interference, this message is fundamentally flawed. All the smiley faces in the world cannot make a false proposition true. If back problems are "definitely" caused by structural aberration, then what about the hundreds of thousands of people, who have completely healed and still have those same aberrations? Why aren't older people the largest groups of sufferers as their backs deteriorate over the years? How could my back problems have been causing my pain since those same aberrations have gotten worse over the years, and yet my pain is gone? It makes no sense. Furthermore, depression does not dissipate after the "physical element" is corrected as she suggested. The physical element exists because of the depression. She has the entire process backwards but she may also have a vested interest in denying TMS—only she could know that. One does not become pain-free and then go out and become happy and active; it works the other way around. You must look inside yourself and change the way in which you respond to life emotionally, and your pain will dissipate because it no longer has a purpose. The physical aberrations have always been a normal part of life that went largely unknown until the introduction of high-tech imaging. Aldous Huxley once stated that "Technological progress has merely provided us with more efficient means for going backwards." It is certainly true that modern technology can save and improve lives, if faced in the proper direction. However, excess information often blinds us, as we are reminded of the aphorism, "I can't see the forest because of all those trees in my way." A little over six months later in the very same pain forum came this final posting from Bernabe.

> Date: Wed, 21 Aug 2002
> From: Bernabe————
> Subject: A hard lesson to learn
> Hi friends,
>
> It has been for a while since I wrote myself a new message. Many of you know me, some more than others. As you know I have always been in doubt about my tms diagnosis. A recent diagnosis using MRI that shown nothing wrong reinforced the hypothesis, but it has not been until today that I have understand the importance of mind in my back pain. I write again to share a wonderful experience with you.
>
> It happens that my father got an illness recently. A fatal diagnosis gave us few hope for him. That shocked me up to the point that my back was hurting more than ever, although I did not relate the increase in pain with my father illness. Then, finally today my father had a new diagnosis using a new test that found nothing about the original diagnosis he was given in first place. The astonishing result was that after hearing the good news my pain ceased!!!
>
> Thanks God for this hard lesson that has allowed me to see the light.
> Bernabe.

"Thanks God" indeed. I often teased Bernabe about his English and about life in an attempt to pick up his spirits. It was ultimately the light of truth that healed him. His pain was shielding him from something unbearable, and he finally found the truth on the **hard road**. To think that this example is an exception is a gross underestimation of the entire process. As long as there are truths, there will be opposers. In every form, in every situation, if there is something that is true—it is a certainty that there will be someone with ego-vested interest standing there in opposition to it. Every day has both light and darkness ...*as the yin chases the yang....*

The Flat-Worlders

When I tell people the healing I personally experienced and have seen happen in hundreds of others, skeptics still sit directly in front of me and tell me that they don't believe it. I always answer them in the same manner, "Just because YOU don't believe it, doesn't mean it's not true." My first thought was that maybe these people were simply too dumb to understand the process, but I didn't really want to project my own shadow onto them. I slowly began to see that it was their **pride alone** that was stopping them from accepting the reasons behind their pain and their fatigue, or dizziness, etc. Some sufferers would unconsciously make themselves worse, creating more dangerous ailments just to prove that TMS was wrong! These people are the door-slammers, the finger-waggers, the eyeball rollers, (the book-across-the-family-room throwers), the ones who doth protest too much, the pride-driven individuals who see vulnerability in their persona—and along comes superego to save their day. The person who coined the insidious and foolhardy term, "all in your head" initiated a world-wide healing catastrophe by challenging people's Achilles' heels: their pride. If egotism wins out, the individual loses in the end, because pride closes the door of healing knowledge forever.

Ego's Shifting Strategies

The overwhelming successes of TMS healing for skin problems, pain, intestinal, and various joint problems—both at a professional and private level—has currently shifted the opposition into recognizing some validity of TMS and begrudgingly into a partial acceptance. What I now hear whispering from the medical field and the lay-opposers is, "Well, yes, there are indeed THOSE type of people (TMSers), BUT, there are also US—the kind with real pains and real body problems." This is a baby step, like in the movie *What About Bob?*, but it is still an ego-denial that is delaying the full acceptance of the truth. It is an attempt by the medical profession to take something very simple and keep it complex—confusing a clear and proven process for the sake of self-interest.

Klopfer

Bruno Klopfer, PhD, a pioneer in the field of health, psychology, and **projective testing** (e.g., Rorschach tests), conducted a survey to predict which tumor types, fast-growing or slow-growing, would most likely form, based on individual personality profiles. From the Simonton's book, *Getting Well Again*, "The variables that allowed the researchers to predict rapid growth (tumors) were patients' ego defensiveness and loyalty to 'their own version of reality'." Klopfer believes that when too much energy is tied up defending the ego and the patient's way of seeing life, the body will not have the necessary vital energy to fight cancer.[86] Ego inhibits healing because it steals energy to maintain itself—diverting energy for healing.

Once upon a time the majority was certain that the Earth was at the center of our solar system and that it was flat (by the way—there are still people who believe it is flat). There are people who still don't believe America went to the moon, or that the Jewish Holocaust ever happened. No amount of truth will ever change the minds of egocentric people with a vested interest in other people's failures. People are free to choose what they desire to believe, but there is no place in science to ignore the truth. Individuals can choose to stay in pain if that is what they still need for themselves, for attention, or to retreat into themselves. However, those who refuse to believe in **The Mindbody Syndrome**, either privately or professionally, should adhere to the Chinese proverb: "Those who say it can't be done should get out of the way of the people who are doing it."

7

Placebo Yo-Yos and Nocebo No-Nos

Placebo: Latin verb, "I will please"
Nocebo: Latin verb, "I will harm"

The placebo is proof that there is no real separation between mind and body.
— Norman Cousins, *Anatomy of an Illness*[87]

Consciousness is an awareness of a situation: an internal knowledge, a perception and understanding of others in relation to you. If you aren't aware of something then it is unconscious to you—beyond your present ability to perceive it. A belief entering consciousness and penetrating more deeply into the unconscious will alter the body, as Norman Cousins articulated so well in his 1979 best selling, *Anatomy of an Illness*. A belief must be strong enough for the unconscious to "accept" for healing to take place, whether what is accepted is from a placebo or from a real therapeutic measure. Cousins knew that the placebo was a powerful tool by which the individual could mobilize his own internal healing resources. He could transform his own power of will (hope) into physiological healing. Nature has given the body what it needs to heal; the body is its own apothecary. But the patient needs to tap into these inner healing forces—and the mechanism is always **belief**. Sadly, people have lost faith in their own healing powers—clinging to healers as guiding compasses.

> *When people are sick, injured, and in pain, they often imagine magical, instantaneous cures.... As a physician who practices and teaches integrative medicine with emphasis on natural healing, I am aware that I am a focus for the projections of the hopes and fears of many patients who would have me play the role of healer. I am also well aware that belief is a powerful influence on the outcome of treatment... the true source of healing is inside us—not outside.*
> — Andrew Weil, MD, *The Healer Archetype*

TMS healing doesn't come from blind belief—it's quite the opposite. It comes from a deeper understanding of what's happening within because the truth is the fastest path to freedom. There is no ritual with TMS healing, or magic, or honestly intentioned deceit—only a new awareness. Credence that TMS healing is not a placebo comes from the fact that pain oftentimes leaves when knowledge is gained. This would be much more difficult if there was a real injury.

Dr. Sarno points out that the fact that so many thousands of people heal through reading his books is proof that the TMS process is not a placebo. There's no physical interjection or personal interaction of any kind in the healing process. So it's not only the mere belief that heals people from chronic pain, it's also an **understanding of the process**. When the physician explains to the sufferer exactly what is occurring, he is in essence taking away any placebo effect. I believe Dr. Sarno would agree that this was one of his most amazing findings regarding TMS—in explaining how the pain process works, his patients began to heal.

With the placebo it's the belief in the drug—or act—that ratifies the body's constitution to free itself. The belief rallies the will to change, which in turn transforms the body. If anything can be taken away from *Anatomy of an Illness*, it's the notion that we are as strong as we believe ourselves to be—no more and no less. The placebo effect pulls people toward their higher potential—but not as high as the truth itself. With TMS healing, the actual truth activates those very same healing mechanisms, but TMS healing has been shown to be more permanent. The truth wins out in the end. But this doesn't understate the necessity of the placebo. Who cares how it goes away if it is so painful that it devastates life? When the doctor erroneously tells the patient he has a bad back, or shoulder, or knee, suffering naturally increases due to the **nocebo effect**. The doctor has now delayed her healing indefinitely with faulty medical advice—and harmed her.

Surgery and Other Types of Placebos

I'm addicted to placebos... I could quit... but it wouldn't matter.

— Steven Wright, comedian

The **ritual** itself is a major factor in determining how well a placebo such as surgery or therapy, or manipulations, or steroidal injections work. Norman Cousins understood that the placebo was not always a pill, but more often "a process."[88]

A 2002 Baylor College of Medicine study[89] reveals how the surgery placebo works as a process. Three groups were created of about 60 people who had osteoarthritis in their knees. Two of the groups received one of two different types of arthroscopic knee surgery. The third group was given a placebo or sham surgery (incisions on their knees with no actual surgery). The final results after a year were that "all three groups reported equal amounts of improvement in pain and function—and the same held true two years after surgery."[90]

Over 200,000 Americans receive the surgery, each year, at an approximate cost of over a billion dollars. The designer of the study stated, "This research indicates that there is an enormous placebo effect for this surgery, but that is the only value in the vast majority of osteoarthritis patients.... We should certainly rethink doing this operation, and policymakers should definitely rethink paying for it."

Surgeon Bruce Moseley, MD, clinical associate professor of orthopedics at Baylor, who performed all the knee procedures in the study, stated that surgery was not the correct treatment for osteoarthritis, a degenerative joint disease causing cartilage breakdown, allowing bones to rub together (often characterized as rigidity). Within the discussion portion of the trial was stated, "This study provides strong evidence that arthroscopic lavage, with or without débridement,* is not better than, and appears to be equivalent to, a placebo procedure in improving knee pain and self-reported function. Indeed, at some points during follow up, objective function was significantly worse in the débridement group than in the placebo group." So—the knee surgeries made some patients worse than the placebo group as it decreased the objective range of function in their knees. This Baylor study is but one showing the ineffectiveness of surgeries. Moseley did state that arthroscopic surgery is still needed for sports injuries or accidents. The same is true for back injuries or shoulder injuries, of course. Acute injury or physical trauma may need outside correction.

Regarding the Baylor study, David T. Felson, MD, osteoarthritis and rheumatology expert, states, "There is a large community of surgeons who do this operation, and what this study is telling them is that what they are doing is worthless."[91] Felson also stated, "There's a pretty good-sized industry out there that is performing this surgery... it constitutes a good part of the livelihood of some orthopedic surgeons. That is a reality."[92] This study has since been confirmed by another study completed at The University of Western Ontario and the Lawson Health Research Institute and reported in the New England Journal of Medicine in 2008.[93]

Back surgery studies reveal similar results as the Baylor knee study. In 1994, within the US Department of Health and Human Services and in what is now called The Agency for Healthcare Research and Quality an article was published on the ineffectiveness of back surgeries entitled, "Understanding Acute Low Back Pain Problems."[94] The survey concluded that 99 percent of back operations were failures and that surgery often created more problems.† As with the Baylor knee study, objective function was sometimes significantly worse in the débridement group.

The surgery placebo becomes effective in disarming or breaking the focus of any conflict—for a short time. However, placebos do not normally last, and the pain, much like Arnold, "will be back." A minority of people told me, "Hey, my back surgery worked." But they are unaware that it was merely their belief it had worked—from the ritual of the surgery—providing means for them to bail out of their tension-filled arenas and enabling them to momentarily escape their spouse, parents, job, kids, and problems. For most, residual pains and fears remain, so surgery did not work.

---

* Debridement is the removal of diseased or damaged tissue.
† The Department of Health and Human Services concluded, "Surgery has been found to be helpful in only 1 in 100 cases of low back problems. In some people, surgery can even cause more problems." (U.S. Department of Health and Human Services, Agency for Health Care Policy and Research, *Understanding Acute Low Back Pain Problems*, Publication No. 95-0644. [Rockville, Md., December 1994, p. 12]

Dr. Sarno wrote that spinal surgery is perhaps the most effective placebo of them all because of the danger involved. Surgery is mysterious and scary and takes time—the ritual's stakes are high—so it can have a more powerful effect on the subconscious. The time spent preparing for the surgery and convalescing gets the individual out of the personal arena that is causing his pain. With surgery, he gets his needed downtime to pull back and regroup and to opt out of current responsibilities. If the surgeon exudes confidence in the procedure, or has a good reputation, it will have a greater impact on the patient's feeling of well-being afterwards.

I hate to tell you this, but surgery may have the biggest placebo effect of all.
— Nelda Wray, MD, MPH, Professor of Medicine, Division of Preventive Medicine, University of Alabama School of Medicine[95]

Societies are just beginning to realize the awesome power, and the debilitating potential, of the human mind. But where there is big money involved, there will always be a tendency for physicians to lean toward the surgical procedure—and, many patients would still rather have the **quick-fix-now** because they don't have the time to stop and examine their lives. Together, they—physician and patient—are making problems worse.

One of my best friends since childhood recently told me he had prostate cancer. His doctor told him he needed his prostate removed—I and others urged him to search for alternatives, such as radiation implants, etc. He replied, "SteveO, I've been bombarded by so many people with alternatives and variations. After weighing them all and including their impact on my busy life, I chose to have the darn thing removed. Radiation might have worked but it would have resulted in a lot of disruption to my already insane schedule." The same holds true for back surgeries of course, "cut it out of me, and let me move on." As Jung had written, negotiations with the **personal shadow** can be long, grueling, and painful—so are avoided.

There is no epidemic of back pain in Asia. Do Americans have weaker spines? No—just shorter deadlines to meet, less time for mending close relationships—and we have fallen harder for the misconceptions and overzealousness of modern medicine. Subsequently, the US back pain rate is far higher than the developing world's.[96]

In *Healing Back Pain*, Dr. Sarno describes a placebo drive-by that involved Dr. Bruno Klopfer and one of his patients. Circa 1957, Klopfer had a patient with lymph node cancer. Klopfer treated the man with an experimental drug called Krebiozen. He writes, "The man had a miraculous recovery with the disappearance of his many large tumors. He did well until he heard news reports of the ineffectiveness of Krebiozen, whereupon he regressed to the same desperate state in which he had been before."[97] Klopfer then told this patient that he would give him a stronger form of Krebiozen, but he gave the man sterile water instead. The man's tumors once again disappeared due to his deep belief that he was being given a stronger drug. However—

once the AMA officially announced its decision that Krebiozen "was of no value," his tumors returned and he died soon after.[98]

The power of belief is awesome, and cuts both ways. Those who believe can flourish, depending on what they believe, and on the depth of that belief.

A second major factor in placebo effectiveness is the **effector**. Stronger placebo results are generated by faith in the performer of the ritual. I had tremendous results the first time I read the work of therapist Pete Egoscue, because I really believed in **him**. His program also made sense and I enjoyed his positive attitude and confidence in healing.

People also tend to have a better placebo effect from surgery when they see a surgeon in another city. The farther people are from us, it seems—the smarter, better looking, and more worth knowing they are.

A key then is the depth of belief in the **ritual** and/or **effector**. I had great results with some physical therapists at first, but my pain came back with viciousness because I hadn't unraveled the mystery of pain yet. It's much like weeding a garden. If you don't pull the root, the weed will come back taller and stronger. Physical therapy does not work in the long run.

My friend Tony talked me into trying acupuncture in the early 1990s. He claimed it had stopped his neck pain of 30 years in one session. So I tried it many times, but it did nothing for me. It was years later that I realized the placebo effect it had on him. He was constantly telling me how much he "liked the doctor." He always smiled wide when he brought up the subject, and spoke of how nice his nurse was and how friendly they were to him and how they understood his pain and what a pretty nurse she was. When people are in pain, a sympathetic ear is healing, and so Tony had been placebo-ized into healing. I didn't care for the doctor. It was obvious he didn't know what he was doing and so acupuncture failed for me. If the person believes acupuncture works, it may—but not because it actually does anything. The ritual simply alters the belief—mobilizing the healing system. I was never much for the sympathetic ear; I always looked for intellectual ears. That acupuncturist appeared to have no idea of what acupuncture even was. He had trouble with the procedure and was elusive in answering any direct questions. He was an ineffective effector to me, and so the process failed me.

The epidural steroid injection (ESI) process is equivalent to surgery. My cousin had a tremendous placebo reaction to his first epidural injection, as do many people. He really liked the doctor because he was kind and patted his hand with a compassionate touch as he listened to my cousin's problems. But the pain returned after subsequent treatments because it missed the cause and attacked the effect. Recent studies confirm this inability of ESI to accomplish anything of value. One study in *Rheumatology* entitled, "A multicentre randomized controlled trial of epidural corticosteroid injections for sciatica: the WEST study," reported, "ESIs did not improve physical function, hasten return to work, or reduce the need for surgery. There was no benefit of repeated ESIs over single injection. No clinical predictors of response were found. At the end of the study, the majority of patients still had significant pain and disability regardless of intervention."[99] The placebo effect of the epidural injection is also quickly waning through increased public awareness, and its application is needle-ess, just as with back surgery, as more sufferers return for more surgeries.

Studies and articles from neurosurgeons and neurologists are increasingly questioning the efficacy of surgery. A newer study in 2006 entitled, "The Spine Patient Outcomes Research Trial or SPORT," has also concluded that surgery has no superiority or equivalence over non-surgery, stating that, "Patients in both the surgery and the nonoperative treatment groups improved substantially over a 2-year period. Because of the large numbers of patients who crossed over in both directions, conclusions about the superiority or equivalence of the treatments are not warranted based on the intent-to-treat analysis."[100]

The 1994 US Department of Health and Human Services survey on lumbar surgery revealing that only one percent of back surgeries are successful is proof enough for most people. However, if you add any of the components I listed above to the surgery, **ritual**, and **confidence in performer**, the surgery may have lasting effects. But this is rare. I personally have never met an individual who has had successful back surgery. That is, there is no residual pain ever again, they don't have to be careful ever again, and are not afraid of injuring their backs again.

New fads like Lordex Decompression Therapy, the large placebo machine that is intended to reduce spinal stenosis (narrowing) by separating the spinal column, can give rise to the benefits of shared suffering. People like to try new things—one upmanship— new fads for new conversations. There are also benefits from the **ruse** of the ritual such as being strapped to a large machine, the time being strapped in, the noises, and the confident utterances coming from the pain brokers. You cannot widen the foramina to ease pain—the absurdity spreads wider than the foramina ever could.

One must not forget that recovery is brought about, not by the physician, but by the sick man himself. He heals himself, by his own power, exactly as he walks by means of his own power, or eats, or thinks, breathes or sleeps.

— Georg Groddeck, MD, *The Book of the It* (1866-1934)[101]

Chiropractic Manipulation—The Therapeutic Sugar Pill

I truly don't believe that most chiropractors are being mendacious—however, it is important to understand that any relief from manipulation is only from the belief that it has worked. The individual has hurt his back or neck* or shoulder, he then sees a chiropractor for adjustments. He eventually feels better at the end of all the visits and attributes the feeling of wellness to the adjustments, or sessions. However, he is healing, with or without the treatments; but he wrongly associates the treatments with the healing ritual. I'm often asked, "How do you know the chiro didn't expedite the process?" The answer is of course he or she may move it along because **you believed it**, and so it can—but that's the only reason it worked… your belief and time healed you, along with the healing touch of connection.

As long as you understand that pain does not come from structural misalignment or degeneration, then there is no problem with having a chiropractic adjustment. It can be thought of as a musculoskeletal massage where the bones and joints are being manipulated—temporarily relieving some tension. A friend of mine who healed using Dr. Sarno's advice still occasionally visits his chiropractor. He knows his pain was never structural but he simply tells me, "I know, I know you can't throw your back out Steve, but it feels soooo good." Therefore, as long as the sufferer knows that there is no such thing as a slipped disc or subluxation—the manipulation may bring temporary relief from pain due to the placebo effect. **But I would do so with extreme caution.** The idea that there is a misalignment or a pinched nerve is deeply ingrained in the collective unconscious. Manipulation often perpetuates the pain by strengthening the concept of misalignment, in the depths of the unconscious, much like physical therapy.

This is a most important point, and a major apex of contention among healers of all sorts. This book is a book about an epidemic called TMS—that causes the vast majority of our health problems. TMS healing does not, and cannot, include alternative physical techniques for healing such as chiropractic, prolotherapy, acupuncture, glucosamine, etc. TMS healing implicitly means to stop these other forms of treatment as they are antithesis to TMS healing—mutually exclusive healing modalities. If you're doing TMS healing, you cannot be doing these other modalities, or you are not doing TMS healing, and Dr. Sarno agrees. True TMS healing excludes alternative techniques because they are a part of the problem, by maintaining body-focus, when none is warranted.

…therapeutic eclecticism is a sign of diagnostic incompetence.
John E. Sarno, MD, Healing Back Pain[102]

---

* Neck and back pain are the same thing and should be treated as such. Dr. Sopher writes in, *To Be or Not To Be… Pain-Free*, "Think of the neck as the northern part of the spine and the low back as the south." [p. 88]

Tapping into the Wonderful, Much Maligned, Placebo Effect

I firmly believe that **ultimately** every healing is mediated by the so-called placebo effect; that is, our deepest beliefs can heal or harm us, even alter the expression of our DNA—as Dr. Lipton implies in the opening page of this book.

So is TMS healing a placebo effect? Yes, "if" the definition of a placebo is predicated solely on your belief—the central mechanism of all healing. I do, though, differentiate between TMS healing (finding the truth about yourself) and healing by being "fooled" through rituals (the list below), all of which may ease the pain of any sufferer and so I cannot dismiss their effectiveness. Below I list what I am simply calling placebos—meaning, they are unnecessary in the healing of pain and other symptoms. The main difference being that TMS healing is more permanent and the treatments listed below may actually delay healing because they reaffirm in the mind that something is wrong with the body that needs fixing. However, if they make you feel better, then by all means use them—but do so with caution, as they may inhibit true healing because they bypass the cause of the problem, which is your history, personality, and present circumstance.

Chiropractic manipulation—Sense of Touch/Snapping/Popping
    (Auditory Placebo Effect)—connection
Acupuncture (for pain reduction only)
Corticosteroid injections (ESI)
Knee or back or neck or foot or RSI surgery
Ergonomic workstations
Drugs (many, but not all, of course), the most well-known placebo is the
    sugar pill
Copper wrist bracelets
True back—orthopedic traction device
Magnets
Ointments
Talismans
Chondroitin
Glucosamine
Prolotherapy—Injections into ligaments to re-grow collagen—it works! But
    pain doesn't come from a lack of collagen, it comes from oxygen
    reduction → TMS. Any positive results are from a placebo effect.
Lordex decompression therapy
Mouth sprays—for pain relief
Intervertebral disc decompression
Pro-Adjuster—A great example of the ritual aspect of placebo combined
    with healing power of touch

Charité disc replacement

Night mouthguards—Stops teeth grinding, but not TMJ—TMJ can begin
    with no jaw movement or grinding.

This is a very short list of the more popular anodyne methods being misused
today—but the concept remains the same, if the sufferer can be made to believe—
healing **can** take place.

> *…much medical treatment today owes its success, such as it is, to the placebo*
> *phenomenon.*
>
> — John E. Sarno, MD, *The Divided Mind*[103]

The power of the mind is infinite in healing and in disabling.

Discernment

> *All creations are impermanent. Strive for your own salvation with diligence.*
> — Siddhārtha Gautama Buddha, said to be his last words

We are different from most animals in that we can discern, reflect, and also laugh.
There often comes that time when the light bulb goes on overhead as a little bit more
comes together and makes sense. My weight-lifting partner recently said to me, "You
know, I think you're right about that anger/pain thing. My boss just asked me to do
something that I didn't want to do, and my shoulder began to hurt." He had made
the nexus between the mindbody and the mind and body—discerning a little more
deeply.

When it comes to your doctor telling you that your pain is from arthritis, disc
degeneration, scoliosis, repetitive strain (RSI), "chronic partial meniscus tears,"
thoracic outlet syndrome (TOS), carpal tunnel, etc., be highly cynical if you have
been chronic or are under severe relationship stress or financial pain. It is critical to
relearn your understanding of pain, through **discernment**. As the Buddha suggested
in the quote above, search for your own truths, doubt everything that you think you
understand about the body and pain. If you think you know all about pain, then you
cannot be taught more about the same subject; find your own light—stop following
the wrong information into further darkness.

Seeing the Light—from Your TV

I've had people tell me that Dr. Sarno is wrong because they saw someone on TV
say he was wrong. I guess if you can't find light from your own TV, where can you
find it? TV can't be wrong, can it? People who fully believe in TMS fully heal. Those
who believe in it slightly, but still have residual doubt, heal a little. Those who don't
believe at all don't heal. They have freely created their realities—based upon their
belief.

I'm frequently asked, "are you telling me that you cannot hurt your back?" The answer is always, "Yes—of course you can!" But it should heal in a progressive manner and within a reasonable time frame. If after a few months, there is no healing, begin looking at an emotional and conditioning process behind the continuing pain.

People will sometimes state that their pain is not chronic because it only comes around two or three times per year and then disappears. This is chronicity! Pain that keeps recurring at various times is chronic—a conditioned response due to a wide array of triggers that come and go reigniting old memories. I also hear, "Hey, I saw **my** MRI and **my** herniated discs, so I know **my** pain is real." The pain is always real, be it from TMS or injury. It can, however, be very difficult to discern between true injury and Phase 2 TMS. Seeing herniated discs on the MRI means little, if anything—the objective function is the more important aspect in the diagnosis. The attorney on ABC's *20/20*, "Dr. Sarno's Cure," had seven herniated discs and was in severe pain; however, his pain left him weeks after experiencing Dr. Sarno's exam and lecture.

Changing the collective consciousness of society is a more daunting and time-consuming task. This book is one step in this lengthy—controversial—process.

An important scientific innovation rarely makes its way by gradually winning over and converting its opponents: it rarely happens that Saul becomes Paul. What does happen is that its opponents gradually die out, and that the growing generation is familiarized with the ideas from the beginning.

— Max Planck, founder of quantum physics (1858-1947)

8

Planting the Seeds, Growing the Pain— Who Is the Gardener?

I think the foot pain epidemic began shortly after Larry Bird's surgery for heel spurs in the early 1980s.

— Marc Sopher, MD, *To Be or Not To Be... Pain-Free*[104]

The quote above is perspicacious; only a handful of family physicians have that ability—or desire—to link cause and effects that determine health and well-being. Dr. Sopher used Larry Bird as an example because Larry was a famous basketball player— a popular international figure of influence and high admiration. Authority figures have power to plant failure or success into the **collective unconscious** (the objective psyche). We tend to look outward for answers; something, anything to believe in, and our beliefs are often guided by a predisposition "to unconsciously follow" in order to remain connected. Beliefs and fears, like common colds, are contagious and universally spread. Jungian archetypal images—eternally repeated patterns—along with social imitation, strongly influence belief and health.

Filling Dry River Beds

The word **archetype** comes from Carl Jung and is loosely translated from Greek as **original model**. Examples of archetypes are the mother, father, drunkard, wise old man, bum, cripple, wounded one, teacher, child, warrior, or even the villain or hero archetypes. Larry Bird may fit the hero archetype to many fans and admirers.

A Jungian archetype is a mental predisposition, a psychic force not grounded in experience, a priori. The archetype surfaces as repeated images or experiences in the **collective unconscious** through time immemorial. Everyone, everywhere, is born with these models or images in their heads of heroes, bums, cripples, wise elders, etc. They are generic, autonomous personalities—preexisting forces of nature that are shared by everybody—spontaneously manifesting anywhere, at any time, in anyone. They govern behavior and perception as a morphogenetic energy.* Jung described an archetype as a dry riverbed that had a preformed impulse to create imagery, outside of conscious forces.

---

* Morphogenetic energy (consciousness fields) is a consciousness that is shared by everything that lives; created by everything that lives—a mass consciousness of information. These fields have been described as "non-physical blueprints" that give rise to forms. One "era" takes on the form of a previous era instantaneously across space-time as the previous era is the embryo for each subsequent era.

146

Archetypes reside within the psychological life of everyone. Archetypal existence along with personal experiences, together, fill the dry riverbeds, which becomes the individual's **personal unconscious.**

There's No Shaman Not Knowing—
The Power of Suggestion Is Covert

> *When Columbus' fleet landed in the Caribbean, we're told that none of the natives were able to see the ships, even though they existed on the horizon. The reason that they never saw the ships was because they had no knowledge in their brains or no experience that clipper ships existed. So the shaman starts to notice that there's [sic] ripples out in the ocean but he sees no ships, [but] he starts to wonder what's causing the effect? So every day he goes out and looks and looks and looks, and after a period of time he's able to see the ships, and once he sees the ships he tells everyone else that ships exist out there...(and) because everybody trusted and believed in him, they saw them also.*
>
> — Joe Dispenza, DC, Life University, *What the Bleep Do We Know?*

The Healer Archetype

Healers determine the health realities for societies, based on their experience and training with causes and effects. When a physician tells the patient he has bad knees or feet, or back or neck, he believes the healer at a deeper level of consciousness—filling the patient's dry river bed, helping to form his personal unconscious. People normally believe what the physician tells them, especially if it allows them to opt out of things they don't want to do—avoid places they don't want to be. Even if the physician is wrong, most people will believe him or her because of their position of influence. If your doctor doesn't believe Dr. Sarno, and you believe in your doctor, then that's it—your healing has been negated.

It's not that the doctor can't see the ships, but in his intense training he hasn't been taught to look beyond his own horizon. He has been conditioned to look for particular patterns, and so what is in vogue is often determined by the perfunctory act of looking only for what one expects to see. It is the sufferer who ultimately heals himself through deeper belief, but he draws his own belief from the healer's belief. If the doctor doesn't believe healing is possible—neither will the patient. *

The Fool archetype is the most symbolic regarding the propensity to believe what remains untrue. Being a fool does not mean one is foolish; it merely means one just does not know. There is hardly a better example of being fooled than the acceptance

---

* "The practice of healing lies in the heart. If your heart is false, the physician within you will be false." —Paracelsus

Jesus sent His disciples out to heal the sick but when they came back they told Him they couldn't heal some of them. After seeing Him heal a sick man that they could not, they asked Jesus how He could do it when they were unable to heal some of them? He replied, "Because YOU have so little faith." [Matthew 17:20]

of the suggestion that back pain or foot pain (neuropathy), or repetitive stress injuries, are caused by normal physiological changes within the body, and that the human body is currently collapsing after 250,000 years of adaptation and survival. As Dr. Sopher writes, "why should incidence of foot pain be increasing now? It makes no sense."[105] He then explains that we have the best footwear ever designed in history to help protect and support the feet and, "Suddenly our feet should start to hurt?"[106] In the 1960 Rome Olympics, Ethiopian runner, Abebe Bikila, won the 26-mile road-marathon race in his bare feet. Our feet can take much—they are strong like our backs. We are as strong as our beliefs, or as Henry Ford said, "Whether you think you can or whether you think you can't—you're right."

Seeding Your Unconscious

In 1993, 10 years before I began to understand the power of suggestion, I was sitting in the clubhouse after a round of golf. A friend asked me if I wanted some spicy chicken wings. I told him "No, they give me heartburn." The next week that friend walked up to me and said, "Dammit SteveO, I have never had heartburn after eating those wings but after talking with you I had heartburn that night!" I was glad to be of help. The process unfolds every day in front of us, and yet goes unrecognized because we aren't expecting to see new ships on the horizon. I also no longer have digestive problems since I've come to understand conditioning and the brain's fervent need for body-focus.

Dr. Sopher writes, "There is a veritable epidemic of foot pain in our society. All of a sudden, everyone has foot problems, from pro athletes to the couch potato next door. This has not always been the case.... When I started my medical training about 20 years ago, foot pain was not a common complaint, now it is in vogue and everywhere you turn.... There is no doubt in my mind that the overwhelming majority of foot pain attributed to plantar fasciitis, heel spurs, neuromas, or other physical causes is TMS."[107] The key words here are "no doubt."

This mystery Dr. Sopher refers to isn't confined to the feet, it also applies to the hands and all the new so-called repetitive stress disorders (RSDs), fibromyalgia, and of course, good old back and neck pain.

Epidemiologists have referred to this passing on of symptoms as **amplification**. In this case, it is shared suffering through shared mistaken beliefs. Television ads, and a very small number of physicians, purposefully plant seeds of fear. Fear-provoking suggestions like warnings of esophageal reflux disease, high cholesterol, high blood pressure, back pain from sitting on fat wallets, erectile dysfunction, prostate enlargement, dry eyes, and so on, all can become chronic conditions if the individual can be persuaded to focus on them—to fear them.

The wheelchair-bound patient was sure she had Parkinson's Disease (a misdiagnosis), but by the end of one session, she was jogging down the hall. A man dies of cancer, yet the autopsy showed there were not enough cancerous spots in his body to have killed him. A priest administers the last rites to the wrong patient, and that patient dies unexpectedly. *

— Cathy Sherman, NaturalNews.com[108]

Dr. Sopher has cautioned radiologists about how they word their reports because they can inadvertently harm the patient. The description of the findings often sounds ominous and threatening, increasing fear—and pain, and traumatizing the victim. The result of a dire report is increased symptoms—the nocebo effect. The attending physician then amplifies the pain by confirming the ominous information. The catastrophe lies in the chain of false information regarding the implications of the report.

Panic and Fear Are Powerful Forces

Norman Cousins stated that every person who goes to a doctor goes to the doctor with two diseases. The first is the disease that is diagnosed, and the other is the disease of **panic**. Norman stated that panic is a "powerful disease" that has been exacerbated by the "great deal of public education" like commercials and overzealous warnings from the medical industry to see your doctor for even the slightest of symptoms. He feared that America had become a nation of hypochondriacs. This may be true, but the final authority is still the self. As Cousins stated, "Your physician didn't make you ill." This is true, she didn't make you ill—your subconscious needs and beliefs did; but she does have the power to help you, or to harm you, through the power of her archetypal presence.

> *...doctors today push all the new diagnostic toys they possess, and encourage patients to have mammograms, colonoscopies, etc., with the explanation "we tell everyone of this age to get one, because such and such a percent of people this age will get" cancer, polyps, etc. Combined with this are the incessant magazine and TV ads for pharmaceuticals purporting to treat the various maladies.... Such seeds sow fear in people's minds, consciously or subconsciously. Where previously the person hadn't even considered the possibility of colon cancer, now he or she starts worrying about it. Every little abdominal pain feeds the worry. Lipton† says that the current high rates of colon and rectal cancers are linked with the amount of information in the media that there is a high rate of colon and rectal cancers.*

— Cathy Sherman, *The Mind-Body Connection:
Fear Manifests in Many Diseases* (Part 1)

---

* "The underlying ancient concept, formalized decades ago by Robert K. Merton, PhD, can be found in Greek mythological stories and elsewhere. Merton further refined its definition calling it the **Self-Fulfilling Prophecy**. According to this construct, once a prophecy or fact is predicted, events are set in motion, that work together to bring it to pass. These events can occur within a person's psyche or develop as part of the situation from which the prophetic statement sprang." [Cathy Sherman, *The Mind-Body Connection: Fear Manifests In Many Diseases* (Part 1)]

† Bruce H. Lipton, PhD, cell biologist, author of *The Biology of Belief.*

I went to a doctor at age 14 and he told me, "Your discs are herniated in such a manner that if you get hit in the back in just the right way, you will be permanently paralyzed." Those words kept me in constant fear of activity and in pain for 30 more years. He legitimized my pain—making it worse—through his foolish warnings of dangers "that could happen"—limiting my life potential and belief in myself. But it was ultimately me who debilitated me, because I trusted and believed in him.

That Which Grows Is That Which Is Planted

What one says, another may believe. When people have been defeated by tragedy, or isolation, or have experienced prolonged periods of pain and sleeplessness, they are extremely suggestible. If they have been conditioned to be good or to toe the line, they are in further danger of falling for anything that comes their way. Goodism—the driving need to do what is correct—creates a vulnerable atmosphere that entertains many false ideologies. Timing is also critical in accepting a belief, and periods of isolation, tension and, stress are open wounds awaiting the emergence of the next suggestion.

> *Illnesses hover constantly above us, their seed blown by the winds, but they do not set in the terrain unless the terrain is ready to receive them.*
> — Claude Bernard, MD, father of physiology,
> created the concept of homeostasis (1813-1878)

A fine example of this power of suggestion appears in Fred Amir's, *Rapid Recovery from Back and Neck Pain*. Fred writes, "I remember a few times when I sneezed at work and was told by my coworkers that sneezing must really hurt. At first it didn't. But after hearing people tell me that it must, I became conditioned to expect pain upon sneezing. Pretty soon every time I sneezed my back hurt, too, and I thought my condition was getting worse!"[109] Fred's need to be good, to do what is right, had created an atmosphere conducive to receptive amplification of thought. A good person tries to avoid conflict, and will often do so by accommodating others' realities at the expense of self. We live in a society that celebrates individual achievement; but regarding our health, we allow ourselves to be pulled into the collective pack. This is evident in the notion of chronic whiplash. Multiple studies reveal that those countries that compensate for whiplash injuries have epidemics of cases, whereas countries that don't compensate have trouble even understanding the notion of post-collision pain. Here, most people are not faking injury for gain—they do indeed experience pain—but they have been led to believe that they **should** have lingering pain because the system is set up to accommodate it through the self-fulfilling prophecy, and so it lingers. The play cannot begin until the stage is set ...**to be or not to be pain-free... that is the question....**

It has been demonstrated, specifically regarding whiplash, that if medical insurance is not available, the epidemic does not develop.

— Marc Sopher, MD, *To Be or Not To Be... Pain-Free*[110]

If the soil is fertile, something will grow. If specific seeds are planted into unfilled needs, that particular information and energy will manifest organically.

The Awesome Power of Expectation

Your expectations can have profound impacts on your brain and your health.

— Tor Wager, PhD, Columbia University, neuroscientist[111]

In 2005, MSNBC ran a medical program on the power of expectation regarding the effectiveness of medication. The scientists in the clinical trials concluded that if the doctor talked-up or increased the expectations of the medicine, the medicine had a much greater effect—creating a physiological change. The placebo effect is more than psychological since it can alter how the body reacts physiologically.

In a University of Michigan study,[112] specific thoughts were planted, which harvested specific beliefs and therefore, specific results. The researchers injected salt water into the jaws of volunteers to create a painful mindbody experience. The men were then injected with what they thought was a painkiller, but it was actually a placebo. Positron emission tomography (PET) scans of the volunteers' brains showed that they were releasing natural pain-killing endorphins. In other words, immediately after the injections, the volunteers' bodies were sending their own natural painkillers to their jaws because they believed the medicine was helping them, even though no medicine was being administered. The mindbody will alter its current state in order to adapt to what it perceives is the reality at hand.

Similar results were obtained by Dr. Fabrizio Benedetti of Italy's University of Torino Medical School. Benedetti connected Parkinson's patients to a morphine machine to help stop tremors and rigidity, but the patients could not tell when the machine was actually administering the morphine to them. In contrast, when a nurse administered the morphine, it was 50 percent more effective. Thus, even though the patients knew they were getting a dosage in both cases, the very same medicine worked dramatically better when they could actually see it being administered. Belief created relief. Similar studies administering morphine to Parkinson's patients who also had Alzheimer's did not have the same results. The testers attributed this to the lack of cognitive ability of Alzheimer's sufferers "to expect" the dosage.[113]

In yet another Parkinson's placebo trial,[114] one of two groups of sufferers had human embryonic dopamine neurons transplanted into their brains, while the second group was assigned to a "sham surgery condition." Of the 18 who received the sham surgery, many reported objective improvements of neurological functioning. One Parkinson's sufferer who had been inactive for several years before her surgery began hiking and ice skating, a year after the surgery. When the double blind was lifted she was shown that she had actually received the sham surgery. Over all, the receivers of the actual transplant showed slightly better improvement, but the point is that those participants who thought that they had received the embryonic neurons reported a better quality of life than those who thought they had received the fake surgery "regardless of which surgery they actually received."[115] This study also maintained the double-blind condition for over 12 months compared to the average length of placebo studies, which is approximately 8 weeks.

In all cases, those who thought they received the transplant reported better scores. Conclusions: the placebo effect was very strong in this study, demonstrating the value of placebo-controlled surgical trials.

— Archives of General Psychiatry[116]

If belief can improve and even heal, it's logical to assume that the mind can even create the disorder—all originating from an **error in thought.** Make no mistake: Parkinson's is a real degenerative disease. But why is it more susceptible to placebo effect than many other diseases? Is there a deeper need at play?

The same concept holds true in a recent German study on the effectiveness of acupuncture. An experiment was performed on 1,100 patients, comparing "real" acupuncture versus both "sham" acupuncture and "conventional" back pain therapy such as physical therapy and exercise.[117] Of the patients receiving the real acupuncture, 47 percent felt better and 44 percent of the patients receiving the sham acupuncture also felt better. The patients who received conventional back therapy did the worst—of course—with only 27 percent reporting feeling better. What I considered the most important part of the article was a side note that stated, "…its findings are in line with a theory that pain messages to the brain can be blocked by competing stimuli."

Changing the Channel on Pain

Addressing these competing stimuli is Dr. Sarno's point, "As long as he (the sufferer) is in any way preoccupied with what his body is doing, the pain will continue."[118] The idea is to focus on something other than the body—some competing stimulus, such as a new life-goal. Emmett Miller, MD, refers to this as "changing the channel on pain." Competing stimuli diverts the brain rendering it unable to process the sensation of pain. Any acupuncture, therapy, manipulation, or surgery merely takes the focus off the pain for a brief time, and redirects it to the current activity by guiding the mind away from the sensation of pain—confusing the individual into believing that these procedures are the source of their healing. This is why identifying a sense of purpose in life, and refusing to feel like a victim, eases pain. Find a way to turn your obsession toward an activity that you love and focus on it, and the pain will slowly leave, as this new, more productive obsession becomes the competing stimulus.

9

What Did You Meme by That?

Piggybacking on the concept of both Jung's archetypes and Darwin's gene replication theory is the theory of memetics. First introduced by Richard Dawkins in 1976 in his book, *The Selfish Gene*, the theory proposes that the meme (rhymes with dream) is an idea, or way of thinking or believing about the world that is passed from person to person, society to society, and generation to generation. A meme replicates information by imitation, using a language of words, sounds, or other symbols (the tune you can't get out of your head that the person who hears you humming, starts humming themselves). Memes replicate in the same manner that organic genes pass down information. To be effective, a meme must infect a host through observation or by thought, and assimilate into the individual's subconscious memory. Then, the meme "must be respectively noticed, understood and accepted by the host."[119] A common example is the notion that cold weather causes colds. Society has collectively and unconsciously agreed to participate in the notion that cold weather causes colds and that slipped discs cause pain. And so they actually do cause these symptoms—if indeed the "infection" is accepted. But these are false realities generated through the unconscious acceptance of a false meme. It strikes at the very heart of quantum mechanics and the reality one chooses to create or accept.

Memetics Is Social Contagion

Paul Marsden describes memetics as the other side of the coin of the "established field of social science," known as **social contagion.** Social contagion, or memetics, is a social infection passed from one individual or group to another individual or group. Hysterical contagion is simply a "stronger representation" of social contagion, a more aggressive form of social contagion spread by person-to-person communication and the awesome power of suggestion.

> *[Hysterical contagion is] "the collective occurrence of a set of physical symptoms and related beliefs among two or more individuals in the absence of an identifiable pathogen."...* *[M. Colligan and L. Murphy] found that it was the verbal reporting of the symptoms that spread in a contagious-like manner rather than the symptoms themselves. Their research also largely confirmed Kerckhoff and Backs' theory that those susceptible to hysterical contagion were suffering from intra-psychic stress.*
>
> — Paul Marsden, Director of The Influencer Marketing Division of Brand Genetics, Ltd.[120]

Memetics & Social Contagion: Two Sides of the Same Coin

Marsden continues, "Because social learning is an evolved psychological trait, it follows that we have an evolved predisposition to replicating the behavior of those around us."[121] Memetics contends that the human infected with the new thought is then the **new replicator** of that thought. Conceptually, the meme is the social counterpart of the gene that copies itself through imitation of other people for self-survival. Memes then are "units of culture" and "social replicators." Germane to the topic of this book is the notion that memes can express themselves in the form of **behavior**. These false notions of the human body's impending demise actually affect behavior because memes alter the brain as malignant parasites by hard-wiring the brain neurologically through imitation.

The meme concept is analogous to gene selection except that it involves **thought selection**. The thoughts that are unknowingly selected are those which enable the individual to survive—to feel connected. Dawkins describes a meme as a selfish gene because memes "…have no foresight. (They are unconscious, blind replicators)."[122]

Back, Hand, and Foot Pain Are Currently Fashionable—"In Vogue"

Mindbody disorders change from generation to generation, and society to society. The need to be connected is universal and everlasting. When that need is not met, the mind turns to the body and away from the personal anguish of separation. Where the mind turns its focus is determined by the new popular disorders. Today the postural muscles are a main area of conscious focus. Ulcers and seizures were once popular, and although they are still manifestations of unconscious rage and psychic imbalance, they are less prevalent today.

What begins a new popular mindbody focus? Dr. Sopher's simple example of Larry Bird was a good place to start in understanding. A revered figure came down with something, or had something—and it spread. That new "bird-seed" is now planted for people who need to focus away from their emotional base and onto a **socially acceptable** symptom. Many people who knew and respected Larry became the new bearer of that symptom—because Larry made it more acceptable to have. If this all sounds bizarre I can only say that I've personally seen it work, and many revered medical doctors have written in the past about observing people getting disorders after they thought they had been exposed to something, when they had not.

Is pain an indicator that the human body is disintegrating? Or is there a survival mechanism at play? What if, as Dr. Sopher has alluded, "the wrong meme" is accepted as the cause of pain—and then permeates the collective unconscious? When I discovered that I could not slip a disc, or that herniated discs were not causing my pain, I removed that meme from my thought repertoire—abandoned the parasites—deselecting them. I now understood that my survival is based solely upon my beliefs. I am what I believe I am, no more, no less.

An "idea-meme" might be defined as an entity that is capable of being transmitted from one brain to another.

— Richard Dawkins, *The Selfish Gene*[123]

The phenomenon of meme replication can be observed in a real life story of a girl named Rachel who had suffered from, and later selected-out, the false meme of so-labeled repetitive stress injury (RSI), using Dr. Sarno's advice. The following is a conversation she had with a person named Alice.

Rachel prefaced her conversation with Alice by stating: "In my case, RSI started as pain in my right hand, followed a week later by pain in my left hand. I then had this conversation with 'Alice,' another girl in my computer science class who had gotten RSI shortly before me."

Alice: *Has it spread to your elbows yet?*

Rachel: *No....*

Alice: *Oh man, that's when it really sucks.*

Rachel concluded: "A week or two later my pain had spread to my elbows, where it stayed for the duration of my RSI. At the time I thought, 'Wow, she really knew what she was talking about!' Now I look back and think she 'spread' it to me by suggesting a place I could legitimately expect to have pain."[124]

Rachel expanded her awareness and began to see the ships on the horizon. Indeed, the thought was planted in her mind to expect the next area of pain. *So it is transmitted, so it shall be done.*

Physicians: Bearers of Meme Authority

Physicians are in essence medical hypnotists. Since the beginning of time, it has been the healer who has been looked to for help, for planting the correct meme for healing. If their guidance is wrong, those in need will be led astray because of the authority that society bestows upon healers, and by the influence that the patient decides to accept from them. The physician is either Clark Kent or Supermeme to his patients.

> *It is we physicians who are responsible for perpetuating false ideas about disease and its cure. The legends are handed along through nurses and fond mothers, but they originate with us, and with every placebo that we give we do our part in perpetuating error, and harmful error at that.*

— Richard Cabot, MD, *St. Louis Medical Review*, 1903[125]

Cabot felt that hospitals were letting patients down by focusing on mere pathophysiology. He wanted physicians to focus on the patients' beliefs, even venturing as deep as their religious beliefs. His hopes went unrealized as the birth of modern medicine followed in what has been called the "start of scientific biomedicine" and the death of "heroic medicine."[126] But as I stated earlier, there is currently a dual-healing modality that some physicians are being coerced into by their patients. The approach a patient chooses depends on whether she wants to know the truth behind her pain, or if she simply wants a quick avoidance-fix. So the patients tug on the **duality** of the physician's human nature, of both light and shadow.

Adolf Guggenbuhl-Craig, Swiss psychiatrist and Jungian analyst, describes the darker side of the physician that can surface given the perfect storm of circumstances. He first describes the good healer as a faithful follower of the Hippocratic Oath, an altruistic healer whose heartfelt desire is to help the sick and suffering. Next he describes the shadow healer, or the quack that he references from Jules Romains' Dr. Knock. Knock is the archetypal quack who "has no altruistic desire to heal,"[127] and who uses his profession merely for personal gain and profit. The patient in fervent desire for the quick fix often entices the Dr. Knock out from the physician's shadow-self by persistently demanding scientific biomedicine. The end result is that if the patient doesn't desire the truth in healing, the physician is less likely to search for it as well, making him a more ineffectual healer—an accomplice who is trapped by the patient's personal motivations.

> *His own patients exert great pressure on him to forego the Hippocratic model and imitate the caricature of Dr. Knock. The innumerable disabilities of unknown origin which he must treat in his daily practice, none with a recognized therapy—disabilities such as chronic fatigue, certain types of backaches and joint aches, vague heart or gastric pains, chronic headache, etc.—he treats them all with a pseudoscientific display of medical know-how. Instead of bringing the psychic components to the attention of those patients whose suffering is largely psychic, for example, he actually helps them turn their psychic problems into physical ones.*
>
> — Adolf Guggenbühl-Craig, MD,
> *The Hidden Power of The Dark Side of Human Nature*[128]

Meme Transmission—It's Like Tag, You Don't Know It, But You're Already It

Everyone gets memed together in a societal whirlwind as false replicator after false replicator gets blindly re-replicated, and it's not just confined to humans. Every being has influence over the other (e.g., morphogenetic fields). My former neighbor's dog even yawns when he sees her yawn. Dogs are just copycats.

> *A yawn is quite catching you see,*
> *Like a cough,*
> *It just takes one yawn to start other yawns off.*
>
> — Dr. Seuss, *Dr. Seuss's Sleep Book*

I became acquainted with a sweet and gentle lady named Jessica who was having terrible hand pain, so much so that she was beginning to use her feet to dial phone numbers, and to change the channels on her TV remote. Her mother walked by and saw her struggling to use her feet in these ways, and warned Jessica, "I hope that doesn't spread to your feet." The very next day the pain spread to her feet. She had been memed by mother, and began a long battle with foot pain. Meming: a painless process that can cause a lot of pain. Once a seed is accepted by the soil, it will grow. What grows depends on what is nourished by the self. Some people see this suggestive effect and feel they are above the process; their egos place them even above themselves. But everyone is being memed in life because life is a shared experience—a nondual consciousness.

This age of chronic pain can be thought of as a mania or **pain-mania**; obsessive-compulsive behavior regarding the body. Why do people succumb to what others around them emit? Tracordification—our basic instinct of the great pull to our shared consciousness that we long to feel connected with, and of course our longing to feel connected to each other. We have the ability to share consciousness from a continuously existing consciousness (consciousness being the present state of mindstream).

Proof of Shared Consciousness

On December 10, 1996, neuroanatomist, Jill Bolte Taylor, PhD, experienced a stroke from a blood clot that disconnected her left and right brain, leaving only her right hemisphere functioning. Her yin and yang were suddenly disconnected. When she lost her left brain, she lost that part that made her individual—apart from others. As her left brain fell silent, it stole her ego, its negative chatter, linearity, language, rationality—all those things that separated her from others. What remained was **nirvana**—the universal connection to everything; the entirety of life. Her emotional baggage was suddenly gone and all that was left was love. The right side of the brain contains the Mindstream that binds us all together, and wields the power of the entire universe. Taylor describes her experience:

> I am an energy being connected to the energy all around me through the consciousness of my right hemisphere. We are energy beings connected to one another through the consciousness of our right hemispheres as One human family.... My perception of physical boundaries was no longer limited to where my skin met air.
>
> — Jill Bolte Taylor, PhD, TED Conference[129]

With the left hemisphere of her brain out of her mind's eye, Dr. Taylor's perception began to change, radically. She was no longer able to discern where her physical body stopped and the rest of the universe began—all molecules blending together into one "magnificent field of shimmering energy." We are linked together by etheric body but ego isolates and separates us—allowing for suffering.

Meme Me Up

Mass psychogenic illness often occurs when masses of people begin sharing the same symptoms after having been exposed to a germ or chemical substance. Mass-mania most often begins with an environmental **trigger** such as a release of a chemical into the environment or awareness of a suspicious substance. People in masses observe others' fainting or dizziness or pain or sickness, and then take on those symptoms themselves, even though "there is no physical or environmental reason for them to be sick."[130] Fear is the great instigator of symptomatology. However these people, just as with TMS, don't have symptoms merely in their heads. They actually do get headaches and nausea and pain, but as with TMS—the symptoms normally fade when they are examined and given a positive prognosis.

A study in Amman, Jordan, "Mass psychogenic illness following tetanus-diphtheria toxoid vaccination" exemplifies this process. In September 1998, more than 800 young people in Jordan believed they had suffered from the side effects of tetanus-diphtheria toxoid vaccine administered at school."[131] The authors went on to explain that the symptoms did not come from the medicine, but were amplified by the fear implanted by local doctors, parents, and media.

Goose-stepping Along

Dr. H. Gold's studies revealed that people with higher intelligence* are more susceptible to suggestion and more prone to the placebo effect than those with lower intelligence.[132] Perhaps intelligent people are more consciously aware, or open-minded, and more easily swayed to new propositions? Whatever the reason, it does show that in the correct instances, ignorance is bliss.

There is an **empathic response** in every Type T individual I have ever communicated with—a deeper personal need to pull others to them. They respond quickly to positive and kind words of hope, encouragement—and touch.

> *Touch is a marvelous and neglected gift.... Few medical doctors use this art of touch enough, and that means that they're losing close and restorative contact with the patient. When most doctors use their hands today, it's to scribble out a prescription. This is such a sad waste of human potential.*
>
> — Robert C. Fulford, DO, *Touch of Life*[133]

Touch is the missing link in many people's lives. Human contact trumps most modern medicine when it comes to healing. People have told me that they healed or felt much better when their physicians held their hands before epidurals, and/or imaging, or during office consults.

A handicapped man and woman I know who have bouts of pain tell me that when pain strikes, if someone touches their back or shoulder the pain immediately stops. This may be why people erroneously feel as though chiropractic manipulation helps them (short-term). The empathetic touch can release the individual from his fixation on his pain by introducing competing stimuli and connectivity that only touch can provide—soothing the sympathetic system—reconnecting with another.

> *It has become clear to me that high-tech medicine, with all its wonders, often leaves out that all-important human touch.*
>
> — Dana Reeve, *The New Medicine*, PBS

---

* It should be noted that intelligence is a highly subjective term.

Knock, Knock, Knocken on Leaven's Door....

I was doing fairly well before I sought medical help.
— Fred Amir, *Rapid Recovery from Neck and Back Pain*[134]

Today, many physicians are mechanically engineering the human system into balance. This is the Gregory *House* (an NBC television series) approach. They are trained to systematically narrow down the possibilities for a particular pain or illness in what is called **differential diagnosis** (DDx), weighing probabilities in order to obtain a diagnosis. The process begins with the patient's history, physical examination, diagnostic studies, etc.; the collective information is then used to deduce a list of possible causes for the symptoms. There is nothing wrong with this; there must be protocol in science. However, as Dr. Sopher questions, "But what if the proper diagnosis is not made?" His point—unwanted emotions are more often the cause of symptoms, but are overlooked because the differential diagnosis doesn't consider a mindbody process. If the proper diagnosis is not made, the treatment may even be doing harm through iatrogenic effect as the 1994 back surgery survey concluded (see Chapter 7).

Dr. Sarno writes in *Healing Back Pain* of a young, strong, healthy man in his 20s who hurt his back while brushing his teeth (this is not a possibility by the way). "X-rays were taken and he was told that there was a malalignment of the lower end of the spine, whereupon his mild symptoms got worse.... He had become disabled, thanks to the structural diagnoses that had been made and all that they implied. He now believed there was something seriously wrong with his spine and that he would never again be able to lift a heavy weight or play sports. When I saw him in consultation he was profoundly depressed. Fortunately, he had TMS. He responded well to treatment and has been living a normal life again (including playing basketball)."[135] This man was iatrogenically affected; the wrong diagnosis from his physician made him worse. When I went to therapy, shortly pre-Sarno, the therapist told me on several occasions it appeared I had ankylosis—sending me into severe spasm. I grabbed his arm once and said, "Stop saying that!" He was increasing my pain by callously throwing around crippling possibilities.

In an advertisement run some years ago by The Cancer Treatment Centers of America, Peggy Kessler is told she has an "inoperable and incurable" pancreatic cancer and is given two months to live by her physician. So her sister wisely contacted The CTCA, which utilizes mindbody healing, high-tech equipment, and **hope**. When Peggy arrived at The CTCA, physicians told her they saw no date marked on her body regarding how long she would survive. They had planted seeds of hope—she accepted the hope—and is now in remission. In her words, "Hope is the mainstay, hope is everything."

Physicians need to stop telling patients that they have bad feet, knees, hips, necks, backs and hands that they will have to live, manage, and die with—callously throwing around arcane techno medical jargon igniting a nocebo response.

I spent a short time helping a woman in Vermont who was in severe hip pain. She described her hip as continuously "locking up" and as being terrifically painful after the death (separation) of her mother. She told me that she healed "80 percent" by simply reading some of Dr. Sarno's *Healing Back Pain* (knowledge therapy). His positive outlook had begun to calm and heal her. When I last communicated with her, she was completely pain-free, upbeat, and happy with her life.

Our well-being has a lot to do with the mindbody connection, in that, we can make ourselves better, and we can also make ourselves worse by that mental attitude.
— Christopher Reeve (a.k.a. Superman), *Charlie Rose Show*, 10/2/02

Gang Mentality

The responsibility for healing ultimately lies with the sufferer. Nonetheless, people are radically influenced by physicians and the ubiquitous others. Mass suggestion and societal imitation are powerful forces that unwittingly pull the individual from his own flight plan into the misguided orbits of others.

There is nothing but atoms and space, everything else is only an opinion.
— Diogenes Laertius, *Democritus*

In his book, *The Power of Thought*, Thomas Hamblin writes that everyone is a "Victim of Suggestion," through their senses, in thousands of ways all day every day. When you see another person sneeze, you are then prompted to believe that "you may shortly develop an [sneezing] attack yourself." Hamblin then describes two famous physicians who set out to prove the strength of the power of suggestion by deceptively telling a man in a restaurant that he looked sick and should be home resting in bed. The man went home, crawled into bed—and died.

Slowly, more and more medical schools are teaching this notion of amplification of thought and the healing power of belief. Martin L. Rossman, MD, with David Bresler, PhD, began teaching guided imagery workshops in the 1980s when approximately 20 percent of the attendees who participated admitted to using complementary/alternative medicine (CAM). At the turn of the 21st century, Rossman reports that 80 to 90 percent of physicians in their classes claim they now practice it.[136] East is beginning to meet West.

It is vital to find a physician who knows how to communicate, and has a hopeful bedside manner. It can make a world of difference because what the patient is told, she tends to believe and her biology follows her belief.

New Horizons: Personal Responsibility

Some 35 years ago, when I created and published the first self-healing guided imagery experiences on tape, I thought the medical profession would sit up and take notice—since it was so obvious that the vast majority of illness that we were seeing in our offices were caused or exacerbated by psychophysiological imbalances. Instead, unfortunately, the field of medicine became more and more institutionalized, and, instead of the direction of medical practice being determined by passionate, caring physicians, increasingly, maximizing the financial bottom line became the dominant concern. They failed to appreciate what people could do for themselves, and the incredibly inexpensive option of giving sufferers from pain and illness simple tools like deep relaxation, imagery and mental rescripting. Their penny-wise and pound-foolish approaches have led us into an even worse situation. Finally, now, as the entire system is on the verge of collapse, they are beginning to recognize the incredible value of these tools.

— Emmett Miller, MD, personal correspondence

Today, the new horizon in medicine advocates personal responsibility for good health, guided by a compassionate healer. While some people resist responsibility, extraordinary numbers of sufferers are seeking alternative or complementary healing methods. A study performed by David Eisenberg, MD, Director of the Osher Institute at Harvard Medical School in1993, and published in the New England Journal of Medicine, was designed to estimate how many people were seeking nontraditional forms of medical care, independent of their doctor's advice. Eisenberg had estimated that it would be approximately 10 percent of Americans, or at the outer extreme 15 percent. When the results came in, the study's designers were astounded: 34 percent of Americans sought alternative or complementary techniques outside their physician's direction. The cost was 10 billion dollars out of their own pockets. Even more stunning to Eisenberg and the other designers of the study was that 72 percent of these people never discussed any of this with their personal physicians. There are currently two different healing methodologies occurring at the same time in America.

The study, "Unconventional Medicine in the United States—Prevalence, Costs, and Patterns of Use"[137] sent shock waves across the country and helped to bring Dr. Andrew Weil's work to the forefront. Weil had been publicly stating the dissatisfaction the public had with their primary care physicians' methods of care, for years—but his statements had fallen on deaf ears. This study revealed the dissatisfaction people had in the care they were receiving from their physicians who were practicing allopathic medicine.

Americans made an estimated 425 million visits to providers of unconventional therapy. This number exceeds the number of visits to all U.S. primary care physicians (388 million).

— "Unconventional Medicine in the United States—
Prevalence, Costs, and Patterns of Use"[138]

I know people who will not go to their doctors for their TMS pain. They head straight for integrative care practitioners (modalities for treating the whole person). When the physician skilled in integrative care listens to them, and works with them, they begin to heal quite rapidly because integrative care blends alternative care with conventional medicine. An understanding and compassionate heart is the greatest healer, because it connects the unconnected—easing symptoms.

Integrative medicine involves treating the patient—mindbodyspirit—not just the symptom. I believe, based on what we currently know, that it is medical malpractice to operate on spinal discs before the sufferer's personal status, history, emotional state, and personality traits have been thoroughly reviewed by a properly trained professional.

Norman Cousins knew that the only reason he survived his "terminal disease" was that his doctor was his personal friend, on his side, during his convalescence. They worked together as a team to heal him. Medical students who persevere through many tedious years of study are not necessarily, or naturally, people-friendly or socially skilled (e.g., TV's Gregory House, MD). A kind word of encouragement, or sign of caring, can balance chemical imbalances, increase immune response, ease pain, mobilize hope, and relax the patient by easing her fears.

> For many, going to the doctor or to the hospital has become an assembly line of tests and procedures and often lost in this examination of the heart and the kidneys and the blood chemistry are the deeper needs of the person suffering from the illness… technology alone is not enough… people's mental state, their level of stress and their capacity for hope can have a great influence on their ability to overcome illness.
>
> — Dana Reeve, *The New Medicine*, PBS

Meming Along, Singing A Song, Side by Side….

In the TMS book, *Rapid Recovery from Back and Neck Pain*, Fred Amir writes: "My family doctor examined my elbows and asked, do your hands feel numb at night? I answered, 'No, not yet, but the way things have been going, that may be next.' And, sure enough, a couple of nights later, I began to have problems with my forearm and hands becoming numb and waking me up in the middle of the night."[139]

> The physical therapist asked (routinely) if I had pain anywhere. I said yes, there was a little place on the back of my knee. By the second time I visited the physical therapist… the pain had gotten worse. I had only even mentioned it in the first place since she had asked me. I wasn't seeing a physical therapist because of pain in my knee. But now that's just what I had!
>
> — Gerre B. Tejas

I recently had new symptoms in my foot, but they are resolving and began to as soon as I recognized it as TMS. An interesting side note is that I had seen an article in the paper two weeks before about how bad wearing flip flops in the summer was. My mind then chose that location as the spot for my TMS!

— Renee

…as we treat illness, sometimes we inadvertently sow the seeds of illness for the future.

— Deepak Chopra, MD, *Body Mind & Soul*

People regularly admit that as soon as they hear someone has new symptoms, they immediately get those very same symptoms. Damn that Larry Bird. Compliant people who simultaneously desire great control, appear to suffer greater in the magnitude and intensity of symptoms, because yielding and controlling are opposing characteristics in conflict. People also get much better; sometimes rapidly, when they discover that nothing is actually wrong with them. This is characteristic of all people everywhere. The more anxious and obsessive and aware they are, the more quickly they assume the suggested symptoms; letting go of those symptoms is often a much slower process. To an obsessive personality (perfectionistic), the illusion and misinformation is disseminated rapidly, and deeply.

Meme Corp., International—Fields of Memes, If You Build It....

Companies, like some physicians, are unknowingly setting up environments for their employees to attract pain syndromes. Through their attempts to prevent future problems with pain and repetitive stress disorders, firms are laying the groundwork for future suffering. I communicated with Barry from Holland who had worked at a firm and had never heard of such a thing as a repetitive stress injury. He then switched firms and things began to change quickly. His new firm was attempting to be **ergonomically correct (EC)** by educating its workers of the dangers of repetitive stress. Within two months Barry developed RSI. The list he sent me of the pain his coworkers were in was fascinating—very similar to the movie *Field of Dreams*, "If you suggest it, it will come." Barry's new firm built an infrastructure for future disasters by implanting in the minds of the workers that they were at risk, and so they became a firm of crippled employees. In Barry's words: "In the company where I worked, RSI WAS A BIG ITEM. When I started the job I got a kind of RSI information session; I also had special software at the PC and there were a lot of people who suffered from it somehow…. In the company where I worked before, RSI was no item [not an issue]. There was no one who I knew who suffered from it, while the company was not that small with almost 1000 employees." At his new firm Barry described the conditions this way:

- My direct colleague (about 27 years old) next to me had back pain.
- There was a girl in the same room who worked very little because of severe RSI.

- There were different people who asked for another type of keyboard.
- There was another man in the opposite room who had severe neck problems.
- There was a girl who came [to the firm] at the same time as I did, who got pain in one arm after several months.
- Another girl from the same room, who I spoke [to] several times, had also RSI complaints and told me to be careful.
- There was another external consultant who worked there for several months who had neck pain which became worse and worse.
- There was a huge absence of people who had colds or other health problems.

Barry told me that the work environments were very similar in the two companies—with the exception of all the persistent and insidious warnings.

All the prohibitions and admonitions were unnecessary. Indeed, they actually contributed to the problem (of pain) by creating fear where none was appropriate.
— John E. Sarno, MD, *Healing Back Pain*[140]

Instituting protective defenses for future problems is a recipe for future suffering. The firm cooks up suggestions, places them in the minds of the workers, and voila— a feast of problems ensues. K-Mart and Wal-Mart and others need to get rid of those back braces they hand out to their employees. Although it's probably done for liability/insurance purposes, it is still planting the seeds for future pain by suggesting that workers should be consciously focused on possible injury—which then will come.

The Law of Attraction

That which is like unto itself is drawn. Vibrations are always matched. It is the basis of our Universe: When it is asked, it is always given.
— Esther Hicks

I remember a doctor speaking about how deleterious having women constantly checking for breast lumps was. He said (paraphrasing), "We have millions of women out there checking for breast lumps, and do you know what they are finding more and more of? Breast lumps!" Many women live with breast cancer and have no problem their entire lives as long as they don't know it is present. They never know they need to fear until they are shown by the imaging that there is something to fear, like with the structure of the spine—once diagnosed, everything suddenly worsens. As with mass suggestion and vibrational matching—there are actual physical changes in matter. That doctor's statement was highly controversial because we have been told there is a better chance for survival if we detect disorders early. So it is imperative to get professional clearance. Or is it? Breast cancer can be tragic, we've all seen it take a precious life away—but why does it form? Why is it now so in-vogue? It could very well be because our fear and focus are now unconsciously riveted on it, in obsession— magnified by the fact that we have better technology in which to detect it.

On October 21, 2009, *The New York Times* carried an article on the American Cancer Society's shift in attitude regarding early cancer screening. In the article, Otis Brawley, MD, chief medical officer of the American Cancer Society states, "But I'm admitting that American medicine has overpromised when it comes to screening. The advantages to screening have been exaggerated."[141]

This is also true with TMS where physicians routinely over-read "partial tears" on MRIs because they feel the need to find a physical cause for pain. The tears are almost always incidental and can normally be disregarded. But they aren't—they are pointed to as the cause of the pain and operated on—needlessly.

On the same topic Dr. Brawley wrote an editorial for *The Journal of the National Cancer Institute* where he spoke of playing to the fears and prejudices of the public. Brawley stated that the early screening "efforts surged" in the 1980s in part because, "Many were eager to push screening because of a financial incentive; some simply did not think too deeply due to the financial gain." Brawley heard a commercial stating that 100 percent of prostate cancers can be cured if caught early enough. The commercial was sponsored by the radio station, a supermarket chain that benefited from drug sales, and a radiation oncology practice that benefited from the screenings. Brawley's reaction to their commercial was, "A commercial like this plays to our fears and prejudices."[142]

> *But finding those insignificant cancers (non-lethal) is the reason the breast and prostate cancer rates soared when screening was introduced.... And those cancers are the reason screening has the problem called overdiagnosis... overdiagnosis is pure, unadulterated harm.*
> — Barnett Kramer, MD, Associate Director for Disease Prevention,
> National Institutes of Health[143]

The tragedy is that, like pain, cancer is an effect of a deeper shadow-need (my personal belief is that most cancers are primarily Phase 4 TMS—through my own observation—a posteriori). So the billions of dollars that people have raised for "the cure" are aimed only at treating the effect and missing the cause altogether. As Dr. Bruce Lipton stated, the cancer gene expresses only when it is "told to" due to deep beliefs—unresolved conflict—and perceptions of the environment. There is no evidence to support that proactive screening and early detection of cancer has saved any lives at all. It makes sense to us collectively, so we accept it as true. But, the irony is that looking sooner for cancer may only be pulling the disorder unconsciously toward self—lodging the notion of cancer deep into the subconscious. It could be the realization of the Law of Attraction.

> *I attract to my life whatever I give my energy, focus, and attention to, whether wanted or unwanted.*
>
> — *Law of Attraction*[144]

We live in a time when people die of bizarre diseases that have never existed on the planet before.... These diseases can be caused or aggravated by constantly and needlessly activating the body's stress response, or in simpler terms, being neurotic, anxious and worried.
— Robert Sapolsky, PhD, neuroendocrinologist, Stanford University[145]

Unfortunately, everyone has witnessed that cancer can be dangerous and, yes, there are a host of mindbody thought processes, as well as, external invaders (chemicals) that can encourage the cancers to flourish. But we also have the ability to attract cancer to us if we consciously obsess on it. It's reminiscent of the Simontons' patient, Millie Thomas, who knew that she had absolutely brought her cancer upon herself. She meticulously explained the thought process that had led up to the transmutation of her dis-ease. She admitted she was deeply unhappy—nearing 70 and mandatory retirement, her students were irritating her more and more. She could no longer tolerate her singleness and her roommate. Her id was suffocating from her superego blanket. With each cigarette she began visually associating the smoke inhalation process with the thought of her life ending. No more hell to pay. As each nighttime came, she felt that it would be one less day of misery for her. She unconsciously linked (vibrationally matched) her feelings of escaping her miserable life to her lungs, and smoking, until one day—she coughed up blood. Cancer asked for, and given.

So, what is it in us that mobilizes the mindbody to seek balance? The short answer is **deep belief** beginning with a thought process. A belief that causes a vibration that permeates the depths of awareness eventually altering matter. Whether it is a sense of serenity, joy, or panic, the body will respond to the perception or emotion—and emotions alter life's vibrations.

The Law of Attraction responds the same way your mind does: it hears what you don't want. When you hear yourself make a statement containing the words don't, not, or no, you are actually giving attention and energy to what you don't want.
— Michael Losier, *Law of Attraction*[146]

Attracting Disease—Fear is Like Honey

I have discerned disease in the human mind, and recognized the patient's fear of it, months before the so-called disease made its appearance in the body. Dis-ease being a belief, a latent illusion of mortal mind, the sensation would not appear if the error of belief was met and destroyed by truth[147]... I name these facts to show that disease has a mental, mortal origin—that faith in rules of health or in drugs begets and fosters disease, by exciting fear of disease, and by dosing the body in order to avoid it. The faith reposed in these things should find stronger supports and a higher home. If we understood the control of mind over body, we should put no faith in material means.[148]
— Mary Baker Eddy, *Science and Health* (1821-1910)

Everyone I know has walked this same unconscious path into TMS—all occurring outside of awareness as meme theory suggests. But the more perspicacious individuals will realize what is taking place—admit it—and take steps to alter their beliefs, adapt, and heal.

> *When I was in medical school, a surprising percentage of the class came down with whatever disease was being discussed. It made no difference what the disease was; it could have been hepatitis, schizophrenia, or syphilis.*
> — Gerald G. Jampolsky MD, *Love is Letting Go of Fear*[149]

Dr. Jampolsky wrote to me that the students normally took on the symptoms of the disease, not always the actual disease; although on occasion he had seen people fear themselves into the actual disease. He informed me that the student's symptoms were temporary and, in his opinion, caused by the fear of getting the disease.

There must be more research and public education as to how a thought permeates the unconscious mind and manifests into the mindbody. Many people ask me, "SteveO, if pain is rarely due to structural decay of the body, then how come more people don't know about all this?" That question can be easily answered with a line from the movie *Tommy Boy*,

> *What the American public doesn't know—is what makes them the American public.*
> — Ray Zalinsky, *Tommy Boy*

10

The Symptom Imperative Phenomenon

He (Dr. Sarno's patient) did well in the program and became pain-free in about three weeks. Shortly thereafter, he began to feel anxious and began to have some of his old stomach trouble again. This was the symptom imperative at work. The occurrence of two simultaneous psychogenic manifestations ... an indication of the power of the unconscious conflict within.

— John E. Sarno, MD, *The Divided Mind*[150]

Obviously pain isn't the only manifestation of subconscious tension, anxiety, rage, fear, or social imitation. Pain is but one symptom of an infinite array of messages revealed through the dissonance of mind and body and spirit.

Dr. Sarno found that as his awareness of the various manifestations of tension expanded, the acronym TMS (where "M" stood for myositis) quickly became obsolete. Dr. Sopher and Dr. Sarno have since concurred that TMS could now refer to The Mindbody Syndrome whether it stands for tension myoneural or any other tension-induced symptom. TMS is now merely a convenient acronym to provide a name to the multiple manifestations. The terms TMS, tension myoneural syndrome, mindbody syndrome and tensionalgia in this book refer to any and all effects of conflict within the mindbody, with no effort made to distinguish among the labels. It's also important to note that pain is not a disease—but a symptom of conflict. However, for explanatory purposes, I made no distinction between the common usage of the term illness and pain because they are both effects.

Why certain areas of the body are targeted is unknown, but **body-symbolism** is often cryptically present. Of course there are illnesses and pains that cannot be attributed to a mindbody process. One example would be acute exposure to extreme levels of radiation that would destroy the body more quickly than it could recover—the result of an overwhelming external influence. Another example would be direct exposure to something like the Ebola virus. The living virus would invade so powerfully and swiftly that it would be impossible for the mindbody to resist, adapt, and recover. So not all suffering comes from within, or does it? The truth always hangs between the absolutes on the left and the right—in the middle.

This book is not a substitute for a physical examination. You must first rule out the most dangerous possibilities. Be certain that you know your life is in your own hands before you decide to place it there. At the very least, follow **The Rule of the 5 Bees:**
Beware… if it is **Bleeding, Bumped, Broken, or Bruised.**

What is a **pain equivalent symptom** or **TMS substitute**? This is a common question, and a very good one. It is an emotional problem that expresses itself physically (somaticizing), identically to pain. Important to understand is that these physical problems continuously shift as the brain attempts to keep the individual focused on the body—away from the psychological. There are an infinite number of examples (see Appendix A for more pain equivalents), but here are a few.

- Your hip locks up, then an hour, or a few days later, you have chest pains, then suddenly your chest pain leaves and your elbow or shoulder locks up—or "freezes."
- Under hidden stress, you develop an ulcer, then you naïvely believe that it is magically cured with medication, but suddenly your blood pressure rises, and when that is under control, your back begins to hurt and you are in surgery having a needless operation.
- You have heart flutters, then suddenly you have heartburn, and then migraines.
- You lose your voice under stress, then you have a panic attack, and then you get restless leg syndrome and maybe some acne or swollen glands or even swollen knees.
- You are leaning toward anorexia or binge eating; however, as you finally get your eating back to healthy, your back begins to hurt, or your stomach aches—when that all goes away fatigue settles in.
- You have back pain, you get an epidural injection—the pain shifts to a migraine or skin problem. Your back pain returns, you have a back operation, but now your knee begins to hurt, and you have knee surgery, then your shoulder begins to hurt, and you're now in shoulder surgery.
- You're under stress, you have an unquenchable thirst, then that goes away and your eyes begin to reduce tear production and dry up, then that goes away and you get a headache up the back of your neck, then that goes away and your heel begins to hurt, then that goes away and you become nauseated, then that goes away… get the picture?
- Etc., etc., etc., etc.; any combination of shifting body symptoms—and you've had them in the past, but have not known why—until now.

Dr. Sarno has called this the symptom imperative (SI), a psychological condition that requires "continuing symptoms." An imperative is something that demands attention or action—the conundrum is that the consciousness within us knows that it is being observed—and so it changes how we react to shifting symptoms. As long as there is unresolved conflict, the mind will continuously shift symptoms to keep fear alive—as a purposeful distraction. The symptoms bounce around in the body to keep you feeling that you have suddenly developed a "real pain" or a "real injury." The brain scans the body until it finds an area or system that you are most fearful of—and then it induces a symptom there and lingers, waiting for your response to it. If you don't fear that area much or don't pay much attention to that particular symptom, it will then shift to another area until it can grasp your attention again somewhere else, all in the attempt to keep you from tending to your emotions. The symptom imperative is a hunter—preying on fear. There it stays—until you realize you've been fooled by your own brain, and then it quickly shifts again—repeatedly—as long as the underlying psychological conflict remains.

Much of the rest of this book is focused on **why** the symptoms become imperative. I believe it all begins with early separation anxieties, and possibly later trauma or multiple "little traumas," that lead to an obsessive, compulsive, intuitive, colorful, and highly creative personality. The symptoms bound around in the body for two reasons: to keep the conscious mind focused away from the threatening emotions, and to send messages of discontent from the unconscious back to the conscious side—to be resolved *... and the yin chases the yang... to cope....*

11

Timing of the Onset:
Don't Beware, Be Aware

You know, at that time I had, for the first time in my life, the feeling to have reached the position I deserved. Strange thing that some months later I had to leave my job because of my illness (pain).

— Bernabe, 12/20/2001

Be aware of current status **during** stressful periods—Phases 1, 2, and 3 TMS
Be aware of life's pauses **after** stressful periods—Phase 4 TMS

It seems obvious to say, "Pay attention during times of overstimulation because you may begin to experience symptoms," but few people are self-aware enough to correlate their symptoms with events. One of the doctors named in our malpractice suit had a heart attack soon after we filed suit against him. Was it a coincidence? Of course it wasn't. Under times of great stress, hidden anger may rise so high that we can experience symptoms in real time, while the cause remains outside our awareness. However, the majority of cases I've seen have been delayed onset of symptomatology—delayed reactions to life changes, as Bernabe stated in the above quote. Phase 4 TMS.

When speaking with people about their lives, people in severe pain often tell me:

- When I was younger my parents divorced or were missing or unloving
- I was adopted
- My mother or father or sibling died
- I was molested or beaten
- I had nightmares of being abandoned
- My parent was an alcoholic
- My parents fought incessantly and were highly critical of me
- I came from a dysfunctional family
- My mother or father is dying
- My child died or is ill

These experiences leave emotional memories, and pave the way for rage to be ignited later on, by a trigger. The scars that we can't see are from the most painful cut; the earlier in life, the deeper the wound. Our childhood development strongly shapes how we cope with stress later in life. When we were sick or ill as children it got us out of situations we didn't want to be in—and brought much needed attention and comfort from someone close. Now, the same stress response, or symptoms—such as colds or stomachaches or pains of all sorts—reoccur when we are once again overwhelmed. The anger and fear of abandonment, trauma, and rejection remain hardwired, and "downtimes" or "new plateaus" reached are perfect opportunities for TMS to surface. All that is needed is an event similar to prior trauma to trigger and reopen the old wound.

Real Time Onset—Phase 1—Teed Off

> World No. 1 Tiger Woods was driven off the course on Sunday with an apparent neck injury.... "I might have a bulging disk," he told a reporter at one point.... Outside of being served divorce papers while standing in the first tee box, the reincarnation of Woods' career couldn't get much worse.
>
> — Steve Elling, CBS Sports, 5/9/2010[151]

The reporter, Elling, was being facetious of course—divorce papers were not served on the first tee box, but Tiger's neck pain was not from a bulging disc either. Divorce was iminent; Tiger knew it not long before his neck began hurting and his hand began tingling—from Phase 1TMS.

I watched as a former coworker rolled around in his hospital bed, in severe back and hip pain agony, minutes before he was going in for a dangerous heart procedure. He was obviously in a state of surfacing rage as the risky surgery rapidly approached. He blamed it on a bad hip, but it was clearly Phase 1 TMS.

I've spoken with several people who had severe back spasms as soon as they saw the hijacked jets fly into the World Trade Towers on 9/11/01. Their sense of security was attacked, and their anger levels rose instantly as the SNS immediately locked into freeze. Their pain was immediate and severe but short-lived because they had previously come to understand and accept TMS.

I sat and watched a man holding his legs in pain in the fetal position on my family room floor after he lost his home and had no other place to live. His security was threatened, as in the **9/11 Syndrome.*** He believed he had a bad back and had had an operation to trim the discs, and it failed → dare I say it? Of course.

When Thomas Jefferson's wife died, he immediately began having severe migraines and didn't leave his bedroom for three weeks. He also suffered a debilitating migraine

---

* The 9/11 Syndrome is a term Dr. Sarno introduced in his book *The Divided Mind*. The phrase represents, as he states, the "dramatic increase in psychosomatic reactions across the United States..." Dr. Sarno says that people who are "prone" to mindbody reactions enjoy complete control of their environments, but on that day the terrorists challenged that control and the result was "inner rage." It must be noted that fear alone does not create symptoms. It is the reaction to the fear, the rationalization of conscious fear in order to try to "overcome its source."

after his mother died, and another right before he began writing the Declaration of Independence. I'm just guessing, but he could have been under some self-imposed pressure at that time; but I'm no founding father. Being consciously aware of tension levels, and also of the shadow-ego relationship, can stave off an attack when accompanied by understanding, breathing, presence, and relaxation.

Many people claim that they get pain during holidays. The **holiday syndrome** has also been called **leisure sickness** by some researchers. The body at work in a stressful job is locked into survival mode and has trouble readjusting to leisure time. Dutch psychology professor, Ad Vingerhoets, has studied this phenomenon. He has stated, "One possibility is a kind of competition for symptom perception. There is a competition between information from the outside world, external information, and information from the body, internal information."[152] In other words, when you are focused on a particular task such as a career or project, you cannot simultaneously focus on your personal needs, and so they go unattended. Once the external focus is taken away, all those internals that were pushed aside come tumbling out. The repressed now demands to be expressed. Vingerhoets also reported that the most common effects were pain, migraines, fatigue, and nausea—and the most common personality characteristic? You already guessed it by now I hope → perfectionism.

> *If you are very busy with external information, then information from your body might be repressed by it. If you are in a boring environment, it is more easy to recognize those signals from your body. When you are in a stimulating environment, you don't attend to those signals.*

— Ad Vingerhoets, PhD, Tilburg University[153]

This is Phase 4 TMS, "away from the battlefield." With the Holiday Syndrome there is also the conditioned response. During the holidays, the abusive or alcoholic spouse triggers their partner's old residual wounds or emptiness with their father or mother or guardian—a **psychological overlay*** that makes symptoms worse. With the holidaze come a higher demand on energy—but most people feel invincible because of the automatic nature of repression, and so they feel as though their backs suddenly go out. Is it possible that an individual's spine will suddenly become weaker during the holidaze, or before the Hawaiian vacation?

Many people get depressed during the holidays. Leisure time allows bad memories, of being alone or of abuse or of isolation, to surface. They feel like outcasts while others are off celebrating, and they can't understand why they don't have a desire to join in the reindeer games. Many actually fear the holidays because they know they will slide into a funk and the pain will come sliding down the chimney. It's clear that they feel isolated, and isolation is separation, and separation is depression, and depression is pain.

---

* Psychological overlay is a medical term for when fear and anxiety magnify physical symptoms.

Pause—Phase 4 TMS

My former coworker was in severe pain and had back surgery within weeks of his wife's death. He would never put two and two together and understand the timing of his pain and its purpose. He had foraminal stenosis surgery after her funeral and remains, continuously, in and out of pain to this day.

In 2006, a news article's headline on singer Sheryl Crow read: "**Breakup Feb. 3, Biopsy Feb. 20.** The singer finds herself battling breast cancer just weeks after her split from fiancé Lance Armstrong." Divorce is ranked #2 on the Holmes-Rahe list of stressors behind death of a spouse. People have pointedly told me, "No… I had this before my divorce." But relationships take time to fall apart, even years. The paperwork is simply the judicial end. Crow's breast cancer may have not begun instantaneously, but relationships also don't suddenly fall apart, they simmer over time and eventually melt down.

I spoke with a man in a restaurant in 2006 about his back pain; he told me it started two days after his divorce was finalized, and it had knocked him off his feet. He asked me if I thought it was due to his getting a divorce. I asked him if he had ever had back pain before the divorce, and he said "no." I guess it's difficult to see ourselves as we truly are, even in our most private mirrors.

Pain can strike during periods of high tension, but in a very mysterious fashion the mind often utilizes after-tension in order to do its bitching and moaning—when it is no longer focused on the task at hand, as Vingerhoets had hypothesized. This is the **nuclear blast** phenomenon—the damage comes from the backlash of the energy expansion.

Smooth Running—Windy Sailing

My friend Graham—as he relayed to me—went into critical TMS post-retirement just one week after he had prioritized his finances and felt relatively sure of a comfortable life. This is the Bernabe Effect. Graham knows that his narcissistic id-child has demands that his conscious mind cannot fully understand. Symptoms often begin when things seem to be going well—at certain levels of life after achievement. Retirement is #10 on the Holmes-Rahe list of stressors. Perhaps we set goals to avoid facing the past and prior rejection? To feel self-worth? Therefore, after-accomplishment can yield time and opportunity for the unresolved to surface—retribution for prior demands, and neglect of internal signals.

Pain often surfaces during periods of boredom or in mundane or repetitive jobs—as familiarity breeds contempt. The mind often has too much time on its hands and the conscientious goodist always feels she can do more. Am I doing enough? Am I a good person? What is left for me now? This is the midlife crisis as defined by Dr. Carl Jung.

I think midlife crisis is just a point where people's careers have reached some plateau and they have to reflect on their personal relationships.

— Bill Murray, actor, comedian, golfer extraordinaire (he wishes)

Triple Bogey in '04

Tiger Woods is a great golfer who serves as a tiger-ific (sorry) example of the timing of the onset of pain. In 2004, he had change occurring, and not for the better. The changes included:

- **Lost his World #1 ranking**—Unconscious anger increases as idealized self-image is damaged.

- **His father (and best friend) had become terminally ill**—Unconscious anger increases from the anticipation of permanent separation.

- **He was about to get married (which in retrospect we know his inner self never truly wanted)**—Unconscious anger increases as a major change in status approaches. Marriage is #7 on the Holmes-Rahe list of stressors.

TMS also baffles people because they cannot understand why the pain arrives during times of fun and excitement. There are a couple of things going on simultaneously. First, there is change, which the inner self doesn't relish, even though the conscious mind may feel the change is warranted—the superego demands more energy to maintain inner control during the change. But there is also the interpretation of the new fun and excitement, since excitement is stimulation. Based on childhood experiences (I don't deserve to have it so good), the mindbody doesn't properly interpret the incoming sensations—and assumes something must be wrong. The inner-child only knows that there is new incoming sensory data, and throws the new stimulation into the freeze mode—the mode it first used under similar stress.

Tiger Woods is certainly not a Type T individual, but he is definitely a perfectionist. His pain most likely came from anger over his father's quickly failing health, and the added responsibility of his impending—and unwanted marriage. He was simply over-stimulated—overextended. Any one of these three changes Tiger faced could produce intense pain in a perfectionist. Add them together and it's no wonder that his symptoms began then. Tiger's upper back began hurting on the way to Kilkenny, Ireland, for the World Golf Championships-American Express Championship. From the Golf Channel's website: "Woods said Wednesday that he injured his back sleeping awkwardly on a plane last week. He played only seven holes in his practice round at Mount Juliet before his back stiffened and he decided not to risk further injury."[154]

Tiger Woods, a month or so later on *The Tonight Show* with Jay Leno (11/11/2004):

> *They just don't make private planes the way they used to (Tiger laughed)… I was just really tired, I played the Ryder Cup, I had to go to New York and on the way home I just crashed. I just fell to sleep in an awkward position and when I got up, I knew my rib was out, it was uh, and actually when I got it worked on they actually found that three rib heads had slipped out. So I had to get that, try and get reworked and my back spasmed up and everything, but that's the way it was.*

An athlete in tremendous physical shape like Tiger Woods cannot hurt his back "sleeping awkwardly." What he doesn't realize is that his unconscious mind is bristling with activity, mostly frustration. He developed a new mindbody manifestation to distract him from his increasing rage. During sleep, his unconscious mind "slipped its rib" (ribs do not "slip in" or "slip out"), because of the changes occurring in his life.

Now those who do not know who Tiger Woods is should know that he is a PGA golfer with a powerful and high velocity swing (and they should also buy a television). His club head speed is up around 125 MPH. The torque on the body's framework necessary to accomplish the swing is tremendous. The doctor that told him he dislocated three rib-heads while sleeping should have his medical license revoked. Sadly, this isn't the most absurd case of misdiagnosis out there—buuut—it's pretty close.

I can see a similar tension-related back pain in LPGA Hall of Famers, Betsy King and Judy Rankin, and PGA players Fred Couples, Mark Calcavecchia, Roco Mediate, Jim Furyk, and the man himself, Jack Nicklaus. I have no doubt that these people could heal their pain if they read Dr. Sarno's books, with an open heart and mind. But they grew up during a time that people believed if the doctor told them they had a bad back, then, by golly, Miss Molly, they had a bad back their entire lives—to be forever managed—never healed. They are all self-driven goodists who smile on the outside. T-it-Up!

Pregnancy

It was such a small window, a peephole really. For years I was this repressed kid, and then there was the briefest of windows, and now... slam... all of a sudden I'm this overburdened mother. I barely got to do it Zack; I barely got the chance to be a person.
— Lane Kim, Gilmore Girls: "Santa's Secret Stuff"

For many women TMS begins during or after pregnancy. The pregnancy is in essence the sudden change from being a girl to becoming a woman, from energy flowing into self as the center, to energy flowing out as caretaker for the new king or queen of the house. The timing of this TMS onset cannot be disregarded, and too often these women have immediate back surgery for no logical reason. A good friend of mine wrote to me after her baby's delivery, telling me her surgeon was going to operate on her back even though she "had no structural problems." I guess it isn't necessary to have anything wrong with your spine to have surgery. Her surgery didn't succeed, of course.

Those Selfish Baby-ids

A woman's baby's birth—and later the lives of her toddlers—invade her proxemic space, creating a great **demand** on her. The anxious individual enjoys people, but not in her face. She loves new people around, but not too close. The new child has now changed this—turned her world inside out. The new mother often feels alone (even surrounded by other people), and helpless as to how to care for the new precious life. She no doubt enjoyed being the center of attention while pregnant, but after delivery, the baby stole her show. TMS would be her id's revolt against not getting enough attention, as well as increased energy demands. Women I interviewed in pain or in postpartum depression often felt alone after delivery—not knowing what to expect from motherhood. This feeling of isolation is enraging enough to create a pain syndrome as a defense mechanism. One woman told me she sat in her closet crying after her baby was born. Not coincidentally, she suffers from TMS mid-back pain.

One can only imagine the fear and rage that a woman must repress during times of pregnancy, both from the little girl inside and from the adult (id-superego conflict)—overwhelmed by the new responsibility about to come forth. I've often wondered if this great responsibility thrust upon them weeks before childbirth is what sends them into preeclampsia as their autonomic systems swing wildly with severe vasculature alterations and accompanying high blood pressure. Preeclampsia could be severe TMS. After all, the cause of preeclampsia is unknown. But we do know that anxiety increases blood pressure, as well as, protein in the urine—the symptoms of preeclampsia.

Even unborn, life is present within her; change is ever evolving, ready to erupt. People in general have a basic need to be taken care of. Now, the mother's id-child will need to make room for someone else, someone more important than herself—yet a part of herself. This is contrary to the id, where self is pleased at the expense of others. How many mothers have children because they feel they should? Whether it is called a biological clock or just societal pressure, there are probably many girls who become pregnant before they are ready—or even truly desire. Deep in their hearts they probably want to remain little girls, free and happy and taken care of, at the center of attention.

The loss of physical shape during or after delivery could also be subconsciously enraging to many. Females attract, and therefore their nature is to want to be attractive. A woman who developed TMS during her pregnancy once emailed me that she felt her body was being distorted and that she was a "reluctant pregnant." Following her baby's birth she said that caring for the baby was a stressful responsibility in a modern world "as one tries to fit the baby in as if nothing has happened." She hit full-blown TMS with a host of nefarious pains and symptoms and ended up totally debilitated. She has since healed after reading Dr. Sarno's books.

The sensation is one of being trapped by the new commitment—and the cause and effect are clear: the depression, demands, and anxiety trigger the pains and chemical imbalance—not vice versa.

Focus Lost—Opportunity Knocks

So—be aware after trauma—after periods of high stress and change, when boredom and reflection pave the way for symptoms. The sympathetic nervous system may not let go because the individual wants to make certain the danger is over.

Greg Beratlis, a juror on the Scott Peterson murder trial, spoke afterwards about the emotional drain the trial took on him. "I mean, it's tough, and it's been tough, and then—now all this burden for us is going now, too... when am I going to finally melt down because we've managed not to be sick in six months, really sick.... And I know emotionally I've been through this, where you're high, like, you know, a season, and, as soon as the season ends, the next day, you are sick. You just—and I'm expecting that to come. I hope not, but I'm—emotionally, yes, we've gone through it."[155] Greg implicitly understands Phase 4 TMS—the gravity of downtime after periods of great demand on the sympathetic nervous system.

Studies confirm what Greg instinctively knew. One such study published in 1964 in the Journal of Psychosomatic Research entitled, "Social Stress and Illness Onset," was designed to examine the "relationships of environmental variables to the onset of illness." The study concluded that a great majority of people develop serious physical illness within two years following periods of prolonged stress. The stress in this study was termed the "psychosocial life crisis" and included such stressors as change in social status, changes in close personal associations (deaths, divorce), changes in residence, changes in pregnancy status, and change in economic status.[156]

Phase 1 and 4 Are Here—Let Me Make One Thing Perfectly Clear

Former President Richard Nixon serves as an executive example of Phase 4 TMS. The exact evening he was pardoned in the Watergate scandal by President Ford he developed left leg pain and was diagnosed with phlebitis as his leg swelled three times its normal size. After he was released from the hospital, however, his attorneys filed paperwork that would give him medical relief from ever testifying in the Watergate Hearings. But when the request to avoid an appearance at the trial was rejected his phlebitis returned soon after; so he never had to testify in the hearings, due to medical reasons. His mindbody had unconsciously found a way out of what he didn't wish to consciously do. Illness has a definite purpose.

Dana GgrrrrReeve!

Sadly, actor Christopher Reeve's wife and caretaker, Dana, also followed the most common pattern of delayed onset after prolonged stress. A few months after Christopher died, Dana began coughing. Diagnosed with lung cancer, she died a year and a half after Chris. Dana didn't smoke—wasn't around secondhand smoke—and lived in a low-risk environment for contracting lung cancer. When a loved one is handicapped or ill, everyone who loves them also pays a heavy emotional and physical price. It wasn't surprising that it was Dana's lungs that were the focus of her rage. The most frightening aspect of Chris' paralysis was his inability to breathe on his own. They both often said they feared he would stop breathing in the middle of the night. Chris' inability to breathe was most likely the thing that she felt most intensely for him, because it also hindered his ability to communicate—frustration! It's possible she may have taken on his symptoms through the Law of Attraction, and also because the competing stimulus was now gone since he had died. All the internal signals she had pushed aside now demanded to be recognized.

When I saw Dana by Chris' side, I knew how she felt. The frustration of seeing a loved one paralyzed is enraging, stressful, and demanding. It is an utterly helpless feeling. I told my ex-wife I wish I could take her place in the wheelchair—every other month—so that we could share the problem. It wasn't long after I told her that, that my left leg was paralyzed.

Caregivers have a high illness rate. Providing for an ill loved one places high demands on the mindbodyspirit. Dana was always described as strong and stoic, an upbeat woman, a beacon of strength. In observing her outward demeanor, she always appeared smiling. She hid her sadness well; however, all this repression finally surfaced in her body when the time was there. It is this super egotistic need to appear strong that is most enraging to the id-self, as true self becomes entangled with persona.

Chris and Dana were married three years before he was paralyzed. My wife and I were married four years before she was paralyzed. The underlying tragedy that Dana and I shared was the knowledge that we did not possess.

People magazine published an article on Dana on March 26, 2006, entitled "Dana Reeve: Brave To The End." In the article were quotes from her, and her friends, that show the path to dis-ease. We know that it is deadly to repress or deny strong emotions. The public persona and stoicism that "everything is going well" is unconsciously infuriating—potentially fatal. We cannot push aside feelings of deep pain without having them revisit us later. I've taken several quotes from the *People* magazine article:

"She set a high bar... no self-pity, in the face of unimaginable tragedy."

"She handled them [challenges] happily, with aplomb."—Deborah Roberts

"After Chris first returned home in his wheelchair, no one knew what to expect... I was surprised how happy the house was."—Adrienne, Dana's sister

"She said that she was glad to know her enemy so she could fight it."—Adrienne

"You have to play the hand you're dealt."—Dana

"I learned a long time ago life just isn't fair... you just forge ahead."—Dana[157]

I fell into the same trap as Dana—act as if nothing wrong has happened—and my symptoms began, like falling dominoes. I needed to fall apart early on, but I never did, and that imbalance in strength eventually weakened me—as Dr. Sarno wrote, TMS occurs because these people "cope too well." The outward appearance of happiness or normalcy only denies self—and self denied is toxic.

The most dangerous thing Dana alluded to was that her cancer was her enemy. As Dr. Weil has described, cancer patients do much better when they accept cancer as part of who they are, and they can get much worse if they treat the cancer as a foreign invader. Just as with pain, the pain is not an enemy; pain exists because of who you are and how you react to life—how deeply you deny your emotional status to yourself. The illness or pain is a part of you—to be embraced and understood. When I was healing, I treated my pain as an outside entity and I suffered much longer because of that fallacy. This isn't to say one should accept pain or illness; it is not a natural state. You are more than these states of existence, which have now become a part of you because you have ignored some truth within you—denied a part of you, giving the symptoms tangible reality—a purpose. Disharmony seeks resolution, as behavior conflicts with belief.

Scientists have a term for when a cancer cell decides to form. It is called **expression**. When cancer unfolds, scientists often refer to the cancer cell as expressing itself. And so the cells in Dana's lungs may have done what she herself would not publicly do, for fear of appearing "not strong." With all she went through, she needed to let her hair down and let out her feelings of loss and rage—openly expressing sadness—discharging her trauma from her system.

Looking Back—It All Had Purpose

In 1990—five years after my wife's handicapping, after a time when I saw the death of my father-in-law, the loss of my mom's best friend who was like a mother to me, the loss of one of my favorite aunts and the loss of one of my favorite uncles, witnessed the cleanup of our town after a tornado, experienced the end of a large malpractice trial and the end of overseeing a new house built, I went out for a golf lesson to try to find a path in life again. During the lesson—I swung—and felt a pop and piercing pain. I was knocked out of commission for nine months, all the while thinking I had pinched a nerve. It is quite a foolish feeling when I look back on it all, but you live and learn. I understood John Stossel when he said he was embarrassed after discovering the real reason behind his pain. He had done it to himself, but John learned; others live, but they do not learn. I had experienced Phase 4 TMS, a reduction in bloodflow after a prolonged period of high stress and tension and goal accomplishment—the window of shadows where the unresolved demons surface. I needed downtime to think, to regroup and to gain the strength to get back into balance. The swing and the pop were only triggers to the onset of the pain—the opportunity for all my coping to finally express itself. It would be 10 more years until I would find Dr. Sarno and see so clearly what had happened to me, and what was happening to those around me. I was still young and naïve. I had to fall so that I could regroup to rise stronger.

Understanding pain is like understanding Goldilocks and the Three Stimulations, where the third stimulation needs to be juuuust right. People live in over-stimulated environments where the desire for quick gratification exacts a heavy toll. But overstimulation for extended periods is simply trauma. Phases 1, 2, 3, and 4 TMS are due to over-stimulated states, where tension breeches the rim of the anger bucket. Phase 4 TMS is a lurker—it is patient.

The question arises as to why we over-stimulate our lives? We are not truly happy and so we look outside to external solutions for internal problems. But happiness— good health and vitality—comes from inside. It doesn't come from a bottle or a drug or surgery or material means or another person. External stimulation is sought to fill the void of isolation.

We distract ourselves from the human condition. We distract ourselves from distraction, by distraction, so that we really don't have to look at our condition.

— Sam Keen, *A Crisis of Faith*

The mind of a driven individual has elevated anxiety-beta wave activity due to predisposed guilt from religious, familial, or societal constructs. Beta is associated with low productivity and high medical bills. By contrast, a relaxed alpha **state of mind** is the goal. Great revelations can be conceived in times of understimulation—if the individual can reach an alpha state of awareness. Unfortunately, the Type T often utilizes under-stimulated times for beating up self. But it doesn't have to be a time of destructive reflection. Understimulation can be a time of tremendous spiritual expansion and creativity.

A Mind Divided

This is a good time to explain, using my own experience as an example, how internal conflict is born, leading to TMS. Although I have seen hundreds of similar scenarios played out, I am most familiar with my own id-superego conflict.

When my wife was paralyzed, the undeveloped and irrational id part of my unconscious instinctual self no doubt wanted out of the situation, to flee and to leave it all behind—to avoid pain. I'm certain that my id-self wanted to kill the physicians for handicapping her. Id **takes**—id doesn't give. Here is where most people get lost in the understanding. Most understand that they have a dark side, or dark thoughts. But what they don't realize is that their shadow-self actually enjoys these sinful or darker thoughts—which bring about a destruction of the ego by uniting id and superego. If we can gratify our primal desires and also fool ourselves into believing it is good to do so—we have successfully destroyed ego—our shadow's sadistic goal.

So, superego, as the moral watchdog, must stop these immoral thoughts, punish them—but it can't—and so it simply diverts the mind's eye's-focus creating the pain we call TMS. The more unconscionable the thoughts are—the more painful the distraction has to be. More precisely, the more you enjoy the unthinkable—the more severely you punish yourself with critical pain—and justice is done as you see it. Evil—or whatever you want to call it—can never be eliminated, only diverted, cast outward onto others in projection, or buried deeply within our shadows. We must have these opposing forces of good and bad for motivation to drive us and make us whole. The person you are depends on which force you decide to nurture. The Indian proverb states: "There are two dogs in every man"—Eros and Thanatos—"which one survives depends on which one gets fed."

Now there is also the adult part of me—Steve, my persona—who gives. This is the conscientious goodist who was taught to be responsible and caring: the conscious me. This is the **rational** side Freud referred to as a matured ego that "obeys the reality principle."[158] This mature side is the beleaguered caretaker who fully understands his duty, obligations, and responsibilities. This Steve is the intellectual decision maker who knows his life is now geared toward never-ending demands of dealing with an injured loved one—the loss of much pleasure. However, along with my id-self, ego and superego, there is also the entire Self—the total consciousness, or Total Being. The Total Being is now conflicted, as the ego tries to satisfy both id and superego—the duplicitous nature of a mind conflicted. The result is conflict—stuck in a freeze survival response, unable to flee or fight.

Suffering insists that we pull back. The **divided mind** is caught in a conflict resulting in pain and illness that demands the individual to either reorganize his beliefs or to punish himself—torn between instincts and moral constraints. When you can push ego aside a bit you may enter alpha, the state of the greatest creativity, connecting the conscious to the unconscious—alert, relaxed and feeling good. This state is creative and resourceful and probably rarely visited by the Type T individual, especially on vacation. Anxiety can actually be reduced by learned increases in alpha wave activity. One method of increasing alpha awareness is to learn conscious breathing. In alpha, mind and body unite and awareness expands. For these reasons alpha has been called the "perfect state of understimulation."

The Alpha Males

In the desert you can remember your name, 'cause there ain't no one for to give you no pain.

— America, *A Horse With No Name*, Kinney Music, 1971

Alpha awareness can lead to great breakthroughs in creativity. It's a type of active daydreaming without calculations that Albert Einstein referred to as "thought experiments." Every prophet (and many great scientists and artists) has gone into some form of understimulation before emerging with a deeper understanding. Whether it is a mountaintop, or a desert, or a master bedroom, or family room floor—understimulation can give rise to greater awareness and original thought because it cuts out background noise. The body gets sick and pained because the individual subconsciously knows she needs to be in that under-stimulated state in order to rejuvenate, regroup, and escape the current turmoil. The body never lies, but the conscious mind will if it needs to protect the persona.

Cat Stevens learned this from the year he spent in a tuberculosis ward that gave him the time and insight to emerge with a fresh attitude and identity. After leaving the TB ward, he published his three best records within 18 months. The solitude of his downtime gave him alpha time to re-emerge stronger and more creative than ever.

Regarding Stevens' contracting TB, in the 1972 article entitled, "The Poets, Cat Stevens," Michael Watts states, "There was probably a strong element of psychology, too, in the fact of his becoming ill." Stevens was very unhappy with his record company and in the direction they wanted him to go. Watts continues, "His body succumbed, his mind dried completely, like a lake. His period of convalescence he spent in refilling it."[159] Illness not only allows us to repair and regroup, but it also allows us to escape a situation that we could not otherwise flee.

If we listen to our symptoms, there can be a new birth, since the suffering reveals the individual's true status at the unconscious level—his truest needs. If pain and illness are viewed as enemies, there can be deleterious effects on health because no one comes to peace with his enemy, thus they are enemies. Befriend your (moon) shadow.

> *Illness has a purpose; it has to resolve the conflict, to repress it, or to prevent what is already repressed from entering consciousness.... But the sickness is also a symbol, a representation of something going on within, a drama staged by the It; [the expression of the human being], by means of which it announces what it could not say with the tongue."*
> — Georg Groddeck, MD, *The Book of the It*[160]

Groddeck's quote is exactly what Dr. Sarno has discovered and elegantly explained. Pain exists to prevent certain emotions or past trauma from flooding back into consciousness. But Groddeck had also written that illness may simply exist to give needed time for the resolution of conflict—so it has at least two purposes. In either the case of under- or overstimulation, emotions work in an antagonistic manner, in the attempt to maintain homeostasis. When the battle escalates into war, the victim is the innocent self.

12

Symbolic Attacks

The part of your body where you have stored your anger is the part that has to express it.

— John Lee, *Facing the Fire*[161]

TMS author Fred Amir writes, "I hated commuting, so my subconscious found a way to get me out of it: numbness in my right leg—the leg that presses on the gas pedal!" He continues, "I have seen this phenomenon in so many people: the professor who coughs and has to take breaks from her lectures, so that she can rest; the programmer whose hand hurts and cannot work."[162]

In *Basic Principles of Psychoanalysis*, A.A. Brill, MD, writes of a woman who had developed a pain in her arm. The medication she was given didn't help. She sought out a psychoanalyst who discovered that she was deeply in love with a man who hadn't proposed to her. Her family had disavowed him and warned her to never speak of him again—to forget about him. Internally she was wrought with turmoil, trying to determine whether he truly loved her. She told the analyst, "He pressed my arm."[163] Apparently, the last night she saw him, he had held and pressed her arm. At that very moment, she thought he was going to propose to her, but he didn't. When the momentous words were never spoken, her internal anger was converted into pain— her focus and anger now riveted on her arm where he touched her.

In the early 1890s, Mark Twain had had enough of writing. He was totally burned out and had vowed only to write for himself. Unfortunately, his continuous bad business ventures left him bankrupt. Twain fell from being one of the country's wealthiest people during the Gilded Age, to being unable to pay his bills. He decided he had to write yet another book in order to get back on his financial feet. The book was eventually entitled *The American Claimant* (1892). He hated writing it—despised having to do what he d(id)n't want. Id rebelled and he soon developed severe pain in his writing arm. The pain was so severe that he could no longer write with that hand, and so he switched to his left, but the pain shifted to that arm soon after (the symptom imperative, it seems, has been around for awhile). Twain eventually finished the rather unsuccessful book using phonographic dictation, the first author ever to use the device. So much for doing what you don't want to do.

I had a professor in graduate school who once told me that every time he had to give a speech in grad school, he would lose his voice (he actually knew where it was, it just wasn't functioning properly). The vocal cords are symbolic of the ability and necessity to express. His brain chose that area, in which to silence his disdain.

One of my favorite examples is in *Healing Back Pain*. Dr. Sarno describes a man who got a rash under his wedding band, but when he separated from his wife the rash went away. However, "Other gold rings did not produce a similar rash."[164]

It's very common for people to get genitourinary infections when cheating on spouses, even when no infection is transmitted—the organ symbolic of the inner guilt. In his book, *The Will To Live*, Arnold Hutschnecker, MD, describes two men having unsafe sex with the same woman. The one with the "stronger guilt feelings" contracts a venereal infection—the more "aggressive" man does not. Marc Sopher, MD, tells me he has seen several cases like this—and I, too, have witnessed it.

In the summer of 2006, I had a conversation with a man about my book and mind and body and symbolic suffering. As we got deeper into the conversation, his voice softened as he began to tell me that his mother was a deeply depressed woman. He confided that when he was a young boy she constantly told him she was going to kill herself. In fact, she would show him exactly how she was going to do it by grabbing him by the arm and dragging him to the vacuum cleaner. She would unhook the cleaner's hose and show him how she was going to hook it up to the car's exhaust pipe, and asphyxiate herself. As a young boy, he didn't fully understand what asphyxiation was. But he knew that somehow when she breathed in from that hose, she would leave—he would be separated, rejected, alone, abandoned—isolated. This is what we fear the most; we spend our lives attempting to avoid rejection and isolation. As an adult, this man suffered from a rare form of lung disease—unconscious focus on his lungs becoming organic reality.

> *It is possible that more severe emotional states are more deeply repressed and that may be a factor in disease choice.*
>
> — John E. Sarno, MD, *The Mindbody Prescription*[165]

Psychotherapist, Lisbeth Marcher, at the Bodynamic Institute in Denmark, has spent three decades studying bodydynamics. She has discovered that every muscle is correlated with a psychological function, or issue—even mapping the correlations out through Bodynamic Analysis.*

Rochelle Gordon's book, *Body Talk*, is devoted to this symbolic process of pain and illness. The book begins with the story of a woman in her 60s who had a large medical dressing on her left leg that covered an ulceration. When Gordon asked her how long she had had the ulceration, the woman replied, "Twenty-five years."

---

* Bodynamic Analysis, BA, deals with measured muscle responsiveness, character structure, shock trauma, and ego functions. BA includes the body within the psychoanalysis process. [bodynamicusa.com/documents/body_map.html]

Gordon soon solved the ulceration mystery when she met the woman's 30-year-old daughter who had developed polio as a young child and had a brace on her left leg.

> *It was as if anguish over the daughter's affliction had ignited a similar suffering in the mother.... Illness is not an isolated event. It is an integral part of the life process in which you actively participate, whether you know it or not.*
>
> — Rochelle Gordon, *Body Talk*[166]

The barking cough becomes the acceptable manner in which to yell publicly; the yawn, a silent shout of disapproval; the cold, a socially acceptable fashion in which to cry; the limp, a physical expression of self-pity. The modern disease becomes a modality by which to fit in with society's woes, and into the collectively agreed-upon reality.

It's not uncommon to actually catch the symptoms of someone close to you. We are connected in some elegant manner and the Type T seems to be a magnet for unconscious infections. This is highly evident with couvade syndrome, or sympathetic male pregnancy, which comes from the French word, "to hatch." It has been clinically proven that husbands can take on the symptoms and pains of their pregnant wives. They will gain weight with their wives, and even feel abdominal pain and queasiness, as well as engage in binge eating and mood swings. Some studies indicate that adopted men are more likely to develop couvade. This makes great sense, since the deeper the initial wound of separation (the more severe emotional state), the more empathic the individual can become in his desire to pull others back together, or to become violently aggressive *...as the yin chases the yang.* The first cut will always leave the deepest scar and the blood from the cut flows from its source.

The flow and mystery of how we influence each other's lives is ever present as females in close-knit groups often begin menstruating together. People close to each other share their lives together—wanted or unwanted—since they have the capacity at fleeting moments in time to share consciousness.

13

SteveO, Do I Have TMS?

I'm convinced that Dr. Sarno is right and that all chronic back pain should be considered TMS until proved otherwise.

— Andrew Weil, MD, *Spontaneous Healing*[167]

I assume that every symptom I have is TMS until proven otherwise because I believe everything our bodies express is due to an unconscious process from conflict (not including dietary deficiencies, or external factors, of course, such as asbestos exposure or anything vile to the system). However, the sure-fire way of finding out if you have TMS is to visit a good mindbody practitioner. Sadly, many sufferers cannot do this—largely due to the lack of "real" TMS specialists and the painfully high costs.

A visit to a TMS-experienced doctor will include a physical exam to check for objective function, look at your imaging, etc., and to seek out any tender points on palpation (trigger points). If the tests show normal herniations and joint wear and tear, you will leave with a TMS diagnosis, which is a great prognosis. The visit will also include an evaluation of your mental position, relationships, family history, and personality, etc. Now—those who cannot visit a TMS practitioner must rely on their own intuition, the Internet, books, and a deepening self-awareness. People sometimes heal more slowly than expected because they're unsure if they are experiencing a mindbody reaction—the source of their pain remains a nagging mystery.

The second most common question asked of me is, "Do I have TMS, SteveO?" It was also a main question I asked of myself. I am not a doctor—I just play one on TV. I can't make a diagnosis—and I won't—but I can point out the obvious. In the absence of a TMS-trained physician, get a general exam to rule out any ailments that may need medical intervention. Then begin asking yourself questions. You can observe your life at a level beyond the immediately apparent, and come to a reasonable conclusion, based on the information in Dr. Sarno's books and hopefully from what you find here, by simply gleaning your house.

The "Do I Have TMS?" Checklist

- Have you suffered from pain on and off for many years, that has neither gotten better or worse? Does your pain only occur at certain times? Does it get worse during certain times of the day, week, or year, and then improve for a time? A back or knee pain or hip or neck pain cannot continue indefinitely unless there's nervous system involvement because the body heals itself—eventually.

- Have you had x-rays, CT scans, and MRIs that show only herniated discs and normal degenerative aging of the joints and body?

- Are you a perfectionist? Goal or performance-driven? Anxious and restless? Irritable or volatile? Compulsive?

- Are you quiet, reserved and yet explosive—insincerely overly friendly, but also harboring a short temper? Or are you anti-social, and quickly agitated by life and people? Are you calm and mild-mannered—smile even when you are angry and in pain? When someone criticizes you, do you walk away quietly and internalize it? Do little things aggravate you? Are you short-tempered with people, or do you let them walk all over you?

- Has there recently been a big change that you are beginning to recover from? Is something major coming up or recently ended? Have you recently achieved a goal or new level in life?

- Do you do things repeatedly and persistently in order to make them better? Obsessive behavior dramatically increases the likelihood of TMS. Do you clean your bathroom floor or house, mow your yard or remodel your home compulsively? Or engage in other acts of repetitiveness (such as hitting lots and lots of golf balls)?

- Do you feel you need to always succeed and win? Do you push yourself hard? Do you fret over little things?

- Do you know when enough is enough?

- Do you avoid conflict at all cost?

- Can you feel your emotions?

- Do you feel nothing except despair?

- Are you suffering from (m)any acronyms such as RSI, RSD, TOS, RLS, TMJ, BMS, GERD, BED, IBS, CFS, UC, CT, or IC or skin problems or migraines or frequent urination or urethritis? Anything, or many things, from Appendix A at the back of this book?

- Is your first thought, "I don't know if my back, or feet or hands or knees can take it," or, "I can't sit on that hard seat"—then you, my friend, have TMS. Your brain is luring you into a distraction because you don't want to be there or go there.

- Do you drink alcohol excessively or take many meds for emotional numbing?

- Do you find yourself crying for no apparent reason? Snapping at people for insignificant things?

- Do you want a sense of control in every situation?

- Do you worry excessively about everything?

- Do you avoid people when you can? Who doesn't, right? This would be a great world without all those people. What I mean is obsessive avoidance of all people. Hermit-like.

- Do you hate your job? Are you bored with your job? Are you worried about money?

- Are you at midlife, and upset about your looks, aging, and mortality?

- Does your pain flare up before athletic competitions, or any type of scenario where you will be observed or judged?

- Do you perspire heavily or hardly at all? Sometimes have trouble breathing deeply without chest or lung discomfort? Grind your teeth at night? Have unidentifiable rashes?

- Did either of your parents suffer from pain and/or tension symptoms? Were your parents heavy negative thinkers? Heavy positive drinkers? Drug addicts? Non-committal? Critical? Absent? Apathetic toward you? Constantly arguing? Ill? Has one committed suicide? Were you adopted or felt abandoned? Did your parents separate or die when you were very young? Was either parent abusive?

- Have you had a major relationship or career **change**? Is there tension in your marriage? Are you going through, or have you recently been divorced? Do you have a sick loved one? Are you in college? Has there recently been a death in the family? New or lost job? Retirement, new residence, destroyed home? Has there been any change that you witnessed with your senses and have **intellectualized** as, "oh well, that's life"? …because you didn't feel anything inside? Well, you should be feeling these things; if not… there's more gleaning to do in your house.

- You can be certain you have TMS if you have **shifting symptoms**—it is the signature characteristic of the disorder as described in Chapter Ten.

If you've checked off any of the above, there is a good chance you have TMS. If you've checked off a majority of them, then you can be pretty certain you have it. If you have symptoms that shift from point to point, knee to back, neck to stomach, fatigue to pain, or back to back, etc.—you have TMS. The movement of symptoms, as Dr. Sarno has described, is the "hallmark" of TMS.

When you "know" you have TMS, the battle of the divided mind has been "one." The difference between thinking you have a mindbody symptom and knowing it, is in the depth of belief and understanding. It is a **gnosis**.

Understanding the Whys: Gathering Knowledge

14

What You Need To Understand to Heal

Every great advance in natural knowledge has involved the absolute rejection of authority.
— Thomas Henry Huxley,
On the Advisableness of Improving Natural Knowledge (1825-1895)

You need to understand that you must **get a physical exam first**. Rule out the need for immediate external intervention. If the exam and reports show only disc bulges or disc protrusions or disc extrusions or disc degeneration (water loss), or spinal stenosis (spinal narrowing) or arthritis, or worn knee joints, or any host of other normal physiological changes, then you are healthy enough to begin TMS tensionalgia healing. The changes shown on medical images may be hard to swallow, but as the old saying goes, "take it all with a grain of salt," and it will be easier to swallow.

You need to **forget everything you have previously understood** regarding back pain and joint pain and hand and foot pain because it is **perfectly wrong**. Pain does not come from improper sleeping alignment, or bad posture, or your weight, or how you move or sit. The general medical industry is looking toward the body for healing, which is 180 degrees in the wrong direction. The current paradigm perpetuates and propagates pain—ironically—by temporarily relieving symptoms.

You need to understand that you must have full belief in the TMS process. You must be fully open to the concept, believe and accept it—or it will not work for you. It is not a passive modality like taking a pill or a drug. A medical modality is the application of a physical therapeutic agent. It's **all or nothing** for complete healing.

You need to understand that **you've repressed the thing that is causing your pain. You don't know what it is.** So if you don't feel angry—when you should be—then this is proof of the existence of TMS. If you feel anger at someone or something, then that is not the anger that is causing your pain. It is the anger that you cannot feel causing your chronic pain, or symptom. Too much intellectualization has led you to a point where you can no longer sense your own emotional state. Emotion is the antithesis of intellectualization. Force the rage to surface through reflective insight and restore the nexus between the pain and the rage. A few sufferers have commented to me, "Steve, I'm not angry, I just have pain." I try to explain to them that the presence of their pain reveals that they are indeed very angry, and that this is the very purpose of their pain, to let them know they have repressed what they so much want to express—but can't. A few individuals come back and say, "Steve, I'm not angry," so I try to explain again:

A Typical Conversation with a TMS Pain Sufferer:

Me: Your pain is revealing to you that you are unconsciously angered inside.

Someone: But I'm not angry, Steve.

Me: I know you don't feel angry, but the presence of your pain shows that you have repressed your anger into your body.

Someone: But I'm not angry, Steve.

Me: I realize that you don't feel your anger, but that is the very reason that the symptom is there, to let you know something you wouldn't otherwise know, that you are extremely angry, but have repressed it—consciously ignoring it.

Someone: But I'm not angry, Steve.

Me: I understand that you don't feel angry, but the pain is there because you DON'T feel angry, to keep your anger from surfacing.

Someone: But I'm not angry, Steve.

Me: I know that you don't feel angry; if you felt angry, you wouldn't have your symptom.

Someone: But I'm not angry, Steve.

Me: Is Clint Eastwood ever going to retire or what?

...**and the vicious cycle continues**... because some sufferers just don't get the concept... yet... and one more for the road. The presence of chronic pain or cyclical pain, or pain equivalents such as those discussed in Appendix A, reveals your latent anger through your body. That anger that you do not feel is revealing itself through your body in the form of pain, or ulcerative colitis, or sinus infections, or heartburn, or asthma, or RSI, etc.; this is why you do not feel angry, this is why the symptom is there, to let you know something that you can't feel—you must become aware that there exists buried emotional evidence. "I know, I know.... I understand, Steve... but I'm not angry...." Ugh—this denial, in stating that everything is fine when it clearly is not—is the superego in super-action and is emotionally unhealthy. The Crocodile Hunter's widow, Terry Irwin, did the loving and intelligent thing when she took their daughter, Bindi, to see a counselor because, as she described, Bindi seemed "so happy" after her daddy Steve Irwin was killed—her anger was too great for her superego to allow her to express it appropriately. She was in too much emotional pain to express herself—so she shut off her emotions. This is dangerous.

You need to learn to **identify when you are TMSing**. What is TMSing? Although Dr. Sarno had originally defined TMS as a pain syndrome, I've obviously expanded it into a **process** to include anything you consciously or unconsciously do to avoid being aware of your emotional status. TMSing is the unconscious mind revealing messages through the body (itself). TMSing is exhibiting myoneuralgia or tensionalgia. **TMSing is the continual distractive search for solutions through the body**—focusing on the body or anything else—in order to avoid unwanted emotional overload. Ironically, the process of continually searching through the body, defeats the purpose of the searching. TMSing would include the following actions or states—**avoidance techniques** for coping with life's anxieties.

I knew I was tense because at night I tight my teeths.

— Bernabe

TMSing Includes:

- The need to fantasize, exaggerate, or to engage in hyperbole
- The belief that you need surgery to heal chronic pain
- The desire for cosmetic surgery—BDD (body dysmorphic disorder), never feeling you look good enough
- The desire for chiropractic or osteopathic adjustments
- The craving for overstimulation, drugs/alcohol/smoking/sex
- The denial that emotions cause pain and illness
- The desire for continuous physical therapy
- The want for comfort devices—soft beds/shoe supports/back braces/ comfy chairs
- The need to criticize (judge) others—projecting your shadow
- The love of money or hoarding
- The need for more and more information
- The seeking of praise by condemning self—playing the victim
- The need to gamble
- Constant complaining of pain
- Pain moving from place to place
- Procrastination—the inability to make a decision
- Workaholism
- Chronic pain or chronic infections or chronic illness, or any of the items listed in Appendix A, TMS Equivalents, more generally:
  - Over-analyzing
  - Chronic fatigue syndrome—CFS
  - Eating disorders—anorexia, or bulimic or binging behavior
  - OCD—obsessive compulsive disorders/repetitive behavior
  - Constant anxiety with accompanying depression
  - Phobias—irrational fears
  - Promiscuity

You need to understand that **you cannot pinch a nerve** without being paralyzed within minutes, if not seconds. This may be the biggest scam currently perpetuated in medicine today. But there are others such as instigating fear over relatively normal cholesterol levels.

You need to understand that **you cannot "slip a disc"** or **"throw your back out"** due to the intelligent design of the spine.

You need to understand that **you cannot therapeutically separate the foramina** to open nerve routes through any type of decompression therapies or machinery. Surgery may indeed open these routes but it doesn't heal the pain and is hole-ly unnecessary because the theory is that the foramina calcifies—keeping the opening from changing or closing any more—as part of the body's natural healing capabilities. Beware of falling for ads and fads and new wild claims that allow people to make money from your su$$ering. Healing is often slow, and it involves dealing, revealing, expressing, and understanding. It cannot come from a machine, no matter how wildly over-exaggerated the claims of succe$$ are.

You need to understand that **you must lean into pain**. Don't pull back from it while sitting down or bending, while in any type of position or while performing any movement. Don't lift certain ways or sit or lie or sleep in certain positions… just live your life as you desire. There is no pinching of nerves, no matter how much it feels like it (it really does feel like it, too). Allowing pain reduces the fear that has wrongfully been instilled in you, that you are damaging your body further. It is an irrational fear that you are hurting your back or knee by the presence of pain, or that you can further hurt yourself through physical movement. Dr. Sarno referred to this phenomenon as a "physicophobia"—a fear of lifting or moving or twisting that is a more effective distracter than the pain itself. As you begin to become active, think of the pain as a ghost memory of a pain that was once there. How do you stand against it? You let pain happen without fear. I asked the veterinarian why our puppy didn't yelp or even blink when she gave him the shot in his furry derriere. He just sat there with that stupid look on his cute face. She told me that when puppies don't expect it, they often don't feel it.

Shaolin monks, as a part of their discipline, test their tolerance for pain through a variety of extreme measures, such as lying on beds of nails while other monks place heavy weights on top of them (they must not have TVs or Wiis for entertainment). They can endure unimaginable pain because they practice **relaxation** before they perform the test of pain endurance. Relaxation raises the pain threshold by calming the mindbody, rendering pain less significant. **Defeat it by allowing it.**

What you resist persists.

— Carl Jung

As you move, think of the body as a whole system instead of a broken part that is perceived to be the area in pain. Feel the entirety of the body moving, and force your mind off the painful area. Don't single out the pained area in thought while moving, which I refer to as "feeding the beast." The pain often defines people, so redefine who you are by viewing yourself as a sum of parts and not just a single broken id-entity. Find victory in spite of yourself.

You need to understand that **your pain is from mild oxygen deprivation**—the result of reduced bloodflow from silent rage.

You need to **think** very **immaturely** when trying to identify the psychological reasons behind your pain. It isn't always necessary to find the exact emotional event that created your now-surfacing conflict. When attempting the introspective approach to healing—think more immaturely—as an id-child would. The child inside will never mature, and so it is important to think like she would. For example, people may search for possible causes by thinking about their father or mother dying, or their boss or their job. These may well be the sources in acute attacks (Phase 1) but it may be as simple as someone not saying hello, or having to park further away in the rain or snow. I once read of a man whose back spasmed due to a leaky faucet. These are examples of **anger overlay**. That is, the leak isn't the cause; it merely triggers a deeper need—magnifying trauma that was never discharged from his system. The aggravating leak kindles his sympathetic system, overreacting to the trigger. Think simpler—look back into yourself through the eyes of a helpless child. Think—what is it that's bothering me?

You need to understand that your pain or symptom is both a **distraction** and a **message**. The distraction is being paid too much attention, and the message not enough attention. You are out-of-balance and the pain is delivering the message.

You need to understand that tensionalgia is extremely **bilateral**. Pain often moves from one side of the back to the other side—one side of the neck to the other. It also moves from back to knee to ankle, all around the body, often fooling the individual into thinking he has suddenly hurt another body part. TMS is a predator. I was told that my back was "highly unstable" because the pain moved from my left side to my right side, alternating back and forth for decades. But this was never true. Sufferers who have unnecessary shoulder surgery often find that the pain moves to the other shoulder. Knee surgery on one knee often forces the mind's focus to the other knee. Elbow-to-elbow, wrist-to-wrist, foot-to-foot.

It's common for the pain to move to the other side, or from top to bottom—very often moving from back to neck. People erroneously feel that the other side is now hurting because they are placing more strain on that side because they can't put any force onto the rehabilitating side. This is a false assumption that is deeply integrated into the collective consciousness. The pain moves for a tactical reason, NOT because of additional pressure placed.

Dr. Sopher writes in his book, "Jack was a former athlete, now in his 40s, with left hip pain. His orthopedist told him that he would benefit from a new hip joint as his x-ray showed 'significant' degenerative changes. After this visit his left hip pain increased and he mentioned it to me at the time of his annual physical exam. When he told me that his right hip felt fine, I asked him to humor me by having both of his hips x-rayed. On x-ray, both hips had the same 'degenerative' changes, yet his right hip did not hurt! I advised him to put off surgery, resume activity and not pay too much attention to his hips. Following these instructions, his discomfort subsided and he successfully resumed exercise and athletics."[168]

You need to understand that **old doctors' tales have morphed into new wives' tales—and vice versa**. People routinely claim that their doctors told them their pain was from their low iron count or low thyroid levels, or that they needed granny's rheumatizz medicine... and these people suddenly healed after hearing this news. Proteins and enzymes are often depleted during stressful periods. The frustration is in the misunderstanding of the proper cause and effect behind the success. These are not cures or causes of pain. Their belief in their doctor had broken their responses to their pain. The blind can lead the blind but only further into darkness. It's a financial and health disaster.

You need to begin to **notice that your very first thought is always directed toward your pain**, and at how badly you need to think about it. The symptom becomes a cognitive reflex. How many times per minute do you think about your body? Notice how your mind shifts to your body when asked to do something that you do not want to do: sit some place you don't want to sit—go some place you don't wanna. Your pain's intensity will rise as your need for your pain rises—to distract. Remove the thinking and the fearing of the pain from the daily process by filling the senses with everything except thoughts of pain. This is a very important tip. Each time you start to think of the pain... at that moment... force yourself to think of the possible reasons for it—never allow your attention to lock onto your body. The focus must shift from pain to message, stopping short of obsessing. As the pain strikes, you can think of a predetermined image, like a baby or funny joke, something pleasurable. By using imagery such as a smiling baby's face, the pain's purpose is diluted; but it may not disappear if you need deeper answers (or if you just hate smiling babies). I used music quite a bit; babies don't smile when you want them to—only when they want to. Ids—what can you do?

You need to **read and reread** Dr. Sarno's books, and then reread them again until it finally connects with you, stopping short of obsession. Several people have told me that they believed Dr. Sarno, but that his books left them somewhat "disconnected as to where to go next." I didn't feel that way, but some have. The answers are there, though you may not fully understand the implications of his message in its entirety the first few times around. Don't reread this book you're reading now, though; instead buy another copy of *The Great Pain Deception* and read that copy. Every time you go to read my book again... go buy a new one! Ask questions of other people who have healed. Go over Dr. Sarno's daily reminders. Then stop reading and listening; cease the quest for more grails. In the long run it is detrimental to healing if it becomes obsessive because obsessing is a distraction. Less ultimately is more. The quest for more details is in itself TMSing because it serves to put off the work that must be done to heal.

You need to **look at what is currently going on in your life**—what has recently happened. Regarding emotional catharsis, James Pennebaker, PhD, writes in *Opening Up: The Healing Power of Confiding in Others*, that you should focus on the current issues rather than focusing on the most traumatic events of life.[169] It's not always the goal in healing to bring THE issue to consciousness to release it, but is more important to understand WHY the individual has disassociated it from his consciousness—what necessitated him to bury the event—not necessarily what the event is. This is true if the pain is nagging, but if the pain is completely debilitating, then it may be time to seek a good counselor or spiritual advisor to begin the metamorphosis of growing inward. Don't look at the distant past yet, the most recent change is germane. Think... think... think. Connect your dots (CYD). However! ... once you've connected enough dots to see your own picture forming, you need to then destroy your thinking mind and allow your working mind to take over. The act of continuous thinking inhibits full healing by blocking the fuller awareness of what "is" in the present moment. Thinking obstructs your healing in the long run because thinking caused your problems to begin with. Therefore, there is no intellectual answer to healing because you can't think yourself out of a hole.

You need to understand that the so-called physical incident that initiated your TMS pain **was merely a trigger**. You lifted or turned and the blood supply was suddenly stopped. The incident was a perfect opportunity for unresolved conflict to overflow in the form of a distraction.

You need to understand that any time you **do something** to relieve pain, such as stretching or exercising, or sit-ups, or talking about pain, etc., that **you prolong the pain**. Perform any routines for the sake of themselves, never for pain reduction.

You need to understand that there are **hidden undertones playing beneath the depth of your awareness**—24/7. This subconscious activity reveals itself in the form of symbols and images that are stored within your mindbody. They remain in the body forever until they are discharged to healthy levels. Even though you love your kids or spouse or job or hobby, at some level it all enrages you. Indeed, many people suffering from TMS symptoms and depression are putting their own lives and dreams on hold so that others around them can remain the center of attention—allowing other family members to move forward. Your brain may deceive you but your body doesn't know how.

You need to **begin exhausting yourself physically**—not mentally. Anxiety results from repression, which is held in the body as energy, an overdose of negative energy. Burn your tension away by staying in motion. Sitting at a desk and stressing out on a job is not what nature intended humans to do. Take the lead and get up and do something you love!

You need to **dissociate your being from your body.** When you move or walk or sit, think of your body as being "not yours"—think of it as an outside object and your spirit as a painless entity that IS you. When I started becoming physical again, I began thinking of my body as an esoteric process—my real self was a spirit moving around pain-free inside my body (this dissociation moved my healing along faster). When the bottom of my feet hurt so much that I could barely walk, I began imagining that my feet weren't attached to me; that they belonged to someone else—not of me—beyond tangible flesh and bone. You are more than your pain, more than your body. When you walk or run or go anywhere… simply **take your body with you.** This is a great insight if you can implicitly understand the concept. The body is only along for the ride in life, to further expand consciousness. Do your work, play and live while using your body as a tool as a means to an end, and not simply as the means.

You need to understand that surgery and steroid injections and anti-inflammatories **do not work** in the long-term because they don't address the problem. If they work for you, you have been placeboed.

You need to recognize **how soon after your relationship ended,** or someone has moved away or died, or your job **ended,** children went off to college, or socio-environmental status changed, that your physical symptoms began. Your under-world is boiling with discontent, your purpose disrupted by these changes. You feel trapped, victimized, frustrated. The pain and digestive tract problems, and skin problems, only add to the frustration and anxiety.

You need to understand **the power of visualization** and learn the techniques of visual guided imagery—envisioning your mindbody moving healthily and happily and pain-free with a perfect spine, or cells, etc. I visualized a virgin-spine, never tested; the most perfect example of a spine. Imagine healthy images—slowly seeping into the unconscious process. I imagined blood flowing into my lower back like a red Niagara Falls of blood. I also used audio "imagery" by closing my eyes and hearing the blood flowing like the sound of a large waterfall into the L4 and L5 area. This will actually entice the autonomic system into letting the blood flow to the deprived area. The body responds to orders from the brain, and the autonomic functions respond indirectly to beliefs and images. It also helped me greatly to think of my lower back pain as a migraine. It gave me a sense of control over my pain because a migraine is "collectively agreed upon" to be an emotional process. Somehow imagining my back pain as a migraine in my back helped my pain dissipate in a more logically acceptable fashion. I implicitly understood the migraine since there were no discs—no moving parts that could deteriorate. The migraine is a tensionalgia paragon.

You need to understand that **if your lower back hurts, you need to walk and bend and move** while forcing your attention to your upper back. If your left knee hurts, walk while forcing your attention onto your other knee, the same with shoulders, feet, etc. Think, as you move, about another area of your body that feels gooooood, each and every time you move. Rivet your attention elsewhere with laser-like focus to break the mind's-eye focus on the current pain. **Do not be surprised** if the pain moves to the area that feels good—it did for me. This becomes a cognitive transversal and is a form of behavioral therapy. Some behaviorists are claiming (unproven) that if you can hold a single thought for 17 seconds, more of the same type of thought will coalesce as the first thought blends into a synergistic mix of thoughts, as in the Law of Attraction. I know when my pain jumped to the spot that I was focusing on in my mid-back that I held my conscious focus for at least 17 seconds. The longer you can hold your focus off the pain and onto an area of "no pain," the higher the vibration, as thoughts of pain-free become organic reality—and old focus fades. This takes some time to grasp, but it will soon be evident that the cognitive process is being redirected and the reuptake slowed. Pavlov would be as happy as a dog.

You need to **become more appreciative** of what you already have, and to stop craving for unmet desires. Appreciation is the highest level of peace and happiness—generating the highest frequencies because it encompasses both love and joy. Take time at night to be thankful for the day. Make a written list if you need to, but the important thing is to really feel appreciative, not to merely write down the things you think you should be appreciative of. If you have trouble appreciating, then **this is part of the problem**. But the work can be done. Invite some old friends over to talk and laugh about the good ole times. These current times need to be put into the past for a fleeting moment. Go visit family and lean on them and talk about life: yours and theirs. Appreciation is not regurgitating what you think others want you to feel thankful for, but rather is a feeling that hits you in the gut. What can't you live without in your life? Those are the "gratefuls." There are so many blessings that fill each day. What moves you? If you cannot see anything, then you have been blinded by self-pity.* Relearn how to have fun because when the laughter stops, the pain replaces it. Go out and belly laugh (or belly dance) with friends, and become a child again—**lose some control**. There is a great art to a light heart. Responsibility has overwhelmed you if your pain has returned. The ability to laugh *and* let go—as a child naturally does—gets lost in midlife. It's eventually replaced with emotional isolation, followed by unhappiness. With the disappearance of innocence comes conflict, because every adult is also a child. Relearn enthusiasm (en Theos, Greek, defined as "in God"). I knew toward the end of my healing that I wasn't enjoying life. But to have fun is to let go, which is difficult for a perfectionist at the controls. So become enthusiastic and find silliness all around you. The mind holds both joy and rage

---

* If you can't find anything to be thankful for watch this YouTube video and relearn appreciation: 29-year-old deaf woman hears her voice for the first time. [www.youtube.com/watch?v=vjU9U81O1n8]

simultaneously—each incumbent upon the existence of the other. They are necessary complements—folds of the same person ...*as the yin chases the yang... and this becomes that....*

You need to understand the importance of **"expressing" through journaling** or **other means** and introspective mental checklists in uprooting possible reasons behind your pain or illness, rather than seeking physical reasons.* It must be noted that talking and writing about deep emotional experiences has worked for many people and has been proven to be effective in studies at The Ohio State and Southern Methodist Universities† Reviewing **possible roots of rage** and purging trauma through **talking it out** or through **writing it down**—works! The reason the exercise is a list of *possible* reasons is that the cause of your pain is unknown to you. Ira Progoff, a student of Carl Jung, is widely considered the father of journaling. Progoff proved that writing is purging, and that purging is healing. The OSU and SMU studies also revealed that people who wrote away traumatic events had better overall health, increased T-lymphocyte production, less absenteeism, and decreased hospital visits. Writing privately reveals our deepest thought processes and "our thought processes can heal."[170]

You need to understand that **you have a hidden temper,** so volatile that superego stifles it through the outward appearance of calmness and control. You keep your temper in check by means of self-punishing pain or an infinite variety of nefarious bodily symptoms. Anger is innately human to possess—it is how you express it that makes all the difference. Most of us have never learned how.

> *This is the symptom imperative at work. When he learned to curb his temper, the back pain begins.*
>
> — John E. Sarno, MD, *The Divided Mind*[171]

You need to understand that **pain is not necessarily a bad thing**—you are on the verge of growth through change—and that you are fighting the needed changes. Part of you wants to see yourself as you truly are and part of you wants to hold strong to your persona that you have so painstakingly constructed for others to observe. There is opportunity knocking at your conscious mind in the form of pain, and you need only to look inward to see what that opportunity is.

You need to understand that **as the pain increases it is desperate.** It often increases its intensity as you ignore it or fight it—it fights your fighting of it. Here is where many

---

* Remember, from Chapter 1, to think psychologically, but to refrain from obsessive focus on the possible roots. Balance Is King. Ease up on your worries.

† JW Pennebaker, JK Kiecolt-Glaser, and R. Glaser, "Disclosure of Traumas and Immune Function: Health Implications for Psychotherapy," *Journal of Consulting and Clinical Psychology*, Vol. 56, April 1988, pp. 239-245. Also, JW Pennebaker, "Writing About Emotional Experiences As A Therapeutic Process," *Psychological Science*, Vol. 8, Issue 3, pp. 162-166. "Talking and writing about emotional experiences are both superior to writing about superficial topics." [p. 163]

people quit and give up on TMS healing because they feel they are further damaging themselves. I began looking at an increase in my pain as a good sign that I was winning because every time my pain increased I achieved a new level of healing—a step closer to pain-free. This, once again, is reversing the way in which the pain is interpreted by the brain. When the pain increases, think, ahhh, tomorrow will be better—my brain is desperate because it's losing its hold on my pretending to be what I am not. You will not heal exactly the same way each day. There will be ups and downs that depend on many interrelated things. Nutrition, exercise, stress, relationship energy demands, delta sleep, motivation, and criticisms are but a few of the many factors that determine the state of the mindbody process on any given day. Life is a dynamic process, and vigilance ever in demand.

You need to understand that it's important to always **reward your physical activity** with something pleasurable to begin the process of reinterpreting movement. The fact that you can move is a blessing in itself, even if it is painful. So whenever you function, reward yourself with something pleasurable to your senses. Please your k-id. The mind remembers the reward, and later, if your backache or headache or stomachache begins, you will eventually be able to stop your pain by simply visualizing the reward. Reconditioning!

You need to understand that **you have an obsessive personality** and may be a **pathological people-pleaser** at your own expense. This perfectionistic compulsion keeps you continually and obliviously angry all day—every day. Your persona smiles on the outside and is royally pissed on the inside. Contrarily, and much less often, you may be the opposite—an agitator—over-arrogant and self-centered with such low self-esteem that you cannot get along with anyone ...as this is ultimately that....

You need to understand that you need to **be less negative and doubtful.** You were likely brought up in a negative environment, but this norm of negativity can be changed into positivity by simply understanding. Things are not always going wrong or against you. But sufferers view things as falling apart because events are screened through a negative prism constructed early in life. The world of pain is a skewed world, distorted by years of low self-esteem and high self-imposed demands.

You need to learn anapanasati. This is the **presence of breathing** in and out. Anapana (defined as "in and out")—Sati (defined as "breathing"). Conscious breathing regulates the autonomic nervous system, which in turn soothes and relaxes the body, easing tension, increasing alpha activity and presence.

You need to understand that **your pain has become a habit.** It's an addiction that can be difficult to break. The limbic (defined as "inner margin") system is the seat of emotions in your brain. It just happens that pain and addiction specifically target your limbic center—sharing the same mechanisms, motivations and triggers. The most important psychological factor in sustaining any addiction is the process of denial. Pain in fact becomes your heroine, your alcohol, your cocaine, your food. The need for it becomes a perceived part of self even though it isn't consciously desired. Pain is often self-induced punishment for the guilty desire for the want of pleasure, for reasons that only the shadow knows. If you're in chronic pain, you are unwittingly a pain addict.

You need to understand that the stage for your rage causing your pain is **built in childhood** from the fear and anger of **rejection** or **abandonment**. The most prevalent early causes are from institutionalized birth trauma, absent parents, or the fear of absent parents, and apathetic caretakers, which create a situation where you want to be liked—for everyone to get along and to come back together.

You need to understand that **your mindbody is overreacting to** the pain due to an obsessive/phobic personality. The obsessiphobe's autonomic system overreacts to pain, pollens, certain foods or other stimuli, creating a more devastating symptom than would normally occur. The Ohio State University once had a phenomenal football running back, who in his entire football career, because of injuries, rarely finished a full season, and not coincidentally, he was a phobic individual. The anxious individual unwittingly increases pain by fearing more than actually necessary. This running back often left the field to take the sideline after getting hit by opponents. Jim Tressel, the former head coach at Ohio State, once stated how his star running back had improved over the season, "…I think he's further along than he was, maybe midseason, he understands how to shake it off a little bit, and he understands that there isn't going to be further injury." Coach Tressel knew the score. He was one of the best college football coaches in history because he "got it." Phobic = Overreaction to Symptoms.

You need to understand that **you have been conditioned to expect pain**, and so it comes.

You need to understand that you need to **get off your own back** when it comes to judging yourself.

You need to understand that the **pain is often symbolic** of the job that you are doing, or the act that you are despising. Wherever the body is seen as **wounded** is where the conflict is being waged.

You need to understand that **you are holding the painful body area in tension**, unconsciously, right now as you read this, but you don't know it. In the process of trying to be all things to all people you've lost your sensation of self.

You need to understand that **you need a break** from your routine (unfulfilled) life. Even if you feel that you don't—the pain tells you indirectly that you do.

You need to understand that there is **often a seasonal effect accompanying pain** and other symptoms. As the seasons change, conditioned memories re-surface—triggering the same responses.

You need to understand that **you need to cry**, but a demanding superego will not allow it. So the pain or cold or flu or cough or sinus infection, intestinal irritation, or skin eruptions, etc., serve as substitutes for what you cannot—will not do—or don't know how to do.

You need to understand that **you may be stuck in a vortex** that you don't understand how to escape. You cannot make an important decision that you need to make—paralyzed by indecision from the conflict. This inability to act or express infuriates you, and the pain exists to give you a sense of control over the lack of direction.

You need to understand that **you need other people** in your life; you cannot do it all alone. Life is relationship. We need others in order to accept ourselves, since we are all bound to consciousness. Whether past or present relationships, they need to be healed either by communicating, or by letting go.

You need to know that **it is indeed possible to hurt yourself.** But that the injury should heal in a few days or months at most. If your back or any pained area is chronic (beyond several months), or has suddenly appeared out of nowhere, then it is more than likely an emotional eruption.

You also need to understand that just because you hurt your back or neck or knee years ago, it doesn't mean that that is the reason for your current pain. That injury has long since healed. If it hurts in the same place now, it's due to conditioning. Back and joint injuries don't last a lifetime, but memories can.

You need to stay away from groups, organizations, books, and people who talk about symptoms! Talking about symptoms enforces imagery that gets deeply imbedded in the subconscious. Talk about life and you steal the need for your symptom.

You need to understand that the **mind and body are one.** There is no difference between mental suffering and physical suffering.

You need to understand that **healing is not an exact process** or done with logical reasoning.* Find your own light in the world, and become the change that you want to see. You have symptoms for your own personal unconscious reasons, and only you can resolve them. If you are not healing—if you're failing—change classes, you don't always need to study harder.

You may need to **get into better physical shape.** The body needs motion, and movement is its sustenance. Good physical shape can reward the emotional state. The two often go hand in hand; however, world-class athletes also get TMS and have to visit Dr. Sarno, so personal conflict comes in many forms.

You may need to **talk to your brain—get mad** at it! I have read and heard about this technique for healing. Dr. Sarno writes that even though it sounds "silly," it has worked many times with his patients. It must have great merit because many former

---

* This is ratiocination, which is an exact reasoning or a logical or precise pathway (in this case, for healing).

sufferers have reported that yelling at their brains for pulling such a deception can alleviate pain instantly. Even though I did get mad at my pain, this technique only prolonged it. It was only when I decided to ease up on myself that my pain acquiesced. Those who feel deep guilt may not need more yelling at their brains. Those who feel overextended, who feel they have given all of themselves, may need soothing. No matter which method you choose, you just end up talking to yourself.

You need to find a daily lifelong **routine that creates a mental transparency**. The idea is to find a routine such as sewing or crocheting, or table tennis or jogging, or singing, etc., that it is second nature to perform it, requiring no forethought as to the mechanics of the process. I play guitar, lift weights, run, and hit golf balls for transparency (you can see right through me at times). This is **active meditation** since it allows varying levels of consciousness to surface while simultaneously being mindful of now. When the act becomes second nature, it allows the conscious mind to release its stranglehold on the body as the mind settles into an alpha state of deepening awareness—the view beyond self-consciousness and ego. That is—we are aware of, but unconcerned about our surroundings; eventually unconscious images and symbols rise to the surface in the form of answers, and daily problems will often roll away or resolve themselves. The routine or activity should be done for its own sake or it is self-defeating. So there should be no sense that something need be gained in the process other than the performance of the ritual itself, or ego is still involved and shielding full consciousness.

You need to become **present**. All the preceding advice, thus far, has been proven to alleviate and release symptoms of pain and disease. But the only permanent pathway out of suffering is by awakening to what is, right now. Through presence, consciousness expands by destroying the stream of thinking that gives rise to the notion of separateness, and to dangerous thoughts and emotional attachments. Permanent healing comes through awareness only, not by "doing things." Although "doing something" can yield temporary relief by shifting attention elsewhere, lasting healing is synonymous with an awakening that only presence can provide through the act of giving attention to the present moment without reacting. Presence means letting go of the past through forgiveness (not thinking about it therefore not attached any more), and by letting go of the false construct of the future which dissolves stress: stress means "not present." Presence extinguishes the desire for fast answers and overcomes fear through radical Love as it increases compassion through deepening insight of the inter-connectedness of all things, being. Presence means allowing the person you are currently pretending-to-be to die, and by default becoming authentic. Tension means "false," relaxation means "real." Presence requires ceasing to try to understand everything and becoming happily comfortable with not knowing, and seeing that you are already who you need to be and that you are already healed. Presence, like healing, is not about achieving something or getting to a certain level, it is coming to terms with your life as it is, right now. Ascended Master Ramana Maharshi stated, "Do not meditate, be, do not think that you are, be, don't think about being, you are." It is not about being good but rather seeing the good that is already in yourself which immediately and simultaneously stops the projecting of the hate in your heart for yourself onto other people which you cannot observe because you are identified with your mind (not present). Presence is an acceptance and complete surrender as your body falls back into being here, no longer craving to be there.

> *"I was gripped by an intense fear, and my body started to shake. I heard the words "resist nothing," as if spoken inside my chest. I could feel myself being sucked into a void... Suddenly there was no more fear, and I let myself fall into that void."*
> — Eckhart Tolle, *The Power of Now, A Guide to Spiritual Enlightenment*[172]

You need to understand that just because you don't believe **hidden rage causes pain**—doesn't mean it isn't true. It has been shown to be true through **repeated observation**. Since denial of the truth is what causes the pain, it is not surprising that you still deny TMS as the cause behind your pain.

Lower your expectations—yield and overcome. You are not having enough fun in your life, which is shown through obsessive body-focus. TMS pain indicates that the demands from life have become greater than the magnitude of happiness being extracted from it. The compulsion of obsessiveness, workaholism, drugs and alcohol is not "having fun." They are numbing agents for emotional pain from prior separation—or lack of connection. The presence of physical pain indicates that joy and appreciation are truant, and that life should be slowed or accelerated—pick it up, or slow it down to rebalance.

15

Conditioning:
The First Cut Is the Deepest

The process of conditioning, or programming, seems to be very important in determining when the person with TMS will have pain. For example, a common complaint of people with low back pain is that it is invariably brought on by sitting. This is such a benign activity one is mystified by the fact that it initiates pain... The brain makes the association between sitting and the presence of pain and that person is now programmed to expect pain while sitting... They (also) have learned to associate activity with pain; they expect it, so it happens. That is conditioning.

— John E. Sarno, MD, *Healing Back Pain*[173]

I found the above statement by Dr. Sarno to be spot-on in my own healing. Whenever I would sit down, the blood would withdraw and the pain would come knocking at my back's door. So it happened that I was in a high-tension state once and had a strike of pain when I sat down. At that moment, I was instantly conditioned to expect pain when I sat, and so it returned every time I did so. Once it's understood that sitting can never cause pain, the brain's conditioned response begins reversing strategy until the tactic no longer works as a distractionary technique.

I began to observe that whenever I moved a certain way or sat or stood a certain way, I was holding that pained area in flexion—contracting my back in a manner that seemed to be protecting that area from further pain, defensively, and unconsciously. Even though the pain was once there, the continuing protection of that area in the form of "tensing it" by the brain is unnecessary and is simply habit. Tensing further reduces bloodflow to the afflicted area leading to permanent and ongoing pain. There must be an unconditioning—a reversal—for healing.

Emotional and psychological pain—in fact all emotional learning—is held in our bodies, recorded on our vast, interrelated neural networks. This is why, when we're scared, anxious, or angry, we have physical reactions like muscle tension, stomach churning, shortness of breath, head pounding, and aching backs.... Until we honestly confront and work through our deeper truths, our bodies will hold us responsible for what we can't "remember."

— Tian Dayton, PhD, *The Neurobiology of Emotions:*
How Therapy Can Repattern Our Limbic System[174]

A common example of this conditioning process is the response to certain medications. The sufferer in pain takes a pain medication and she believes it works. But is she coincidentally having a better day? Or perhaps she lay down to rest after she took it, or her doctor has hyped-up her expectations of it, and her pain eases due to her deep belief, or to good timing. She now believes that this particular medication makes her pain go away. The next time she takes it, it works swiftly because the trigger-conditioning process has been recorded in her neural network—her information highway paved from the first time the information drove it. She has been conditioned to believe that her favorite medication worked the first time, and so it does, every time. She swears by the medication to all of her friends. If it hadn't worked the first time she would not believe in it and would not have taken it again. This is typical. I have seen this conditioning work with ritualistic endeavors such as the use of chondroitin and glucosamine, as well as the Cox-2 inhibitors.

I was conditioned to feel sharp pain whenever I straightened my leg and lifted my toe in the air. The first time I lifted my foot and had pain—voila, the pain ensued each time. Conditioning is immediate and powerful, and it is the process of being continually victimized by your own memory. The same sensory experiences generate the same results, in perpetuity, until new experiences replace existing ones, until the conditioned response has been **repatterned**—an experiential makeover.

> *I am the driver of my memories; memory is not the driver of me.*
> — Ayurveda, Vedanta philosophy sutra by Sharakacharya, *Science of Life*

Deepak Chopra, MD, restated the above as, "I use my memories, but I don't allow my memories to use me." We need memories to function every day, to remember who we are, where we need to go, what we need to do. But old memory patterns can also disable us. There are ways to use memories, and there are ways that memories can use us ...*and the yin chases the yang... as this becomes that....*

Positioning for comfort promotes a conditioned response by binding the pain to the individual like a drug. For over 20 years, whenever I would place a pillow under my right leg, my pain would ease. Once it eased my pain the first time, it always worked. As I look back, I now see how insane it all was. I was conditioned to believe that a 2.934° change in my leg angle was working to keep my hips or spinal discs in line to help stop the pain. It is a silly thought, but the brain runs with suggestions, and for a long time, doctors had been telling me to put a pillow between or under my legs for comfort. They were right; it helped, but only because I believed it did.

This concept is extremely important to understand for recovery. You bend to tie your shoes, you have a back stab: you have now been conditioned. It's like playing yet another game of tag—now you're it. It happens instantly. I've referred to this as "pain's thumbprint" on the brain. Phantom limb pain is very common among amputees. The brain remembers the pain; after all, the brain created the pain defensively from the signals it first received—and memory is born. Now you begin to expect pain because of memory, and the expectations lead to chronicity. Dr. Sarno gave a great example of the silliness of expecting pain from one of his patients. "A woman who could bend over and touch her palms to the floor without pain, told me she always felt pain when she put her shoes on."[175]

A few people have told me that their backs hurt when they tilted their heads forward. I also had this response. It, too, leaves with TMS healing (the pain, that is, not the head) and is a conditioned response.

Conditioned responses can take many forms and are infinite in number. They are similar to triggers. A trigger is more often an event, place, or substance that precipitates the beginning of symptoms, a catalyst that initiates a symptom or set of symptoms. The conditioned response can be considered the brain's **auto-memory** initiated by a trigger.

Robert Scaer, MD, describes in his book, *The Trauma Spectrum: Hidden Wounds and Human Resiliency*, a conditioned response that Robert Tinker, PhD, witnessed while working through an EMDR session with a physically abused woman.[176] As the woman began to consciously recall a traumatic memory with her abusive husband she began to cry; suddenly a handprint appeared on the left side of her face, four fingers of his hand from the slap—a stigmatic reaction. Her **autonomic system reproduced** the trauma as the memory reentered her consciousness—reproducing the original effect of the handprint. This is conditioning.

Ailsa

I had become acquainted with a belle named Ailsa who had written a fascinating synopsis of her journey from being wheelchair-bound due to pain, to full recovery. Her healing journey began after reading Dr. Sarno's *Mindbody Prescription*. Before she had become wheelchair bound and while she was still able to walk, she had been conditioned to believe that she had only one pair of shoes (sandals) that didn't hurt her feet. When she put on any other shoes, or her favorite expensive boots, her feet hurt badly. In her story she writes, "It seems crazy now, but I believed that I only had one pair of shoes that didn't cause damage to my feet. Of course I'd worn them non-stop for three years and they were almost worn out, and I was starting to panic because I couldn't find a replacement.... On reading *The Mindbody Prescription* I suddenly made the connection that this could be association. I went and dug out my shoes. I put them on. Much to my shock I found my heart racing in fear. And my feet hurt a lot." So Ailsa began setting goals and rewarding herself each time she wore her shoes a little longer—to dilute the fear. She acted on her new knowledge and began to reeducate her brain from fallacious admonitions to enlightenment. Today she wears any shoes she wants—walks as long as she wants. Through the knowledge that she could not further harm herself, she healed. She even went back to playing piano, which she had given up due to foot pain. In her words, "...I've been playing the piano without trouble ever since, playing whatever I want. In fact I've just given two ninety-minute concerts in the last couple of months (wearing my boots of course)."

Ailsa's is a beautiful story of the human will to overcome through expanding awareness. Adding to the joy of her recovery, her allergies and asthma of 40 years also disappeared simultaneously. This is not uncommon in tensionalgia healing, since allergies are a conditioned overreactive response triggered by pollens, and other external stimuli. It's also not uncommon for tension sufferers to have their food allergies suddenly disappear along with their pain as conditioning reverses. Fear must be overcome to break any conditioned response.

We place glass ceilings on our own endurance, strength, and abilities. Once those ceilings are removed through knowledge and self-determination, there is an unlimited world to attend to. Why do Olympic athletes narrowly break the world records from the previous year? Why don't they annihilate the previous records? Why does the next generation consistently come along and break the previous records? The answer is clear; **people need benchmarks**. They need to know how far they need to go. Once they know how far they need to go, that is all the further they will go. They won't go any more than they have to, because it takes more of life's precious energy than they're willing to part with. Life is relationship, but energy is life.

> *Patients are usually conditioned to expect pain with physical activity and so they must not challenge the established programmed patterns until they have developed a fair degree of confidence in the diagnosis.... Losing one's fear and resuming normal physical activity is possibly the most important part of the therapeutic process.*
> — John E. Sarno, MD, *Healing Back Pain*[177]

The Dynamic Mindbody

In my own healing, I never considered the mindbody to be an entity, but rather a process. I understood the concept of how persistent thinking patterns yielded persistent mindbody manifestations. In *Body, Mind & Soul*, Chopra speaks of the body renewing itself approximately once a year through cell replacement, as cells continually die off and are replaced by new ones. Thus, the body is essentially an entirely new one about every year or so. Dr. Chopra is often asked, "Why then, do I still have my arthritis and clogged arteries?" It's clear that conditioning patterns, that cycle pain, and other mindbody symptoms are the result of the same ouroboros circle of patterned information, or as Chopra phrased it in *Body, Mind, & Soul*, "Through conditioning, we generate the same impulses of information and energy... which is not merely the same thoughts and feelings, and emotions and ideas, but also the same behaviors, the same dietary habits, the same sensory experience of the world. And as a result of that, we, of course, engender the same states of information and energy that transform themselves into the same biochemical events, the same physiological events, the same behavioral patterns, and ultimately the same outcomes of disease."

This process is identical to chronic and reoccurring pain, whereby the chronicity is incumbent upon the generation of similar quanta of information and energy. Perceptions and realities also change as the perception of the reality changes the reality. Every time you view something, you alter it. The problem is that people aren't viewing or reviewing their lives and so they never change—resulting in the same symptoms. The surgery, injections, drugs, and therapy allow them to continue on their same conditioned paths. So how does one fundamentally change awareness? It happens only through a deeper understanding—by breaking associations. Nothing can grow until something first dies and new soil is broken. I tell people to write left-handed, get out of bed on the other side the next morning, drive a different way to work, etc., etc. Break the daily patterns—change your life!

Cold, rainy, damp weather used to hurt my back and joints. But the weather only acted as a trigger for a conditioned response through my misguided belief. The tightness of a body area that is already held in tension can worsen with constricting weather. Society has collectively agreed that cold and damp rain can actually worsen ailments, and so it often does. One of my pet peeves is now the soft versus hard mattress argument. Pain levels are not correlated to a mattress's flexibility. I tried them all. I can sleep on a bed of nails now and have no pain. I was conditioned to believe that a hard mattress would help me because I was told it would, early on in life. Anyone can sleep on any surface, anytime, without any pain if they are tense-less. Only the firmness of the belief is relevant. But most do not realize it yet because they fear the pain, and have fallen for a false meme. This particular meme needs to be put to sleep.

> Don't be fooled by people telling you that you need to stand a certain way, or lift a certain way, or sit a certain way. I was told that my iliopsoas muscle set was too short on one side and that this was causing my pain. These are fallacious—insidious—misguidances that only propagate and perpetuate pain.

General (George) Pattern

A typical example was a patient who, through compulsive hard work, established a very successful business and became the patriarch and benefactor of his large family. He enjoyed the role but felt the responsibility deeply. Throughout his entire adult life he experienced low back pain, which resisted all attempts at treatment. By the time I saw him, the pain patterns were deeply ingrained and part of his everyday life. He understood the concept of tension-induced pain but was unable to erase the patterns of a lifetime.

— John E. Sarno, MD, *Mind Over Back Pain*[178]

I am a living testimonial that the patterns of a lifetime of pain can be erased and replaced with new impulses of information and energy—if the deep desire is there. Be of great cheer. This man in the above quote was unwilling to change. His refusal to change was his own choice, based on his personal motivations and on his unconscious need for his pain. Change is often more frightening than pain. To challenge familiar patterns was to leave his comfort zone and walk an unknown path. Patterns are conditioning in disguise. The common long-term patterns of my pain had been during post-accomplishment, OR triggered by a new demand. Every time that I had completed a hard-fought goal or raised myself to the next level, at whatever I was doing, pain would appear so that I could recover from the demands that I had earlier placed on myself.

I met a man in the summer of 2006 who sneezed only in multiples of three. He either sneezed three times, or six times, or nine times in a row, never any other combination. It was amazing to witness. The brain loves familiar routes. Old neural pathways are the smoothest, fastest roads on the synaptic highway—formed instantaneously.

The Pop Heard Round the World

She said it began when she was bending over and "felt something snap." This is a common description of onset and invariably suggests to patients that something terrible has happened to their back, though we know in retrospect that this is not the case.
— John E. Sarno, MD, *Mind Over Back Pain*[179]

I sometimes hear popping in my back or knees but think nothing of it anymore. It's some type of ligament movement or synovial fluid expanding and popping across the joint, ligaments, or bones. Who cares? The popping indicates to me that I am under some stress and my tension levels may be elevated, nothing more.

He steps up to the plate, swings the bat, hears a loud "pop"—and falls to the ground. He is taken to the hospital where the MRI shows herniated discs. The herniation may or may not be near the injury site but that won't matter to the physician. The doctor (doctor, defined as "to teach") will teach him that his pain is from those discs. The herniation was most likely preexisting but there was no reason to take images before. Surgery or bed rest or medication or therapy is ordered and he has been further conditioned to believe that his back is now somehow damaged—his spine weak. What he doesn't realize is that he would have healed without the surgery, but he heeds his doctor's advice because he needs time away from his tension-filled arena—the reason for the triggered-response. He then erroneously links the surgery to his healing.

Related to this "popping" phenomenon and a conditioned response is the chiropractic adjustment. When the individual hears and feels the sudden pop and the chiropractor says, "There, that got it!" the brain thinks it was "gotten" and so the brain momentarily relaxes that part held in unconscious tension—from relief and belief. But it was not got. Nothing happened except a sound being made, and with it a positive statement of reinforcement from the chiropractor or osteopath. But the relief rarely lasts because the reason for tension still exists. If a back makes a sound, and there is no doctor to hear it, does it make a pain? Understand—nothing has gone in or out in the spine with an adjustment.

You can't have conditioning without a trigger, something that pulls the brain back to the past; thus, they are triggers (Dutch trekken, defined as "to pull"). The **suggestion process** can take time to integrate, but conditioning occurs instantly. The trigger initiates the conditioned process, so one is incumbent upon the other.

Pain Clinics

Never tell a lie—P.S.—except to keep in practice
— Mark Twain, Mark Twain's Autograph, *Atlanta Constitution*

Show me a chronic pain sufferer who has been helped by a pain clinic, and I will show you a person who is under the direct influence of a placebo. Treating the pain is not an option for healing in the long term. It may sometimes be necessary, however, to bring a sufferer back into balance temporarily with the use of analgesics, anti-inflammatories, increased movement, or through planting the seeds of confidence.

My wife, as a paraplegic, had spent many hours in a local pain clinic. I'm always surprised by how few people realize that people paralyzed from spinal cord injuries are in chronic pain. The paralysis is only one of their many problems which stem mainly from their inability to move around. The spinal cord injury that causes the paralysis often causes pain, but not due to the paralysis itself because those nerves are dead and no longer sending pain signals. The pain emanates from the "edges" of the injury where healthy nerve tissue attempts to communicate with scarred nerve tissue, resulting in unconscious rage from the injury. The body revolts in its attempt to become whole again—mind and body angrily separated by the loss of communication with one another.

The pain clinic physician we were seeing at the time had decided that he should perform an epidural cortisone shot in her spine to help ease her pain. I asked him what his success rate was and he quickly replied, "76.4 percent." Point four percent? The injections didn't alleviate any of her pain. The next few times I spent in that pain clinic's waiting room with Susan, which amounted to about five to six hours "a shot," I began asking the patients if the shots were working on them—all said "no." No one I spoke with had gained relief from the treatments. A nurse who worked at the pain clinic whispered to me after hearing me asking the patients—"they're not helping anyone." I believe that the stats claiming such high rates of success have been injected with steroids.

Another woman who had worked for a pain clinician once told me, "It's clear they aren't helping anyone—and they know they aren't." They are treating the symptoms and not the cause. There is no 76 percent success rate. It is a lie in order to keep in practice. There's now a new fad that claims to alleviate back pain through decompressing the spine with large machines that pull apart the foramina to allow the nerves more room. They are currently advertising success rates in the upper 80 percent range. It is not possible to separate the spinal foramina to ease pain. In fact, it isn't even necessary since the pain is not due to narrowed foramina—even if it was, the machine could not help in any fashion.

> *The idea is to make the holes larger so the nerves won't be "pinched." But we have said before that the idea that they are being pinched is usually fantasy and, once again, there is much ado about nothing.*
>
> — John E. Sarno, MD, *Healing Back Pain*[180]

Pain centers are multiplying rapidly around the US. It's difficult to know how many are in operation because many chiropractors, MDs and massage therapists are simply calling themselves pain clinics. Pain.org estimates there are around 4,000 pain clinics currently in the US. To quote Dr. Sarno, "Pain is, has been, and always will be, a symptom. If it becomes severe and chronic, it is because that which is causing it is severe and has gone unrecognized. Chronicity, in the case of these pain syndromes, is a function of faulty diagnosis."[181]

The best benefits the pain clinic can deliver are analgesics to dull the sharp edge of the most cutting of pains, as the body begins to realign and heal itself. The danger is in the addiction to the avoidance of any buried conflict, and for the desire of the pleasure through analgesia.

> *The pain clinics are a part of the problem. They perpetuate the belief in infirmity. Most of the patients I see who have been to pain clinics are forever lost. They have been so completely conditioned to believe they have a physical/structural problem that they cannot open their minds.*
>
> — Marc Sopher, MD, personal correspondence

The key words here are "perpetuate the belief in infirmity"… and "forever lost."

16

T–Wrecks, The Painful Personali–T

The key word in tension production is personality.
— John E. Sarno, MD, *Mind Over Back Pain*[182]

Everyone carries physiological manifestations of their emotional processes. Emotions generate energy, altering bio-physio-neuro-chemical balances. Individuals' state of health is in large part, the effect or lack of expression of this energy—because of ego. Emotions such as anger and fear or guilt alter the physiology as they respond to id-superego conflict—the stifling of impulses, instincts, and emotions. Other emotions such as love, joy, and happiness also have tremendous healing power through their effect on physiology. The scale below is a graphical representation of emotions and physiology and the T-persona. Note that there is no zero on the scale since all humans naturally generate energy when conflicted.

Emotional Health Scale

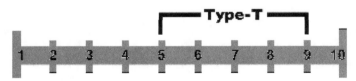

On this scale a 1 indicates that the individual is by and large a non-repressor. She has some worries and therefore, some physical problems, but she moves with balance, she quickly forgives or expresses her concerns—lets them go—and her physical problems quickly dissipate. A 10 is at the other extreme. She is strongly conflicted. She would suffer many emotional and physical problems becoming debilitated to the point of her being unable to function around others without medication and counseling. She may suffer from serious neurosis, psychosis,* schizophrenia, post-traumatic stress disorder, or a host of potentially deadly diseases as a result of her inability to recognize

---

* Neurosis is simply having some emotional issues under stress—a restabilizing of self. These issues would include phobias, perfectionism, anger, low self-esteem, etc.—all within acceptable norms of society. Psychosis is the loss of contact with reality and is outside of any acceptable states of mental health. Dr. Karl Menninger noted that psychotic patients "as a rule enjoy the most robust health"—and when the psychosis began to wane physical health problems returned. [Arnold Hutschnecker, MD, *The Will To Live,* p. 3] So—the Type T are truly grounded—overly-sane people. The neurotic need for the appearance of "normal" is the very thing that generates so many health problems.

or purge any toxic emotions. She doesn't know how to let go of criticism aimed at her. She has an extremely demanding/controlling superego due to residual separation anxiety from childhood. These Ten-ers need in-depth counseling and are genetically or environmentally challenged by sensitivity. I would still consider them as TMSers, but they are beyond the scope of this book—needing complex professional intervention.

Here, I want to identify the specific region on the emotional health scale where the Type T personality resides. The T is characterized by a region somewhere between nine and five. The nine-ers are on the high end of a typical T—often abused, molested, or abandoned, and have experienced early separation trauma. They crave the approval of others, and are **trouble healers**—more unconsciously resistant to change. But they can heal if they desire, and can resist the cravings for modern medical techniques by finding the self-preservation instinct within themselves instead of allowing for the self-destructive instinct to dominate. The five-ers on the scale would have fewer "issues" but would still experience unpleasant symptoms from unconscious anger.

The nine-to-fivers are goodists, hyper-responsible, worriers, empathic, competitive (although many would deny it), and non-confrontational. They fear making mistakes. They possess low self-esteem and high-tension. They function reasonably well in society, for the most part. They have, to varying degrees, repressed anger problems— they unconsciously use pain or a host of other symptoms to control situations that enrage them. They are the perfectionists of the perfectionists. They obsessively poke and push at their pained limbs and joints, hoping the pain will suddenly be worried away.

Perfektionizm: The Child of Sensory Processing Disorder

No one is perfect. Yet many people measure themselves—and others—against impossibly high standards. The result: guilt, anger, depression, and disappointment.
> — Harold S. Kushner, PhD, *How Good Do We Have to Be?*
> *A New Understanding of Guilt and Forgiveness*

Perfectionism is born in childhood along with the first layers of the persona. It can follow the need for parental approval or acceptance that never comes. The child feels that if he becomes more perfect the angst will cease—rendering rejection an impossibility. However, connection (tracordification) doesn't require perfection, nor does perfectionism ensure connection. Perhaps he was praised by parents once when he did something well, and that becomes his modus operandi, for life—to never fail. Children only want their parents to be happy, to stop fighting, to stay together, for everything to be perfect, and to feel secure. To live happily ever after.

Parents/caretakers are everything to the child. Children also need boundaries in order to know that their parents love and care about them. However, the fear of making a mistake for fear of parental reprisal is just as problematic as not having the parent engaged at all in parenting. No matter which scenario, the child still needs security.

Children can sense even low levels of tension in the household, and will often turn inward, relying on perfectionism, fantasy, or TMS to save themselves from deeper heartache. Former actor Michael Landon's daughter, Leslie, became bulimic after Michael made an off-hand remark about her getting fat. This was shortly after Michael had abandoned her and her family and started another one. Leslie, feeling to-blame, began self-punishing bulimic cycles hoping that losing weight would somehow bring her mom and dad back together. But the child who adapts to please parents is becoming something other than what she truly is, and her own conflict is born—leading to obsessive, self-punishing behavior. Eating disorders, drugs, depression, compulsive cleaning or working out, etc., taken to the extreme, are their means of coping with angerziety. They are mechanisms of avoiding our greatest fear: rejection.

Perfektionizm is the dominant behavioral characteristic behind mindbody syndromes. It is a form of neurosis. It is not knowing when to put limits on behavior. How much is enough? When to let go? Is it too little or too much? Am I going to be accepted or rejected? Am I good or good enough? I don't know—so I will continue on my obsessive path to get it right, to avoid that next sting of rejection. It's a hybrid cocktail of low self-esteem and increased narcissism (with a twist of lime).

Me? I'm No Perfectionist! Or is it Perfectionistic?
Or is it Perfectionalistic? No Wait....

There's the occasional individual suffering from tensionalgia who doesn't appear to be perfectionistic. Even their friends or relatives tell me that these individuals don't appear anal or perfectionistic. But people can deceive even themselves. Denial is a fundamental aspect of continuing TMS. We get mad at someone, we smile. This is denial. We are hurt by a criticism, we smile. This, too, is denial. We become so hurt that we become detached, and at times compulsive and repetitive, as rage battles with goodness. Even denial is an avoidance mechanism—a means of control. These people have perfectionistic tendencies, but have never looked or just don't have the self-awareness to sense it. To be a perfectionist doesn't mean to be perfectionistic at everything or in every matter. It is being perfect with those things that matter—during times that matter. The more things that matter to her, the more control she desires, and the more pain or pain equivalents she must experience as a penalty for maintenance of that control.

I Can't Believe My Bad Luck!

I have a difficult school speech to prepare and my lower back has just slipped a disc, and I have a graduation party to plan and my ankle has swollen. And can you believe it, I have to attend a boring PTA meeting and my sinus infection has returned! Now on top of all these things I have to make a doctor's appointment. I have so much to do, so much to control—I don't need all this right now. Deep down I don't want to HAVE to be nice all the time. This is the purpose of the aphorism, *never trust a man who doesn't drink*, because everyone carries a shadow; if his shadow isn't readily apparent, then it is darker than the unthinkable. Truth has already shown throughout history, that if he doesn't possess some type of visible vice or maudlin personality—if he appears as perfect—then he owns an even darker shadow, because everyone has the cravings of his/her undeveloped self, a curiosity for pleasure that must be squashed by the moral superego in order to satisfy and protect others.

Deep within ourselves we already know we are powerful beyond our means, and so we fear this knowledge because of moral-worldly expectations. Our fear of our own power then acts as a boundary, since we already know that once we move beyond our wants and desires, we will become our-Self—no longer needing mortal distractions to contain us. To expose our shadow is to become so powerful that we fear what we may ultimately become, what we despise most, as societal norms have defined. The conflict between allowing our shadow-self to be revealed and also restraining our limitless power is what generates our suffering. It is this fear that keeps us TMSing, anxiety-ridden, OCDing, and failing. We know we are more than we are; so much so, that we fear what we may become, and so we sometimes self-punish and fail—fearing we may be unable to control ourselves. Just take a look at how badly people treat one another across Internet discussions—the hatred, with only the small power of anonymity. Given much more, even unlimited power, we know what we could become—and fear it.

So, physical suffering then serves as punisher for the unthinkable. Our darker side (Thanatos) is somewhat curious and desiring of the ideas of suicide, rape, murder, torture—things of such unimaginable horror to our conscious being that they must be imprisoned in the dark (the body), never allowed to fully develop into a conscious thought. Pain and illness once again arrive to save our day, as we self-inflict wounds that don't meet our conscious codes of morality. Sick pleasures of death wishes and of doing harm to others begin to surface when moral responsibility overwhelms us.

Everyone carries a shadow, and the less it is embodied in the individual's conscious life, the blacker and denser it is…. If you imagine someone who is brave enough to withdraw all his projections… then you get an individual who is conscious of a pretty thick shadow.
— Carl Jung, *Psychology and Religion*[183]

So, Jung means that if you appear squeaky clean on the surface—grounded—watch out for the dirt below! If you can stop for a moment and listen to yourself criticizing, judging other people, ridiculing them, nit-picking their looks, traits, and lives—you will see it is YOU who has the problem. Then you need to begin to understand why you need to do and say these things—eventually seeing in yourself a very dense shadow.

An example of a **shadow eruption** would be Winona Rider, the wealthy and famous actress caught shoplifting $5000 of items at Saks Fifth Avenue in Beverly Hills. She could have easily purchased the items, but she needed to satisfy a deeper need that had gone unattended. Shadows often erupt at the most embarrassing times, which are always problematic for ego. However, these eruptions have a balancing effect between the conscious and the unconscious, and the ego and the shadow. The shadow eruption can be thought of as emotional purging—once over, you feel so much better because containing what was within was so poisonous to the spirit. An eruption reveals the repressed or darker desires of the true person, the chink in his armor of persona that suddenly bursts through to consciousness—an act that reveals a small part of what he truly desires. People who don't think New York Governor Elliot Spitzer wanted to get caught in a prostitution ring don't understand shadows or shadow-work. Tiger Woods also proves Jung to be correct in that the less the shadow is embodied in the conscious life, the denser it is. Tiger's squeaky-clean persona had created an even darker shadow because it wasn't readily apparent in his daily life.

We all carry a shadow. This is important to understanding TMS for two reasons. First, the individual is not as "perfect" or "good" as she thinks she is, and second, it is normally more important to understand WHY she has repressed something than it is to know what she has repressed. We have to repress—but why do we repress certain things is the more relevant question. If you can answer this you can understand the person.

> *Sometimes the source of the tension is not obvious. I recall a young married woman who reacted to the diagnosis of TMS with great surprise. She denied being tense or nervous and said that she was not particularly conscientious or compulsive. The friend who accompanied her confirmed this and said she was known to be a very jolly, easygoing person. Only after a long discussion did she reveal that her strategy for coping with life's problems was to put them out of her mind. She simply would not allow anything to bother her.*
> — John E. Sarno, MD, *Mind Over Back Pain*[184]

The key words here were, "Only after a long discussion." Superego can be very controlling.

I've had people tell me that they aren't worriers. But in deeper discussion with them, it's obvious that they worry so much that they have fallen for a false image of themselves. They are often procrastinators, and the first to fall asleep at night. Sleep is their way of coping; they hide behind the sheep while the Type T counts the sheep all night *...and the yin chases the yang... as this becomes that....*

I once had a conversation with my neighbor and back pain sufferer extraordinaire, who at first denied being perfectionistic. But after a few minutes he admitted that after raking leaves in the yard, he couldn't stand it if he saw one leaf blow back into the yard.

It is sometimes difficult to define who a perfectionist is, since to avoid rejection, people may simply avoid life's problems by pretending they don't exist.

Intellectualizing means independence from emotion. Nine-to-fivers often justify away feelings; in doing so, they distance themselves so far from their emotions that they eventually no longer experience the magnitude of their emotions, except through bodily symptoms—substituting intellect for instinct, emptiness for happiness—lost in intellect, they are neither happy nor sad, only emotionally constipated. The body takes the heat for trying to appear cool. The pain or illness is the messenger. Don't kill the messenger; invite him or her in for an intimate conversation.

The T Is Good Enough—Sometimes to Self-Detriment

All TMSers are of Type T—not all Ts are TMSing.

The TMSers evidence a number of qualities, some of which would normally be healthy and admirable, but to the TMSer they can develop to a point of self-detriment.

- The TMSer can be very honest, to a point of self-detriment.
- The TMSer is very conscientious, to a point of self-detriment.
- The TMSer is very loyal, to her self-detriment.
- The TMSer is never happy, to his self-detriment.
- The TMSer avoids confrontation, to her self-detriment.
- The TMSer pushes himself, to his own detriment.
- The TMSer always feels like an outsider.
- The TMSer is a loner at heart, even though he enjoys company—he still prefers being alone.*
- The T-wreck is more often very private, most likely due to low self-esteem and for the desire to avoid overstimulation. There is a big giant beast in all of us. Those who won't admit to it, or can't recognize it, often suffer physical problems because their energy is tied up in the struggle to hide the beast within, to appear "perfect."

Key Characteristics of the T

The Type T personality can be characterized as an **absorption personality**. They often take on the problems, emotions, and dreams of others, in order to get along, go along, and belong. Their intention is not to mislead. They are actually too committed, afraid to take that chance. They use rationale to control the situation, and while others

---

* Being a loner or desiring privacy doesn't mean that the person is not well-adjusted or is unhealthy. Some people just prefer to protect (and enjoy) their sensitivity or to simply be alone with their thoughts and be under-stimulated. They may enjoy the opportunity to be alone for creativity and to seek deeper awareness. It can be normal and healthy behavior, but it can also reveal a deeper need.

are off saying and doing what they wish, the TMSer is holding down the fort. An absorbing personality survives by taking on any persona as a chameleon absorbs its surroundings in order to fit in. The problem is that attempted maintenance of emotional homeostasis is paid for by a physical non-homeostasis.

At a party, the T will be the one enjoying herself with one eye on the door. She needs and wants people close to her, but not in her face—proxemic space delivered in moderate portions. Her own pace is her means of controlling the rate of her absorption of external stimuli.

The TMSer can also be **overly social** to the point of obsequiousness as the dire need to be accepted dominates truest desire—stifled by a repressive superego— adapting to feel the emotions of others as substitutes for their own emotions. The chronicity of symptoms reveals the inner turmoil, as low self-esteem is born from the sense that others' opinions are more worthy to embrace.

TMSers can be highly **empathic**—acutely aware of their surroundings and how others feel at any moment in time. It may sound odd, but people often begin to despise the people they depend on because codependency is threatening to ego. Ego does not like needing people and so our first reaction is often to get mad at those taking care of us because we can sense the demand we place on them. Thus the Type T rarely asks for help, since they're normally too busy giving it.

The TMSer is driven to achieve and unable to relax. Relaxation is a puzzle to Mr. T—I pity the fool unable to achieve a relaxed state of mind and body. He may sit and watch television, but it is lost time to him. Chronic guilt and mental goals (tyrannical shoulds) keep him going from morning till night. If a goal is achieved, he feels empty because he feels he can always do more. If the goals become overwhelming he can become gridlocked, unable to accomplish even the smallest of goals. If he nears his goal, he may stop short of achieving it for the initiation of yet another goal. Closure is death to him, because there will be unwanted time for reflection. He stays busy as an avoidance mechanism.

In his ever-evolving life, perfectionist and Type T, ThoMaS Jefferson never finished the construction phases of Monticello, continuously overlapping new projects as others neared the end—for over 40 years. Monticello was symbolic of his personality and of his inability to ever be satisfied—never able to accept relaxation or closure; it is a phobia of resolution because if completed, the underlying motivational forces must finally be confronted (Dr. Sarno referred to this type of person who starts toward another goal before the first one is reached as an ultra-perfectionist). Contentment to a TMSer is viewed as failure, since, in his mind, more can be done and "time wastes too fast." Jefferson often regretted socializing and wasting time early in his college career at William and Mary and vowed to never let it happen again, eventually becoming a "miser" of his time due to earlier guilt from having fun in his life. As Dr. Sarno wrote, "TMS occurs because they cope too well." Those who have healed care less about details and criticism. They care, "but not that much." Once the anchor is raised, the ship can sail freely. But the anchor can be so deeply buried under the unconscious waters that it dare not be raised for fear of moving forward.

It's rare to find a chronic pain sufferer who doesn't feel disenfranchised by life somehow. It's also extremely difficult to love someone who doesn't feel they deserve to be loved and so a Type T can be difficult to love—thus they often find themselves alone, or lonely.

They more often feel undeserving—believing they will have to pay later for present happiness, so they often shun joy. American Civil War General Stonewall Jackson was a poster child for TMS who always felt that current happiness had a price tag. In a letter to his wife he told her not to love their baby "too much," fearing that something bad would then be needed to offset the additional love. Jackson suffered from a multitude of TMS mindbody manifestations—holding false notions—afraid of the revenge of happiness—fearing balance would need to be restored through tragedy.* This is very common among the Mr. and Mrs. Ts. They expect happiness to be taken from them, and so they accept anxiety where serenity could be. They move ahead of the light instead of basking in its brilliance, imagining the fall that will follow the current climb.

Many T-personalities have told me that their parents were very austere or indifferent, even though their parents took good care of them. Often one or both parents were not tender or touchy-lovey with warmth. They were rather stoic, phlegmatic, or undemonstrative; more inclined to protection, discipline and rule and following the lead of others than tending to gentle kindness and compassion. A man who once suffered severe back pain as well as other TMS equivalents, pre-Sarno, told me his mother's friend told him, "Your mother was a good woman, too bad she didn't like children." It should be reiterated that of all the needs that the child might have, lack of **touch** is the most painful, leading to stunted emotional growth. The security of touch and human contact outweighs the need for words and deeds, as seen in the emotional deprivation exhibited in psychogenic dwarfism or in feral children.

The TMSer's parents invariably had a parent or parents who suffered symptoms. Their parents' parents had low self-esteem, may have been highly critical, negative-thinking worriers. Their parents' parents also feared, and were also perfectionists and untouched by the loving warmth that they too yearned for. The cycle continues until someone does the work required to heal—esteem is restored—the cycle is broken and a new cycle begins in a higher plane of consciousness.

TMSers feel a deep need to be cared for and for things to go perfectly. Ironically, due to their responsible nature, they often end up taking care of others instead. The inner-child then rebels—showered by the storm of conflict.

The T takes everything personally, but hides the fact—pretending it didn't hurt, generating tremendous potential energy, and ANS problems.

---

* General Thomas "Stonewall" Jackson was a hypochondriac—often riding into battle with one arm raised above his head because he felt it balanced out the blood in his body.

In the end, it is the false personas that drain the most energy, and so generate the most rage—producing the most chronic of symptoms. The covering up of true identity is most enraging because it demands more of what we are not, and reveals less of what we truly are. Acknowledging she has needs makes her feel vulnerable to an outside world, and so her needs are buried in her body—to be exhumed at a later date when opportunity arises.

What Drives the Model—T

Narcissism, **goodism** and **perfectionism** are the primary character traits driving the T-persona.

Narcissism—is the love of one's self; everyone has narcissistic characteristics. When narcissism coexists with stunted self-esteem, it creates conflict. Malignant narcissism is the inability to feel the pain of others, and is most often observed in people who have never been down and out—the "golden spooners."

Goodism—is the unattainable desire to do "what is right" all the time, never ceasing.

Perfectionism—is the need to never fail in the eyes of others—demanding energy for the persona and unwanted responsibility.

The Introverted

The overwhelming personality type of the TMS sufferer is the introvert. You could look at former TMS sufferer, entertainer Howard Stern, and say that this personality type doesn't hold true. But a deeper look will reveal that it does. The word personality derives from the persona, which translates as "mask," not only for how we would like to be perceived by the world, but also by what we would like to hide from the world. Howard hides behind a mask of obsessive extraversion, but I don't believe what he reveals to the public is his truest self. This was illustrated by the existence of severe TMS in him. A peek at his autobiographical movie, *Private Parts*, is further evidence of the man behind the mask. Howard found Dr. Sarno and was open-minded enough to see himself as he truly is, and healed; his parts no longer private.

Therefore, introversion is often masked by extraversion. The late Robin Williams is a tragic example. Conflict needs to be buried which is sometimes accomplished through extraversion, a way of openly coping with anxiety—a TMS equivalent. Introverts are defined through the process of personal revelations. They remain aloof and are not nourished in the external environment around them. Thus, through their personal revelations, according to Jung, "crowds, majority views, public opinion, popular enthusiasm, never convince him of anything but merely make him creep still deeper into his shell."[185] The typical TMSer avoids cacophonous situations. The super-TMSer extrovertly masks the fear by actually becoming the noise *...and the yin chases the yang... as this becomes that....*

The Type T Can Be a Stubborn Mule

Marc Sopher, MD, believes that faster healers are more easily able to uproot old patterns and beliefs and replace them with newer ones. They "get it" more quickly and are able to reprogram their minds more swiftly than others. Long protracted periods without healing can indicate a fear of lifting the mask to reveal what is underneath. This inner stubbornness is often accompanied by tinnitus. I was astounded at how high the correlation between slow healing and complaints of tinnitus was when first communicating with tensionalgia sufferers. Years after talking with many of these people I found a book called *You Can Heal Your Life*, by Louise L. Hay, which displays a list (taken from her book, *Heal Your Body*) of correlations between dis-eases and probable causes. In that list under tinnitus she cites, "Refusal to listen. Not hearing the inner voice. Stubbornness." Louise Hay must be listening to the people she works with. The slowest healing TMSers are stubbornly resistant to accepting new belief systems, extremely recalcitrant to change as to how they see themselves—only partially accepting TMS—clinging to drugs and other excuses for their continuing symptoms. They hold strongly to their own ideas of what is wrong with them—their own concepts of healing and perfection. But imperfection is the only thing that brings us deeper consciousness, as Jung wrote, "There is no light without shadow and no psychic wholeness without imperfection."[186]

The Perfection Disconnection

As long as the detached person can keep at a distance he feels comparatively safe.
— Karen Horney, MD[187]

One of the more common threads woven into the fabric of those who have the T personality, leading to perfectionism, is that as young children they were taught it was bad to show anger. They were told that it was not good, and so to be good they developed a method of hiding anger inside the body in compliance—and the foundation for the persona is laid. But if she knows she isn't being true to herself, she may cope by becoming detached—which also detaches her anger—containing its expression. A famous example of this is the late Princess Diana of Wales, described by historians and biographers as an American woman trying to live for England. The unhappiness behind her beautiful mask was becoming more evident, as her true self began struggling with her persona. To grow is to shed the mask that was once worn in order to please others, as the wrong assumptions come from a right person. In attempting to infinitely please, the TMSer finds herself feeling alone.

Be good and you will be lonesome.
— Mark Twain, *Following the Equator*

17

Goodist-itus—Inflammation of the Low Esteem

When a person doesn't really know who he is, a major portion of his life's energy usually ends up going into a struggle to be what he thinks he ought to be. The unfortunate result is that he gets ever further from discovering his true self. The more he makes himself like someone or something outside of himself, the more dissatisfied he's going to be deep within. This dissatisfaction in turn drives him on to even greater efforts, taking him even further away from that which could ultimately bring fulfillment; the honest expression of who he truly is. This is the kind of vicious circle so many of us are caught in. In fact, this can never set you free; it can only enslave you, because you are dependent on their responses, on their behavior. To feel that someone, or their behavior, is necessary for your happiness, for your here-and-now contentment, for your acceptance of the world, is to feel, and in fact—to be helpless.

— Emmett Miller, MD, *I Am*

Dr. Miller has been a pioneer in the field of mindbody healing, and continues to this day. Early in his career, he learned that in order to best assist people in their healing, he needed to move beyond techno-medicine and reach into their hearts and minds. I was intrigued when I first heard his words above because they are in essence the context of this book. The concept is rooted in Jung's work on the human psyche in his Principle of Equivalence and in humanistic psychology: when we're not being ourselves, more energy gets poured into our shadows, draining us of our potential—increasing anxiety—ingraining helplessness.

Dependabili—T

To feel that living for someone else can somehow yield an advantage has been classified as low self-esteem. Some Ts tend to let themselves be used by others since they don't have the control over their anger to say no. She implicitly knows she must say yes to bury her disdain and fury. Type Ts are normally highly dependable, which infuriates them, as undependable people use them in order to conserve their own time and energy.

Paradoxically, there are the extreme Type Ts who refuse to submit to guidelines or time frames or schedules. They do their best to remain undependable to avoid being asked to help. These people are socially challenged—they don't know how to deal with people. They refute everything asked of them, or told to them. They run from life, never committing, never helping, always wondering what's behind Door Number 2—often hiding extreme sensitivity and impatience with drugs, alcohol, and cigarettes.

The classic TMSer is not an anti-socialite, nor is his behavior pathological. TMS is, however, a close cousin to obsessive-compulsive disorder (on the mother's side). With anti-social disorder, people will tend to blame others for their own behavior— lashing out—releasing their frustrations and anger onto society. The classic TMSer, contrarily, will blame self and take the appropriate measures to teach self a lesson by feeling guilt where none is appropriate.

Emotional health is based on the strength of personal relationships. Knowing when to take a stand in relationship, when to draw boundaries, when to yield and when to change—knowing when good is good enough—are all important to understanding that being accepted is not that important in life. You're not adding any value in this world if you aren't making enemies. The Type T will tend to wait for someone else to tell him how much is enough—or good enough. The non-T says, "That's it—good enough," and he stops what he's doing. The T says, "Where are you going, this horse is still alive, keep beating!" There's always more to do.

Please, Won't You Be—My Neighbor?

The compliant type will be prone to overrate his congeniality and the interests he has in common with those around him... he becomes sensitive to the needs of others.... He becomes compliant, overconsiderate—within the limits possible for him— overappreciative, overgrateful, generous. He blinds himself to the fact that in his heart of hearts he does not care much for others and tends to regard them as hypocritical and self-seeking.

— Karen Horney, MD, *Our Inner Conflicts*[188]

In the Seinfeld episode, "The Masseuse," George Costanza is irritated by the fact that Jerry's girlfriend doesn't like him.

George: She didn't like me?

Jerry: Look, it's not like you're going to be spending a lot of time with her.

George: So she doesn't like me?

Jerry: No.

George: She said that?

Jerry: Yes.

George: She told you she doesn't like me?

Jerry: Yes.

George: What were her exact words?....

Jerry: [interrupting] I don't like him.

George: Uh-huh. Why didn't she like me?

Jerry: Not everybody likes everybody!

(George, the goodist to the end.)

Karen: What difference does it make? Who cares if she doesn't like you? Does everybody in the world have to like you?

George: Yes! Yes! Everybody has to like me. I must be liked!!

As I have said, people who tend to get TMS tend to be hardworking, hyper-responsible, conscientious, ambitious and achieving, all of which build up the pressure on the beleaguered self.

— John E. Sarno, MD, *Healing Back Pain*[189]

I have labeled TMS the **smiling disease** because the attempt to appease the unappeasable only serves to anger the already beleaguered self. Hiding steadfast behind a despised persona creates imbalance—or TMS.

He tries automatically to live up to the expectations of others… often to the extent of losing sight of his own feelings. He becomes "unselfish," self-sacrificing, undemanding—except for his unbounded desire for affection.

— Karen Horney, MD, *Our Inner Conflicts*[190]

Trying to be too nice—all things to all people—is a self-denial that sends increased energy into the shadow. To deny that one has been sexually molested, abused, or abandoned, and that there is no hatred toward the one who did these things gives great power to the shadowy complex. To deny that one hates his job or spouse or life has a shadow-building effect. The denial is a **complex** or a formational cluster of pent-up thoughts and feelings. Each time you say to yourself or to others that your life is going exactly as you had planned, when deep inside you know it is not, energy is sent to the shadow—manifesting either mentally as in nightmares or schizophrenia or physically as in TMS, or worse. People in great pain often tell me that their lives are great! But a little probing beneath the surface brings tears, then deep sobbing, as their shadows break down in the light of truth. They begin to heal through the therapy of knowledge.

Facing the T—ruth Can Burn Like Holy Water

I know a man whose wife left him and his child, to be with someone else. He was unemployed, and struggling to raise his kid alone. He was on several anti-depressant medications. When I told him that he could not be happy, he bluntly told me, "My life is great, it came out exactly how I had planned it." He was soon in surgery having his discs carved out of his back to stop the pain and paralytic episodes. It failed, of course.

In *Mindbody Prescription*, Dr. Sarno tells the story of Helen who was bedridden, "paralyzed with pain," as her shadow began to possess her. At 47, she had remembered being molested by her father, and joined an incest support group to try to heal her wounds. As she entered the support group her symptoms began to worsen (the TMS exorcism). She couldn't understand why she was getting worse but her husband insightfully pointed out "You're talking about forty years of repressed anger." His words suddenly triggered an emotional catharsis (the compassion trigger) as she cried harder than she had ever cried in her life, as she described, "out of control tears." She began blurting out words such as "let me die," "I feel sick," "I'm so afraid," "please take care of me." Her shadow began to fade in the light of truth. She described her pain leaving her like a pipeline from her lower back through her eyes, pouring out of her. Her pain initially began to increase—as it often does—to prevent certain emotions from entering consciousness. In the end, the truth set her free as her pain had no more purpose, since it only existed to suppress the denial of her fury.

> As I cried, I was that child again and I recognized the feelings I have felt all my life which I thought were crazy or at the very best, bizarre. Maybe I removed myself from my body and never even allowed myself to feel when I was young. But the feelings were there and they poured over me and out of me... I knew—really knew—that what I was feeling at that moment was what I felt as a child,* when no one would or could take care of me... the shame, the horror.

> — Helen, *The Mindbody Prescription*[191]

Raw, self-honesty is essential for recovery. But, the persona holds strongly to deeply held views that "things are all ok" and "I am appearing perfect." This is not saying that TMSers feel they are perfect; on the contrary, they never feel good enough.

We Are Both Light and Dark

Those truly free in spirit are the happiest and healthiest individuals. They understand they have opposing forces within, and that they aren't perfect. We normally don't notice our shadows because we don't look for something that we don't want to find, and it's difficult to find things that are deeply hidden.

The free-in-spirit understands opposites exist within them from black to white, love to fear, anima to animos. They have Split the Adam. We are therefore defined by what we do know, our conscious-light, (Latin, conscio, "I know") but even more so by what we don't know, our unconscious-dark, (Latin, un-conscio, "I don't know").

On the ABC *20/20* show, "Dr. Sarno's Cure," an attorney whose MRI showed he had seven herniated discs admitted that his back pain dominated his life. John Stossel said to him, "I notice you're in pain but you're smiling." The attorney answered, "Anybody who knows me says I'm always smiling, even if I'm in pain, I'm smiling." Self knows deep inside that there exists deeper feelings of conflict, but the ego stands between the light of true self and the wall of persona, casting a shadow. If fake-niceness rules, then there must be an equal counterbalance—and that counterbalance is pure

---

* The McKenzie **Two-Trauma Mechanism** discussed in more detail later.

rage. The opposing psychic force to feigned niceness is blinding rage which happens to be the root of TMS pain, and most likely all illness. So, life is a constant dance for balance between intellectualization and feeling—repression and expression.

Dr. Sarno wrote of the mother who stopped her child from throwing a temper tantrum by tossing cold water in his face. But what the mother doesn't know is that she immediately conditioned her child to repress rage. This can result in a life of chronic suffering if the child never learns how to express anger again—automatically casting it into his body.

I found no correlation among Type T individuals as far as political or religious ideologies. All races, religions, and ethnicities share the same life. However, those that were further toward one end of an ideological spectrum were the ones who were healing the most slowly, or not at all. Those who were more ready to see both sides of the issues tended to be healing at steadier rates. Those rigid in their own positions—seeing everyone else as wrong—suffered the most.*

---

* I noted a disproportionately high number of TMS sufferers were agnostic or atheist. But most of them also healed with TMS healing.

18

T n A—Major Personality Types and Health

With one lecture, Sarno cured me of 20 years of back pain. It's so embarrassing; I can't believe I'm telling you about this. But apparently, I didn't have a back problem, I have a personality problem.

— John Stossel, "Dr. Sarno's Cure"

The Type A and Type B personalities were introduced in 1960 by San Francisco cardiologists, Meyer Friedman and Ray Rosenman. The Type T is a quasi-combination of personalities A and B.

The Type A is characterized as being:
Belligerent—aggressive outward expression of self
Impatient—time is his enemy; no patience for patience
Tempestuous—constantly agitated and tumultuous
Competitive—aggressive assertion of self, arrogant
Hostile—externalizes self at the cost of others

The Type B is characterized as being:
Reasoned—thinkers, more creative and imaginative
Easygoing—patience, even under strain
Less ambitious—lets life unfold as it will
Accommodating—friendly and generous
Cooperative—works well with others
Kicked-back—carefree
Sangfroid—unflappable under stress

Friedman and Rosenman became medical icons when they identified the Type **A personality** as having an extremely high correlation with heart disease. Early on, an astute secretary of theirs noted that "those with coronary disease were rarely late for appointments and preferred to sit in hard, upholstered chairs rather than softer ones or sofas. These chairs also had to be reupholstered far more often than others because the front edges quickly became worn out. They looked at their watches frequently and acted impatient when they had to wait, usually sat on the edges of waiting room chairs, and tended to leap up when called to be examined."[192]

Dr. Rosenman also indicated that the Type A had an "unusual preoccupation with time."[193] They have a compulsion to accomplish as many tasks as possible in the shortest amount of time (workaholics).

Aristotle once stated that the heart was the center of all emotions. Indeed, emotions are felt in the heart, not the brain. It's easy to understand why the Type A would have heartaches powerful enough to damage the precious pumping system. The rage-filled A personality treats time as an enemy, and for this skewed perception ultimately pays a higher price at the pump.

The following is a memo found on the desk of a Type A man who suffered a fatal heart attack while rushing to catch a train that day.

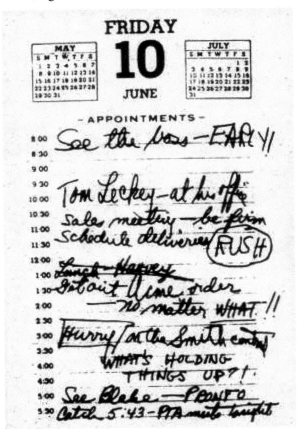

American Institute of Stress [reprinted with permission]

More recently, a third type of TMS-prone individual has been identified that can be considered to be a Type AB—a blend of the A and B—labeled the **Type T**, or **T(e)**. The T is prone to chronic pain, fatigue, digestive tract problems, skin problems, and anything else that may be in vogue. (See Appendix A).

> **The Type T is characterized as being:**
> Narcissistic—the love of life and self
> Internalizing—automatic repression of things that don't go perfectly
> Controlled—uses control, creating conflict and by default, creativity
> Easy Outward Appearance—hides true feelings from self and those around
> her; smiles through her pain

Joe-T internalizes anger like Joe-A. But Joe-T has been taught to be good and that complaining and showing anger is a bad thing. He has never learned to express anger appropriately; he suffers from terminal niceness dis-order. Ts are do-gooders who often come from households that adhere to a strict regimen: lack of affection, and religious doctrine with accompanying threats of eternal punishment.

Both A and T personalities suffer from anger overload. However, Type A is extraverted, publicly proclaiming self, where Type T turns inward to bury the proclaiming of self. "A" forcefully moves forward, "T" politely pulls back. In *Healing Back Pain*, Dr. Sarno writes that many Ts describe themselves as Type As, but it is evident that the Type A is more hostile, while the T feels the need to be gentle, "accommodating and helpful."[194]

As always in life, there aren't always distinct lines of demarcation. There are Type As with chronic back pain that meander over into Type T territories, and Type Ts who have heart problems. These wanderers I have identified as **Special Tease.** These Special Tease are arrogant, overbearing, bitchy, and self-centered. They purposefully criticize others, hoping for retaliation, which will assure they are being heard—their need for attention unparalleled. Their egos dominate everyone else's lives. They are intentional agitators. They aren't quite whole Ts—they're closer to A-wholes.

Both the T and A are competitive. Perhaps competitiveness is their way of proving self to others, of being heard *...and the yin chases the yang... as this is already that....*

The Type A has an unusually high rate of coronary disease; the T a high pain rate and a lower rate of coronary artery disease.[195] Perhaps it's merely the degree of anger that is held since it is healthier to get things off one's chest? If this reigns true then the Type A should have the healthiest hearts among us. But they don't. One can only wonder what anger lies underneath, compared to that which is seen. I believe the differences in symptomologies lie in **where** we store our anger. Also, each of us responds differently to how we observe others around us who are struggling with their own symptoms (memetics or contagion). Deepening awareness may alter the predisposed physical state by telling the cells what they should do, as they act more like programmable computer chips than predestined entities.* We can change much about our physical destinies. This is a fact, as proven by TMS healing, as well as by the results seen from guided imagery and learned relaxation.

Also interesting is the difference in personalities' breathing patterns, since the rhythm of breathing is an emotional expression. In an interview for the American Institute of Stress, Dr. Rosenman described the Type A as having "unusual breathing patterns"[196] in that they take in too much air and tend to let it out in the middle or end of speaking pauses, in the form of sighs. I have seen this type of "A-breathing"—it looks like a blowfish out of water. This is in direct opposition to the Ts who are breath holders—exhibiting frozen breathing. Ts tend to be shallow breathers, taking in too little amounts of air, and repressing emotions, along with the breath.

> As Dr. Sarno has shown, you do not need to change your personality to heal. The understanding of the TMS process and full belief are all that are normally needed to heal, but not always. Sometimes your life needs to be dissected and specific memories discharged to heal.

Tyranny of the Shoulds

This is where tension often comes from: the battle that goes on in the subconscious part of the mind between the "should" and the "don't give a damns."... One of the worst aspects of TMS is that the process seems to be self-generating.
— John E. Sarno, MD, *Mind Over Back Pain*[197]

I should be calling this person, I should have spent more time with that person, I should have told that person off, I should be exercising more, I should have gone to school, I should have stopped eating, I should have visited them, I should really stop worrying, I should stop thinking that I should stop worrying, I shouldn't be worrying about stopping thinking about worrying, or should I? Pssst... deep within, I already don't care at all—but I know I should.

Twentieth century psychoanalyst, Karen Horney, felt that these inner shoulds prevented the individual from ever achieving self-actualization. She referred to this simultaneous behavior of "pretending to be perfect and hating themselves" as a battle of the tyranny of the shoulds, which taken to the extreme, becomes neurotic behavior.[198] This conflict-of-the-shoulds adds to the anxiety—making symptoms worse.

---

* "Simply stated, there is no cancer gene; illness is not inherited. Rather, cells become cancerous because they were told to do so. Fear is often the operative that drives such instruction." [Cathy Sherman, *The Mind-Body Connection: Fear Manifests in Many Diseases*]

Introverted iNtuitive Feeling Perceiving

The closest personality-type to that of the Type T would be the INFP—Introverted iNtuitive Feeling Perceiving. The TMSer can fall into any "type" but the more common symptom sufferers are the INFPs—the idealists. Generally:

- Hard-driven perfectionists with extremely high standards.
- Do not relax well.
- Tend to avoid conflict.
- Often unaware of their own needs.
- Reticent in expressing their emotions.
- Genuinely care for other people and are good listeners.
- Excellent problem solvers.
- Make loyal friends to others as confidants with true compassion.
- Their main goal in life is to make the world a better place.

These people are idealistic, self-sacrificing, and somewhat cool or reserved. They are very family and home oriented, but don't relax well. You find them in psychology, architecture, and religion, but never in business.

— C. George Boeree, PhD[199]

As I mentioned earlier, a common complaint of severe symptom sufferers is that they put their own lives and dreams on hold for those around them in a silent and controlled manner. Those who are being taken care of just "expected" to be taken care of—never acknowledging the sacrifices made for them.

The Quest for the Holy Detail

Our life is frittered away by detail…. Simplicity, simplicity, simplicity.
— Henry David Thoreau, transcendentalist,
Where I Lived and What I Lived For (1817-1862)

The classic TMSer has an unparalleled thirst for information. They are information junkies. They would be happiest if they could just plug an Internet connection into their jugular vein and Google everything. It's a classic survival response.

ThoMaS Jefferson is once again a paragon of the perfectionistic personality. His thirst for detail and the suffering of mindbody disorders that he brought upon himself is recorded in history. He maintained a perfect outward image for all to see—he is described by historians as having walked perfectly upright with arms folded neatly across his chest. He showed no emotion, and when he spoke, it was so softly that people could barely hear him. He was a highly sensitive redhead with a speech impediment that may have made him self-conscious. When his wife died, he burned all the letters they had written between them, leaving nothing for history to see of his private side. At times he would have 20 open books lying around his desk and floor, always needing to know and understand more, and yet he remained hidden and private. Jefferson was the founding father of modern perfectionism and he endured many psychosomatic manifestations as he hid his personal pain behind "monticellos" of intellect and achievement. He was stoic, goal-driven, and a hyper-achiever. Even though he only helped found one nation, it ended up a pretty good nation.

> *Thomas Jefferson was a shadow man... his character was like the great rivers whose bottoms we cannot see, and make no noise.*
> — President John Adams, old family letter to Biddle

Learning how to stop looking for **all** the answers is one of many keys to healing. Over-intellectualization is a declaration of independence from emotions. Therefore, through diminishing returns, the quest for more knowledge beyond what is needed is, in itself, TMSing—and slows deeper understanding.

> *Many people try to accumulate knowledge, and one day they may realize that the knowledge they possess has become an obstacle to their understanding.... If you are not ready to let go of your knowledge, you cannot get deeper knowledge of the same thing.*
> — Thich Nhat Hanh, *Going Home, Jesus and Buddha as Brothers*[200]

19

Separation and Rage at 26 Months

A child's life is like a blank piece of paper where everyone leaves a mark.

— Chinese proverb

Now—where do anxiety, depression, neurosis, anger, and perfection originate? The deepest patterns of conditioning occur very early in life. Psychiatrist Clancy McKenzie's extensive research has shown that, "Early separations and early trauma—when the infant is most helpless—sets the stage for enormous rage later in life." He continues, "99 percent of trauma that I identified had one common denominator: physical or emotional separation from the mother, as experienced by the infant." Separation (rejection) at any age can have a profound impact, but the earlier in the brain development the more intense the rage because of helplessness. According to Dr. McKenzie's findings, the peak age of origin of the most intense self-condemnation and depression is 26 months.

German-born psychoanalyst, Karen Horney, developed a crush on her own brother at age nine. His rejection of her "…led to her first bout with depression—a problem that would plague her the rest of her life."[201] Karen's rejection by her brother left her feeling unattractive; this along with other personal problems led her into the study of psychoanalysis—her main focus, the study of neurosis. While she fought depression throughout her life, Karen's anger from rejection had directed her towards a meaningful career.

Those who feel they were never abandoned must look closer. They were born and so were abandoned. More generally, according to McKenzie, abandonment can be interpreted in many different ways by a child, but it always results in separation anxiety and guilt. He writes, "Thus the human infant is very sensitive and can be terrified or overwhelmed by what it experiences as a threat of separation from its mother. Not just the obvious separations such as the mother dying, but subtle ones such as the family moving to a new house, the birth of a sibling, or an older child getting sick and requiring all the mother's attention for a period of time. And if there are five older siblings there is five times the chance of this happening. There are literally thousands of events that can cause the infant to experience a separation trauma and feel threatened—by physical OR emotional separation."

*A child in its greed for love does not enjoy having to share the affection of its parents with
its brothers and sisters; and it notices that the whole of their affection is lavished upon it
once more whenever it arouses their anxiety by falling ill. It has now discovered a means
of enticing out its parents' love and will make use of that means as soon as it has the
necessary psychical material at its disposal for producing an illness.*
      — Sigmund Freud, *Dora: An Analysis of a Case of Hysteria* [202]

An intensive study by Dr. McKenzie* included 9,000 patients who exhibited some
form of schizophrenia, post-traumatic stress disorder, or separation trauma. This
study revealed that a perceived abandonment at any point in life will cause the
individual to revert back in her mind to the very first traumatic separation—AND—
the earlier the first trauma, the greater the panic and anger generated when perceived
abandonment occurs again. In a "normal" individual, a traumatic flashback may
return to an early separation trauma that occurred, at say, 12 to 20 years old; however,
in the patient with the more severe disorder, there will be a reflection in abandonment
memory all the way back to infancy.

McKenzie proved in his massive study that the same regions of the brain were
reactivated—the same brain cells ignited—all still hard-wired to the rest of the body
as though stuck in the past.

More simply—a perceived abandonment in later life triggers the brain back to the
earlier stages of brain development when the first perceived abandonment occurred.
For example, a woman's husband leaves or dies—she shifts brain activity to the region
of her brain that was developing at the time of the initial separation to sometime
during infancy, and away from later developmental brain structures. How far back
her brain reverts depends on when the first perceived trauma occurred; and how severe
the implications are depends on how young and helpless she was at the time of first
trauma. She becomes the helpless little girl once again, developmentally: the same
neurotransmitters and all. This is the McKenzie Two-Trauma Mechanism. Everyone
has an inner child that will never mature with unresolved conflict from early
separation panic. However, as Dr. McKenzie showed, the earlier that the separation
trauma occurs, the more it sets the stage for enormous rage later in life.

Why is this important in understanding TMS symptoms? I noticed that the more
severe TMS sufferers had early disconnects with their mothers—some, so
overwhelmed by the next fear of separation that they found themselves curled up in
the fetal position, unable to move or speak. They had reverted back to an earlier,
preverbal state of brain development. Most everyone I communicated with who was
suffering from chronic pain had admitted that they had experienced early
abandonment fear, or rejection. So there is some form of residual panic in TMSers
from infancy—childhood separation anxiety, causing a chronicity of anxiety—most

---

* The powerful mechanism of ontogeny recapitulating phylogeny.

likely mother's absence due to her attention being directed toward younger siblings, or an infinite number of other reasons.

If you suffer from TMS, it would be wise to ask yourself some questions: Were you deathly afraid of abandonment? How many years are there between you and your siblings? Where were your parents when you were between one and three or even five years old, and what was happening at that time in the family? How many siblings do you have? If you have four siblings there is four times the potential for depression as mother's attention continuously gets subdivided. If you were an only child you had the parent's entire attention lavished upon you—needing constantly to be the center—constantly panicked if not.

20

Neurosis: Affectional Needs Gone Haywire

Any incompatibility of character can cause dissociation, and too great a split between the thinking and the feeling function, for instance, is already a slight neurosis. When you are not quite at one with yourself in a given matter, you are approaching a neurotic condition.
— Carl Jung, *Analytical Psychology, Its Theory and Practice* [203]

Psychiatrist Karen Horney didn't think that it is always abuse or neglect that led a child to develop neurotic behavior later in life, but rather that other causes were parental apathy or verbal criticism. She classified three broad categories of behavior the child may fall within when she feels rejected by indifference or callous and thoughtless remarks: **compliance**, **aggression**, or **withdrawal**. The compulsive lack of affection is seen by the child as indifference.

- **Compliance:** This is the more common form among TMSers. This is the tracordifying of others due to the overpowering need for acceptance from them. This includes "the self-effacing solution... the need for affection and approval, which is the indiscriminate need to both please others and be liked by them; the neurotic need for a partner, for someone else to take over one's life, encompassing the idea that love will solve all of one's problems; and the neurotic need to restrict one's life into narrow borders, including being undemanding, satisfied with little, inconspicuous." [204]

- **Aggression:** I have occasionally observed aggression among pain sufferers, whereby, "...children's first reaction to parental indifference is anger or basic hostility." [205] This is somewhat rare because these people are rebels, while most Type Ts are self-abusive and compliant.*

- **Withdrawal:** If the child cannot get the parent's attention through compliance or aggression, or if she wishes to circumvent their arguing, abuse, or indifference, she attempts to become self-sufficient or independent through accomplishments, with the intention of becoming unassailable by achieving goal after goal in order to deny her feelings for—OR—need for

---

* The movie *Good Will Hunting* is a perfect example of early separation/rejection rage using Horney's **aggression** classification for coping followed by an emotional catharsis when a compassionate listener enters the picture.

others. She turns inward and may later get misdiagnosed as having ADD, but this is only the anxiety-coping mechanism she has chosen in order to hide from the overwhelming tension, and needs.

This is where the term tracordify stems from, the most basic need to reduce the pain of early separation through **complying** (becoming perfect by falling in line), or **rebelling** (becoming antagonistic—to gain attention), or **self-sufficiency** (becoming perfect through the fervent desire to be independent).

Neurosis is merely the need for affection gone haywire, since everyone needs affection in some form. The severity of the neurosis is in the degree of need for affection and approval. The "normal" individual just tries to survive and cope, while the neurotic "makes the need to control central to her existence."[206] The true neurotic has a greater need for power, control, exploitation, admiration, achievement, independence, perfectionism, and unassailability. The Type T can be borderline neurotic under this definition, if the need for control is too central. Remember, Horney believed that most of these patterns of behavior stem from "parental indifference."

Dr. McKenzie wrote to me that he once witnessed a man upside-down, head first in a toilet bowl trying to get back into his mother's womb to experience rebirth—a tragic need for affection. On the other end of the neurosis spectrum, teenagers may just say the word "like" too many times in a sentence. "Neurotic" is a highly subjective characterization.

Intellect versus Feeling

If a man is perfect in his thinking he is surely never perfect in his feeling, because you cannot do the two things at the same time; they hinder each other.

— Carl Jung, *Analytical Psychology*

Thinking and feeling are polar opposites. Thinking is impersonal, analytical, and logical, and its opposite—feeling—is based on empathy, values, and harmony. Logic versus Empathy. If you attend the funerals of people who you care deeply for, and bury all unconscious emotional pain, but substitute rationalization by saying, "Oh well, that's life, we all die," then you subjugate your feelings to thinking. She thinks instead of hurting—rationalizes instead of valuing. This is how she prefers to make her decisions because she is overwhelmed by her feelings—an **inferior function** as far as she is concerned. An inferior function is the function that is the polar opposite of an individuals' dominant function. If she is predominately a "thinker," her inferior function, as Jung noted, would **always be** her feeling function because they are dichotomous by nature. Feeling is deeply buried under the unconscious, and is now far outside of awareness as long as thinking is the dominant function. Jung based this concept on the scientific Principle of Equivalence, under the assumption that there is only so much energy to go around. The individual's entire personality is incumbent on the dominance or inferiority of these functions over one another. With each trauma, each life stressor, each feeling of helplessness where she must rationalize her emotional pain away—she neglects to properly discharge the rage she has experienced because her feelings are inadequate to her. She then seeks information to "think" instead of feel. In this way, she avoids her emotions because she fears them and cannot control them.

A thinker cannot control his feelings, and so is absolutely possessed by them. It's not that he doesn't have feelings, but that he has no conscious control over them, they're primal and undeveloped and therefore, desperately avoided. How are they avoided? Through intellect—by pouring more energy and focus into the decision-making function in which he is most comfortable.

But one can feel "correctly" only when feeling is not disturbed by anything else. Nothing disturbs feeling so much as thinking.   — Carl Jung, *"Psychological Types"*[207]

TMSers are intellectualizers, great suppressors of feeling. By attending only to conscious affairs, they bury the ability to feel life; they are too busy running around robotically rationalizing to avoid further pain. If you don't absorb life through your intuitions or feelings, but live through conscious thinking alone, then you can't be hurt any more, and as author John Lee wrote, "The intellectual escape is our first conscious refuge from anger."[208]

Feeling will get you closer to the truth of who you are than thinking.
     — Eckhart Tolle, *The Power of Now: A Guide to Spiritual Enlightenment*[209]

The intellectual type is afraid of being caught by feeling because his feeling has an archaic quality... he is a helpless victim of his emotions. It is for this reason that primitive man is extraordinarily polite, he is very careful not to disturb the feelings of his fellows because it is dangerous to do so.... Nobody can attack them in their intellect. There they are strong and can stand alone, but in their feelings, they can be influenced, they can be caught.... Therefore, never force a man into his feelings when he is an intellectual. He controls it with an iron hand because it is very dangerous.
     — Carl Jung, CG Jung, *Analytical Psychology*[210]

Is Goodism Neurotic Behavior?

Show me a sane man, and I will cure him for you.

                                                        — Carl Jung

Jung understood neurosis to be a restabilizing state—an attempt at a "self-cure"— a self-regulating psychic state to restore balance. He also knew that if he had enough time with any individual, he could find a problem with him that necessitated his persona. So the answer to goodism versus neurosis is merely a matter of degree to which you aren't being true to yourself, which can be observed by the intensity of the TMS—a reflection of the magnitude of the conflict in trying to appear as normal. But, as Jean Houston, PhD wrote, "A normal person is someone you don't know very well."

Not Out of the Woods Yet—Is Perfectionism Neurotic Behavior?

There are other ways of interpreting neurotic behavior. Would anyone consider Tiger Woods to be neurotic? Probably not, but his life has been one of constant repetition—to be the number one player in the history of golf. Hitting millions of golf balls and spending tens of thousands of hours on the chipping and putting greens to be the very best is neurotic according to many definitions of neurosis.

However, if a housewife cleaned her kitchen floor 100 times per day as in obsessive-compulsive disorder (OCD), she would be considered neurotic. People see no worthy records or success in her actions. So the diagnosis of neurosis can be highly subjective. Is the goal socially rational? Obsessive-compulsive disorder is the need to repetitively perform certain acts or various ritualistic behaviors in order to alleviate anxieties. OCD is a **coping strategy**—repetitive behavior utilized as an avoidance mechanism. TMS-prone individuals often bounce their legs in the air when sitting down, or check and recheck locks and windows, or clean repetitively in order to cope through the moment. My brother and I laughed about a man he saw in New York City who was walking backwards and also talking backwards as he walked by. Is that neurotic behavior? Judge be the you.

What does this all have to do with pain and illness? There are first traumas that set life in motion and keep it in motion, starting before, or with, birth, as anxiety and motivation are born simultaneously. Subsequent traumas or major changes reflect us back to each earlier separation. But that initial perceived trauma sets the stage for how we deal with emotional problems later in life—depending on when it occurred in our brain's development. With each new fear of rejection or separation, intellect comes along, as a way of coping, to save us from dealing with overpowering emotions that threaten to trap us because we aren't very good at expressing feelings—so—we use "facts" to communicate, avoiding that which we fear most—that our emotions may erupt and pull the mask off our personas.

Little Miss Perfect

In the first episode of The Golf Channel's special series, *"The Big Break III— Ladies Only!"* one of the women contestants called another competitor Miss Perfect. Miss Perfect's name was Danielle Amiee. Danielle fussed over her hair, her clothes, her makeup and every aspect of how she looked and acted. The other women wondered if they would get a chance at the mirrors in the one bathroom, as one woman stated, "if Little Miss Perfect got in there first." Danielle had been cursed with beauty and she obsessively worried about appearance.

The lucky amateur winner of this Big Break competition would get a chance to fulfill a lifelong dream by receiving a pair of exemptions to play with the LPGA golfers in professional tournaments. Danielle didn't play perfectly, but she ended up winning that challenge and got her big break to play on the ladies' tour. Fast forward to May

26, 2005, before the Corning Classic, after Danielle had won the Golf Channel's competition and was now about to play in the big league under stressful conditions with the women professionals. The following is from golf.about.com.

> *"Big Break III" winner Danielle Amiee withdrew from her second appearance on the LPGA Tour, citing a bad back on Thursday at the LPGA Corning Classic.*[211]

> *"I'm trying to loosen up a bit; the muscles are a little on the tight side," she said while on the practice range Wednesday afternoon. Unfortunately, the 29-year-old Californian was unable to work out the kinks prior to her 1:40 p.m. ET tee time. Upon withdrawing, she headed back to her home in Newport Beach, Calif., to see her doctor.*[212]

Unfortunately Danielle will never know the truth behind her back pain, unless her doctor is of the caliber of Drs. J. Sarno, M. Sopher, E. Miller, A. Weil, D. Schechter, P. Gwozdz, P. Zafirides, D. Colbert, N. Brosh, J. Whiting, or A. Leonard-Segal. Danielle had been over-stimulated from the pressure she was placing on herself in order to succeed—an affectional need. The pain arrives to hide her anxiety and to control a situation where she may be criticized—redirecting her mind's eye away from a panicky side of herself that superego wishes to remain hidden.

Criticizing Is Shadow Casting

> *Show me the stone that the builders rejected: that is the keystone.*
> — Jesus, Ha-Nozri, *St. Thomas,* 66

Tensionalgia sufferers react badly to criticism—by not addressing it. They are quickly angered but slow in expressing the anger appropriately, if at all. They can't quite feel or express their anger, since they're conditioned repressa-holics from childhood. They just end up frustrated, and with symptoms. Their pain can be transformed—and eased—if the sufferers understand that those people who condemn and judge them, who think they are somehow superior to the sufferers, are projecting their own flaws onto the sufferers, because such people's egos are threatened by their own shadows.

> *Thus, instead of befriending and integrating our negative traits, we alienate and project them, seeing them in everybody else but ourselves.*
> — Ken Wilber, PhD, *Meeting the Shadow,*
> *The Hidden Power of the Dark Side of Human Nature*[213]

This projection is necessary due to the relationship of ego and shadow. The shadow is the **alter-ego**. In order to keep this darker side hidden, the individual must cast her fears and faults outward. In Alcoholics Anonymous there is a mantra, "If you spot it, you got it." Everything the criticizer says, or projects, about another person, he himself also is and has. **Criticizing is scapegoating.** Carl Jung believed that the shadow is most often encountered through these projections. When you call someone afraid or a chicken or stupid or lazy, you are revealing your own shadow-self—your own fears of encountering those same flaws that already exist in you. You can't recognize something in someone else if you don't understand it, and you can't understand it unless you also have that same trait. Throwing criticisms at others keeps the criticizer's shadow "out there;" if he did not project onto others, his ego would be forced to recognize that what is wrong with others is also wrong within him. Criticism that stings the ego often creates an animating force, a motivational energy that drives people's careers and life choices, such as with Karen Horney. It drives some people to action—others to inaction.

A criticism or a word of praise may have an accelerating effect as a motivational force driving the individual in one direction or the other. Needless to say, the person deeply hurt through criticism is not the only one who needs support—the individual who receives constant affirmation may be the one to really worry about. Praise can be severely damaging (as with an only child receiving all the attention), creating co-dependency and lowering self-esteem.

> People who criticize you do so because they are envious of your courageous attempts at trying, and angry at their own fear of trying. They are projecting their own low self-esteem onto you. So is everything we "direct" at others always projecting our own flaws? Philosopher Ken Wilber, PhD, contends that it depends on whether what we perceive interests and informs us, or whether that "person or thing" affects us and brings forth a reaction from us. If it informs and interests us, such as an observation, it is most likely not projection—if it induces a reaction from us, then it is most likely projection.

21

Highly Sensitive People — HSPs

The unconscious sensibility of an hysterical patient is at certain moments fifty times more acute than that of a normal person.

— Carl Jung, on Alfred Binet[214]

The Type T chronic symptom sufferer is an extremely aware, or sensitive, personality. What many would consider as simple things bother highly sensitive people (HSPs—or somatically sensitive). They take criticism more personally and will dig deeper caves to avoid confrontation. I have known people who try to avoid all people because they were once criticized by one person. It hurt them deeply enough that they dropped out of social relationships altogether. If the avoidance of social life isn't enough protection, they often turn to self-numbing counter forces—anti-depressants and more glasses of courage—to be able to face other people. They are hyper-responsive, generating more stress, making muscles more rigid and tense.

Many people don't recognize they are hyper-responsive because they only know their own experiences, and have no reference point. A chronic pain sufferer told me that she wasn't sensitive, but that she didn't want other people to wait for her when she was driving her car, so she never made left turns. A man suffering symptoms once reported that he avoided "any situation that could possibly turn confrontational." He too denied being sensitive to me. But it is his temper that he fears because he cannot control it—so the "situation is avoided." Extreme sensitivity, contrarily, can make people appear to be insensitive—cold and distant and sometimes arrogant—wearing an aggressive public persona. Entertainer Howard Stern is once again a good example. Howard is a self-confessed obsessive who suffered greatly from TMS. Few people would call Howard an introvert but that's the purpose of a persona, to hide the deeper self.

What fulfillment can HSPs gain from life? What makes them feel productive? In *The Highly Sensitive Person*, Elaine N. Aron, PhD, writes that finding the right **vocation** for the HSP is the hottest topic in her seminars. This makes perfect sense since a large group of chronic pain sufferers are either unemployed, working part time, hate their jobs, or have recently been forced to leave their jobs, or retired. They don't know how to move forward—in career-coma—feeling unproductive and empty.

Aron explains that HSPs "don't thrive on long hours, stress, and over-stimulating work environments." Their difficulty in finding a satisfying endeavor stems from "their not appreciating their role, style, and potential contribution." These people are often gifted artists or writers, teachers, consultants, counselors—people of great intuitive talents stuck in mundane and externally draining environments. They only find true satisfaction when matched with the right career—only truly happy when they are "liberated" from the first half of their lives and finally begin listening to their own voices. Aron continues, "Being so eager to please, we're not easy to liberate. We're too aware of what others need[215].... Often their intuition gives them a clearer picture of what needs to be done. Thus, many HSPs choose vocations of service."[216] When I read this line from Aron's book, it reminded me of a story in *Guideposts* I had read in October of 2003. The story was entitled "Back in Shape," and the cover of the magazine read, "How a Back Problem Led to a Breakthrough."

The preamble of the *Guideposts* story reads: "Sometimes the best treatment for body and soul is change. A breakthrough—in attitude, in lifestyle. Meet this young man, who lost his job to debilitating back pain and found his calling by overcoming it."

This true story was about a 23-year-old man from Oklahoma City, Oklahoma, named Marcellous Hurte (yes, his name is Hurte). Marcellous was stuck in a mundane and unfulfilling job rebuilding transmissions. At the young age of 23 he had become totally debilitated and had lost his job when his pain spread from his back to his left arm. A back brace only made his pain worse (of course). His doctor gave him the worst possible advice, of course. That advice was, "no physical activity. And absolutely no lifting." From the physician's ill-advice, over the next 2½ years, Marcellous went from partial functioning to total debilitation.

It's not by accident that Rick Warren, author of *The Purpose Driven Life*, was once selling nearly a million books per month. People need direction, and purpose, or they wander aimlessly, punishing themselves with depression or pain. The topic of purpose may be the most important topic in understanding Phase 4 TMS, and experiencing a healthy life. If you believe your purpose is to make as much money as possible, then you don't understand how big a camel is or how small the eye of a needle is. The best things in life are not things, they are relationships.

The soul needs meaning just as much as the body needs food.
— Richard Rohr, OFM, *Quest for the Grail*

Pain serves as a message. It was the messenger that let Marcellous know that he was unhappy. He began reflecting on his life and decided to start anew, one small step at a time. He became reflective—more spiritually aware. He also did what Dr. Sarno said was possibly the most important thing of all—he became much more active. A year or more later, **It** happened, as Marcellous explained in *Guideposts*. "I woke one Sunday morning with the strangest sensation—nothing hurt! The pain in my back, gone. Same with my right leg, my left hand." Today Marcellous is a personal fitness trainer who helps other people get their own lives back into shape.

I couldn't have dreamed up a better job. You should hear me push my clients.... It's not about the pain, I tell them.... It's about rebuilding your body. Rebuilding your health. Rebuilding your life. You can do it! I know. In a way, that pain in my back was the best thing that ever happened to me.

— Marcellous Hurte, *Guideposts*, October 2003[217]

How you react to your sensitivity is everything in how you proceed in your career. I saw the young phenom golfer, Michelle Wie (pronounced "we"), say, regarding her recognition of the importance of criticisms aimed at her, "If they just praised me all the time, I would just sit back and relax." Even at a young age, Michelle knew that you cannot learn from constant praise. As stated before—constant praise can be detrimental to the health of a child. It makes him dependent on the opinions of others in order to feel good about himself. Michelle, however, turned the negative energy from the critics into positive action.

Michelle Wie may be a highly sensitive person; only she knows because her public persona is all wie see. Patience does have its limits, though; Michelle later stated that she hopes the critics realize that there is "a person" at the other end of the criticism. While most people are sensitive to criticism, the great ones know how to use it, and when to lose it. The greatest female golfer in history is Sweden's Annika Sorenstam. Annika was so shy and highly sensitive when she began golfing that she would purposefully hit bad golf shots at the end of tournaments to lose—to avoid giving a victory speech. But Annika had found her vocation, her true love was golf, and today she is currently the most successful lady in LPGA history. Frank Nobilo, a Golf Channel analyst and former tour player, stated in August of 2008 that Annika "turned fear into motivation… using the fear she had as a child for her success." Tremendous insight by Nobilo. Annika used her shadow (fear) to enable herself to grow— discovering the gold within her, to shine.

Highly sensitive individuals often tell me that they fear hearing of a certain ailment because they "fear they may just get it." Ailments can indeed be induced by fear of those same ailments, as Attraction becomes the Law. However, fear can be turned into a vehicle for success, as proven by some of the greatest.

I'm here to tell you that the fear of failure is the engine that has driven me throughout my entire life… People are always surprised how insecure I was… I wasn't the most physical or the fastest receiver in the NFL, but they never clocked me on the way to the end zone. The reason nobody caught me from behind is because I ran scared. That old fear of failure again.

— Jerry Rice, induction into the Pro Football Hall of Fame,
— 8/7/2010, the greatest receiver of all time

Ways Your HSP Trait Affects Your Medical Care:

- You're more sensitive to bodily signs and symptoms.
- If you don't lead a life suited to your trait, you'll develop more stress-related and/or "psychosomatic illnesses."
- You're more sensitive to medications.
- You're more sensitive to pain.
- You'll be more aroused, usually over-aroused, by medical environments, procedures, examinations, and treatments.
- In "health care" environments your deep intuition cannot ignore the shadowy presence of suffering and death, the human condition.
- Given all the above, and the fact that most mainstream medical professionals are not HSPs, your relationships with them are usually more problematic.

— Elaine Aron, PhD, *The Highly Sensitive Person*[218]

A major factor regarding chronic pain comes from not feeling productive, and if the individual's true gifts are not matched to his vocation or purpose, he suffers—and society loses a valuable asset.

22

CFS: Chronic Fatigue Syndrome

A long and hazardous course lies between me and my goal, how could I travel alone? How could I force this fog of half-understanding, that confuses my sense of direction?
— Hans Selye, MD, *From Dream to Discovery: On Being a Scientist*

Stress: Latin, verb, "To pull apart"

Hungarian-born Hans Selye (pronounced, SELL-yay), endocrinologist, is widely considered to be the father of stress. He didn't create stress, but he did spend his lifetime studying it, and writing on the subject; he even coined the term stress.

Selye understood stress to be a nonspecific response on the mindbody to the demands made of it. From my communication with chronic fatigue syndrome (CFS) sufferers, it's clear that their chronic fatigue is indeed a response to demands made on them—placed there by them. Selye's research is germane to the understanding of what is occurring during times of stress that catalyzes bouts of chronic fatigue—which is TMS on steroids. *CFS is a TMS equivalent; they share the same emotional bypass mechanism.* CFS = TMS + more continuous repression (adaptation).

Selye identified a three-stage mindbody response to stress. The first stage stress response he called **alarm**. Alarm is the initial recognition of the stressful event that evokes the fight or flight response. Perception is the most important characteristic of this stage. A perception of danger engages the body for fight or flight—releasing the appropriate hormones. Remember, a perceived event has the same effect on the mindbody as a real event, the mindbody makes no distinction between real or imagined, even releasing the same neurotransmitters.

The second stage stress response Selye called **resistance**. If there is no fight or flight, but rather freeze, and the situation chronically continues, the mindbody faces the likelihood of both physiological and psychological consequences as it struggles to maintain homeostasis. These consequences are TMS equivalents—Selye referred to them as "diseases of adaptation." Physical effects include stomach/intestinal disorders, headaches, hypertension, back pain, muscle aches, etc. The psychological effects resulting from resistance include resentment, depression and anger. The irony is that there is no need for the resistance since it's often a false perception of danger.

Selye's third stage is **exhaustion**, or fatigue. If the individual feels never-ending self-imposed pressure to do good, be good, or appear good, she will eventually fall into the long-term effects of fatigue. The long-term effects of this can only be characterized as chronic fatigue.

I was fascinated to discover that, in most people, their fatigue would increase as their pain lessened, and that their pain would increase when their fatigue lessened (the symptom imperative). Their perception and anticipation of future events froze them into an often prostrate state; stuck between fight and flight. These people were in hyper-TMS—the effect of increased energy (anger) overload due to an oppressive superego. This steady build-up of unexpressed energy now must be contained by superego—demanding even more energy. The analogy has been made of trying to hold a beach ball underwater—energy needing more energy to futilely try to hold something down (hint: that "something" is the anger). This overload of energy sends the body into a state of quasi-mental-physical paralysis. Note that apart from the obvious stressors, such as criticism or jobs or health, social status is also considered a stressor. Needless to say, financial worries play a large part in fatigue and pain.

Much like a circuit breaker that trips when there is an overload of current, the breaker trips to protect the entire system when it can no longer contain the anger-energy overload—or hold the beach ball underwater. The circuit that breaks is the hypothalamus, not due to an energy deficiency—but to TMS—an overload of energy. So, once again TMS becomes controversial because it tests current beliefs about CFS. It is the repression of energy, the imbalance that triggers the hypothalamus' reaction, not an energy deficiency—rather it is the opposite. There are other major factors involved in the CFS process as well, such as nutrition, and delta sleep irregularity since the hypothalamus also controls the sleep-wake cycle—all of which is involved in the repression of emotions. CFS is TMS—the disowning of the shadow-self.

CFS is a classic freeze response survival mechanism, and should be treated just like TMS. If she can't quit her job, or pay her bills, or argue with her husband, and cannot run from her colleagues, or classmates, or neighbors—she has no way out of her current situation so she ends up in a freeze state—or fatigue. Each time she encounters a similar scenario where she feels helpless, she falls into sleep mode, much like a computer—dissociating herself from the situation. She even unconsciously begins to use freeze, when she actually could fight or flee, because it has become her way of dealing with problems—imprinted in her memory.

An illustration of this concept can be seen in the movie, Awakenings. Malcolm Sayer, portrayed by Robin Williams, discovers that his paralyzed patients are frozen in a state of physical paralysis because their mindbodies were actually moving so fast that it rendered them statue-like with encephalitic lethargica (a.k.a., sleeping sickness—but not the kind transmitted by the tsetse fly). Dr. Sayer, whose real name is Oliver Sacks, MD, brought them out of their paralytic states by giving them doses of L-dopa in order to slow their mental activity—enticing them out of their frozen states. This is only an illustration of a similar process, not the CFS process.

CFS is a syndrome in that it, too, manifests itself in a variety of ways. Recent studies show heart involvement in chronic fatigue, no doubt from brain-heart dysregulation—signal flow interruption as the autonomic system struggles to adapt to the stressors such as threatened proxemic space, over-developed sense of responsibility, financial worry, and of course relationship worries. Therefore, a calming agent would most likely yield more energy to the chronic CFSer, by slowing the incoming sensory and improving mood. Several former sufferers told me that sedatives did indeed increase their energy levels.

I know people with this particular syndrome who have been successful in easing and shortening their symptoms by becoming aware that stress and emotional overload were the instigators. Elaine has shortened the frequency and longevity of her attacks by applying Dr. Sarno's TMS healing knowledge. Her mindbody sometimes rebels against her challenges to CFS, but overall she has greatly improved. Elaine's pain leaves her when the "fog of CFS" kicks in. The more severe her fatigue the less her pain, and vice versa (that symptom imperative again—see Appendix A for a list of common symptoms), as her mindbody struggles to hold two simultaneous distractions. Others have told me their TMS pain stays about the same during episodes of CFS. Thus, CFS is confusing and complex and by default, a syndrome. The good news is that people are beginning to understand the emotional cause behind CFS and that it is a mindbody imbalance, so half the battle is already won.

> *I strongly believe CFS to be a psychosomatic disorder, and this belief is supported by my success in treating a very large number of cases. A further indication that we are right is that many people suffering from CFS have recovered from it simply by studying one of my books.*
>
> — John E. Sarno, MD, *The Divided Mind*[219]

It is clear and has been proven that fatigue and pain serve the same purpose. When we get overwhelmed or angry because we can't escape a situation, we give ourselves symptoms—fatigue being a common one from an infinite variety. So, CFS is no doubt a distraction by the mind from overwhelming stress, anxiety, and repressed desires (the deferring of immediate gratification). Freud often referred to the chronicity of fatigue as neurasthenia, a term coined by American neurologist, GM Beard in the late 1800s. Today neurasthenia is called dysautonomia— "autonomic dysregulations" in the autonomic nervous system, or TMS. While the terms CFS, and fibromyalgia are often used interchangeably, fibromyalgia is CFS with multiple pain sites. They are all part of the mindbody syndrome.

The US Center for Disease Control and Prevention (CDC) has recently announced that chronic fatigue syndrome is not psychological, but rather "a disease." This proclamation can only have negative consequences, since the new classification of "disease" will literally close the door on all subsequent understanding as to how to stop it. **CFS is a symptom—NOT a disease.** The CDC's announcement will encourage sufferers to dismiss the psychological component that drives the disorder—the truth can now be "officially" ignored—as with herniated discs.

Now, viewing it as an "official disease," scientists will try to dissect it biologically like they're still trying to do with ulcers. And they will find all kinds of fascinating things in their research: cell changes, heart involvement, brain inflammation, abnormal cortisol levels, potassium deficiencies, adrenal malfunctions, everything but the cause. So the new classification by the CDC will most likely set healing back by decades, since the syndrome is now taken from the psychological to the physical realm because many people would rather not own their own responsibility (a cultural meme). It would be best to label such syndromes as disorders rather than diseases. The word disease is even a self-fulfilling prophecy. It connotates a sense of helplessness that cannot be overcome—something that needs to be corrected from the outside.

The fatigue syndrome is psychological in origin, although it is certainly not imaginary. It is real. The process begins in the mind and permeates the body. I can well imagine why so many CFS sufferers get frustrated that some people think they are imagining or faking their fatigue. CFS, like TMS, has a specific purpose—to pull back from stress, adapt (as Selye has put forth), recharge, escape, and regroup in order to be able to face life anew. This process naturally takes place outside of awareness. The question is: why does the mindbody overreact? The simple answer is that it perceives itself to be overloaded, and so it is. The more detailed answers for this psychological phenomenon lay in the thought/emotional experience, and of course, the sensory-genetic and conditioning albatrosses—that is, those things we have learned "wrong" behaviorally or to which we are "overly" sensitive due to our genetic makeup.

> *The more energy we invest in holding back these energies, the more drained we become, physically and psychically.... Exhaustion and fatigue, more often than not, are a function of strong instincts that are being disowned.... She discovered she had disowned her anger so totally that when she was deeply irritated by her husband, she experienced not anger but overwhelming desire to go to sleep. When she learned her drowsiness was a substitute for natural aggression, she began to search for the anger concealed by her overwhelming fatigue. As soon as she became aware of her anger voice, and learned what it wanted, the drowsiness disappeared.*
>
> — Hal Stone PhD and Sidra Winkleman PhD,
> *Meeting the Shadow, The Hidden Power of the Dark Side of Human Nature*[220]

23

Anxiety, Depression, and Metanoia

My father died at 102. Whenever I would ask what kept him going, he'd answer,
"I never worry."

— Jerry Stiller, *Married To Laughter*

Where there is pain and fatigue there is anxiety and often depression. The pain is revealing their existence to the sufferer who thus far has been unaware of their intensity. Freud believed that anxiety was a sign of impending danger—a result of unexpressed emotion. No matter the mechanism, given the choice, most people prefer pain to anxiety, and so they unconsciously give themselves pain to be able to persevere.

Depression manifests following a traumatic separation or the feeling of isolation. Depression—like back pain—is also extremely common during what Jung had labeled the midlife crisis. In midlife the individual transitions from concern over the outer world, in the first half of life, which Jung called the "natural phase," to placing more of his energy into understanding his inner world or the "cultural phase."* It is within this transition period that the transcendence of ego normally begins.

In between these stages a crisis can occur when an individual feels isolated and becomes so lost and confused that she turns deeply inward—left with no means for self-expression. If she has access to counseling, a compassionate family ear, friends, and a stage to openly express her isolation, the depression has no place to grow. But most deeply isolated people feel they have nowhere to turn, or their egos won't admit they have needs, and so adaptation becomes chronic and isolation spreads. The need to express, and to share, becomes elusive as night settles in. But this can change with the understanding of self-worth. As irrational as it may appear, depression has an evolutionary purpose, which is to inhibit aggressive behavior. Depression is a survival mechanism when she cannot fight her way out of, or run from her life—leaving her self-esteem nonexistent. The result of inhibition of expressive behavior is depression and anxiety.

Anxiety

Anxiety should never be viewed as an inherent weakness, but rather an out-of-control strength. It takes tremendous strength to never act out rage; to take that

---

* Jung used the term **individuation** as that act in the cultural phase whereby the individual transcends her ego-complex by peeling away her layers of persona in search of what he called the "true individual."

energy, to repress it inward where it becomes anxiety—so as to not harm anyone else. Anxiety then incapacitates the individual when he can no longer function due to his steadfast desire to maintain an ongoing image. It takes even more strength to explore this process and to undo it.

Sometime around 1994, entertainer Donny Osmond began feeling a sense of anxiousness in himself that he had never experienced in his lifetime as a performer. Superego's stranglehold over time can overwhelm an individual in the form of social anxiety—and even panic. Donny commented, "I was always trying to be perfect. I was crippled by social phobia." In an interview he admitted being so caught up in the complex of perfection, and the barrage of being constantly judged by others, that he couldn't decide what shirt to buy in a store, standing frozen in mindchatter-gridlock. The anxiety had crippled him to the point of paranoia—unable to move or function. So Donny began working with therapist Jerilyn Ross who taught him to face his fear and to give it tangibility, a face or name or color, and to never run from it. Donny had what is called social anxiety disorder, the effect of always feeling the need to be → perfect. Today, through cognitive behavioral therapy, he is doing much better since he has learned that he will make mistakes, and that it is okay to do so. We must eventually begin to transcend ego and live beyond our concern of outside observers.

Ever since I started in the business, I knew at least somebody in that audience is looking at me all the time.... So I've got to be perfect.
— Donny Osmond, CBS News, *48 Hours*, August 10, 2000

Over time, people get worn down by outside observers. Actor Laurence Olivier, after 40 years of acting, developed stage fright during a stage performance of Othello. Famed actress Jean Arthur also developed stage fright in her later years. People can only expel energy to maintain their personas for so long before they begin to mentally breakdown.

Anxiety comes first, and then pain. If the pain never forms, anxiety has carte blanche to run rampant. So the bodily symptoms serve to control the anxiety by giving it a holding cell. When anxiety hits threshold highs, people sometimes feel they are going crazy or losing their minds. Even though it is a common feeling, it is never true. If she is going to lose her mind, she will never know it. So don't worry.

Anxiety is **pushing ahead of the light**—not having faith to wait for the light to unveil itself in real time—the attempt to thwart any future possible disaster by being pre-ready, pre-worried, and locked in survival mode. Planning may head off disaster but it usually breeds worry, because its foundation is anticipation—causing muscle contraction. Worrying about health destroys health because the focus remains on health. If we live only for today, our worries simply go away.

Depression

Suicide is not chosen; it happens when pain exceeds resources for coping with pain.
                                                                              — Metanoia.org

Anxiety and depression are folds of the same person, anxiety being the lighter side of anger, and depression the darker side. Depression is the **absence of light, the opposing state of vitality.** The individual sees only the bad—eventually giving up on his anxious attempts to see any light at all. His light has burned out from anxiety— he falls prey to darkness. If the darkness is black enough for long enough, irrational thinking enters—ego begins to despise superego.

The fear of death in melancholia only admits of one explanation: that the ego gives itself up because it feels itself hated and persecuted by the superego, instead of loved... the same situation as that which underlay the first great anxiety—state of birth and the infantile state of longing—the anxiety due to separation from the protecting mother.
                                            — Sigmund Freud, *The Ego and the Id*[221]

Suicide is the most desperate need to be heard of all—the creative instinct succumbing to the destructive instinct. When she doesn't know how, or to whom, to express herself, she expresses her sadness through her actions. Suicide is that final expression of the unexpressed self that she feels could end all her pain. But we know from TMS healing that she can heal and become much happier. The signs of depression are usually clear to the outside observer but the depressed individual often remains in the dark. You can feel hope and love again if you have the courage to just hang on—just a little longer. You are not alone. Together with many others who have gone through TMS—you will come through it a much happier person. There are former TMS sufferers out there everywhere online who will help you.

Deep depression is not always rational. In fact, people who seem to have everything have a very high rate of depression because purpose fades when motivation ends. They find that money and material things do not bring happiness—once obtained, it no longer excites them. Depressed people need purpose, a sense of connectivity, to bring back that flicker of light—a motivation. If you are reading this book for someone you love who is depressed or in chronic pain, then go intervene in their life now. If you love them, take over and hear them before it is too late. If you yourself have entertained the idea of leaving this world, STOP! TMS knowledge gives hope for a brighter tomorrow. The pain will leave—if you believe.

The Depressed Chicken or the Anxious Egg?

In my experience anxiety is always the first to appear before depression. When the superfluous anticipation of future events becomes chronic, she can't sustain a continuous adaptation response. The fight eventually begins to wane, as more bad perceptions of outcomes bring more focus on the bad, and finally she abandons any possibility of hope. As darkness settles in, her pain intensifies to keep **the unthinkable** from rising out of unconsciousness. Exacerbating the problem is the fact that perfectionists are always mildly depressed because life is never perfect.

I watched an interview with Mel Gibson and Diane Sawyer where Mel was speaking of his own trials and tribulations and self-doubt as whether to continue in this life or to leave it by suicide, which he referred to as "the height of spiritual bankruptcy." In his words, "...whenever I hear of suicide, I just want to die, I want to cry... because there's something better if they can just hang on a little longer."

Courage is fear holding on a minute longer.

— General George Patton (1885-1945)

Two people I met while writing this book admitted to me that they had made the plans for suicide, but they couldn't "pull the trigger." They, too, held on for that minute longer, and it has paid off a thousand times over as they both live much happier lives. Your pain will leave you, too.

> Depression and anxiety occur FIRST, and then the pain arrives. It does not work the other way around. People often tell me, "if the pain would only go away, I would not be depressed." No!! The TMS process is diametrically opposite. You do not get better emotionally and THEN go become active in life. It's all about courage and hope. You must jump in and get back on the Reeve's horse first, and the pain will eventually fade into productivity—getting back in the saddle being the most difficult part.

Metanoia

Metanoia: Greek, defined as "change of mind". From metanoia.org:

Imagine you are standing in a circle of people. In the center of the circle, there is a source of light. But rather than facing the center and the light, you are standing with your back to the light, facing outward.

When you stand this way, facing away from the light, all you can see is your own shadow. You cannot see the light. You can only look into your shadow. You cannot see the others in the circle with you. From what you can see, you are disconnected and alone in the dark.

Now imagine that you turn around to face the light that is in the center of the circle. When you turn toward the light, you no longer see only darkness. When you turn toward the light, your shadow is behind you. When you turn toward the light, you can now see the other people who are standing with you. You can see that the light is shining on everyone and that you are all connected in its radiance. Making the decision to turn around, to turn away from shadow, to face the light—this is metanoia.

— Metanoia.org

This is why friends, counseling, and support groups help so often. They enable people to see that there are others standing with them—connected—as depression slowly fades, and light reenters the body.

Scenario Analysis—What if?

The greatest griefs are those we cause ourselves.

— Sophocles, *Oedipus Rex*

A tree's age is determined by the number of rings it contains, just as an individual's personality can be measured by the number of branches on his **decision tree**. Branches grow as an individual chooses between several courses of action. Decision trees are used in a process called scenario analysis, which is more commonly known as what-if thinking. What-if thinking is the curse of the tension sufferer. Formally, the decision tree process serves the individual as a tool for fight or flight. "Scenario analysis is the process of analyzing possible future events by considering alternative possible outcomes (scenarios)… allowing more complete consideration of outcomes and their implications."[222] Meditation experts often refer to this what-if-thinking as **negative chatter**. It's simply noggin noise that resembles the branches of a tree, as each bad possible outcome is relived and reviewed, growing branches and increasing tension— the antithesis of **presence**.

Conceptually:
A Decision Tree—the mind making a decision.

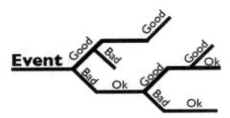

Non-Anxious Individual:
He has a few doubts and lets them pass quickly.

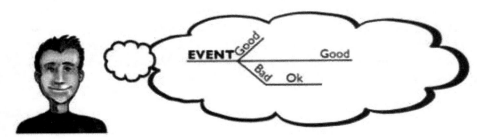

Anxious Individual:
He has a few more doubts but functions in his daily routine.

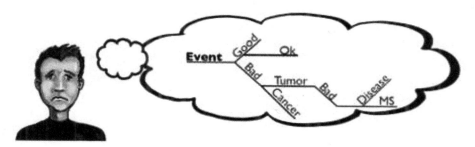

Highly Anxious Individual:
He cannot let go of any doubt—gridlocking him in the pursuit of his life goals and paralyzing his decision-making. He becomes his own curse.

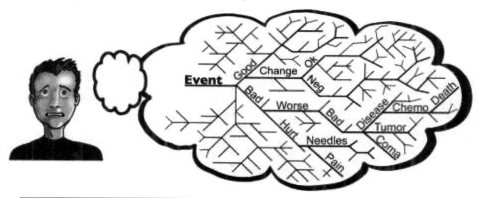

The growing of the branches is TMSing through "stinken thinken"—side-stepping feelings, keeping the individual distracted from his emotional base.

The way to stop the what-if branches from growing is to change the what-if to **SO WHAT!!!** Pruning the tree takes courage and faith.

Today is the tomorrow that you once worried about, and yet today came anyway. Events in life do not cause stress. It is the emotional attachment to the event that causes stress—the reaction to it. Worrying warriors use what-if thinking as a weapon to head off possible bad future outcomes. But no one has ever made a future event better by worrying about it.

Who of you by worrying can add a single hour to his life?

— Jesus, Ha-Nozri, *Matthew*, 6:27

Ockham's razor is a mitigator with regard to the worry process. William of Ockham's principle states that "an individual shouldn't make more assumptions than the minimum needed to explain anything." This is sometimes referred to as The Principle of Parsimony—also called the KISS principle, "keep it simple, stupid."

I always tell people to get off their own backs when healing, because if enough chaos enters the thought process through doubt and trial, doubt and trial, the size of the anxiety tree is such that nothing gets accomplished. Just Do it! The individual worries herself into a state of paralysis through procrastination. Here dreaming of being there, and there dreaming of being here. The worrying-branches incapacitate the worrying-warrior—and a problem is only a problem if one perceives it to be a problem. Over-analyzing life only adds more complexity, adding further demands to the already besieged self. Ease up on you!

Me—My "self" and "I"rene

People sometimes name their TMS pain in order to bring a sense of identity and control to the syndrome.* When I finally understood how pain occurs, I began referring to my pain as Hank. I got the idea from the Jim Carrey movie *Me, Myself and Irene*. I'm fairly certain I wasn't suffering from advanced delusionary schizophrenia with involuntary narcissistic rage, but I do believe Hank personified how I felt life had treated me. One man I got to know very well named his TMS pain Nancy, for narcissistic child. And a woman I spoke to who asked to be nameless called her TMS back pain, Mom. I later understood that this might have been another reason my pain was so protracted. The personification of it can give it life and meaning. The concept in healing is to render pain meaningless and without tangibility. Never discuss your ailments by name.

Financial Pain

I don't care about losing all the money. It's losing all the stuff.
— Marie Kimble Johnson, *The Jerk*, 1979

Many people have physical pain when on the edge of financial crisis. Instinct tells us that money will keep us safe and that it will secure our stature. The threat of the loss of cash is a threat to self-survival and image. It isn't the finances themselves that create the anger that is generating the pain, but rather the threat to security, survival, and status. This is currently being labeled as **debt stress**. A 2008 AP-AOL poll of 1,002 adults showed that those with high debt had twice the heart attack rate of those with low debt. They also had over five times the cases of severe depression, over seven times the cases of severe anxiety, three times the number of migraines (or other headaches), over three

---

* This is not the same as a phobia where a sense of identity is important. With pain, it is more important to never give it a form; the idea is to render it useless—innocuous.

times the number of digestive problems, and that, "More than half, 51 percent, had muscle tension, including pain in the lower back. That compared with 31 percent of those with low levels of debt stress."[223]

Proxemic Space Invaders

When crowding becomes too great... interactions intensify, leading to greater and greater stress.

— Edward Twitchell Hall, *The Hidden Dimension*[224]

It's easy to feel the sensory effect that others have on you when they enter your **proxemic space**, as your back, neck, colon, or chest tighten. TMS symptoms spike when our space is invaded—and are magnified if phobias are present. Your language changes from how you speak to your friends, or to the minister, or to a member of the opposite sex. Some of the most hateful rage is now spewed across the Internet because there is complete anonymity of the shadow. This vitriol aimed at Internet authors, and ad hominem attacks against people who are subjects of articles, is the shadow erupting, due to unlimited "space" between the criticizer and the subject. People become awfully tough when they're anonymous, their dark sides surface accordingly. As this vast territory shrinks, however, and others begin to get closer to their physical bodies, they alter their thought process by pretending to be kind and respectful, and the body reacts accordingly by tensing because of pretense (they don't want to have to be nice—it demands more energy). Maintaining a measured distance allows them a sense of freedom to be themselves, but if their perception is that their space has been overrun, they defensively tense necks, backs, shoulders, knees, and hearts. Many people tell me they get chest pains, migraines, and joint pains when they go out to dinner and mingle with the public.

The space-invader causing TMS is most likely a family member, mate, boss, or client, but it may also be a job, or project. As people violate **intimate**, **personal**, or **social space**, the senses begin to chatter with stimulation as the sympathetic nervous system fires with incoming information, dulling full awareness due to increased brain wave activity. To a highly aware individual, social or intimate space is precious territory. A commonly reported problem is being out in public and having increasing pain or dizziness as the senses are heightened in the public eye, due to social anxiety— the drain of outside observers (the hall monitor superego always on guard).

Great prophets always went into some form of seclusion to free themselves from the drain of others. There they can reach deeper into their own humanity—to discover what sustains them beyond the ego's watchful eye. As proxemic space narrows, our superego demands more energy, our senses become overloaded, breathing shortens, anger rises, and tension mounts—a classic survival response.

As the Tao Te Ching puts it, muddy water left to stand will clear, the mud will go to the bottom and we can live in a clear ambient. But we are so harassed by the avalanche of distraction and demand and duties, many of which we impose on ourselves, that there's no time to know thyself... what one ultimately lets go of is the ego, this clamorous ego with its demands.

— Huston Smith, in *Portrait of a Radical*[225]

Lost in Space

Personal space allows muddied waters to clear—decreasing angerziety. People freely fulfilling each other's needs use little energy because there are no false facades (French, façade defined as "face"). The sympathetic nervous system eases down when we feel secure and safe and can wear our natural faces—relaxed, confident, aware, and healthier.

Anger and frustration are almost always relationship-based. The first place to look when pain appears is toward your spouse, parents, or children. Blood pressure rises, cholesterol rises, and chest pain increases as symptoms magnify from the sensation of proxemic-imprisonment. If the individual senses entrapment due to his circumstance, his body reveals the price paid for his silent compliance. A friend of mine going through a divorce had his systolic blood pressure rise to 190. Within three days after his divorce it had dropped 60 points to 130. Hypertension is also caused by the anger of aging, life-crisis, diet, and genetics.

A good relationship is one where each person gets to be more of who they are.
— Deborah L. Schuster, Job Search Coach, Certified Professional Resume Writer

24

Drugs

The desire to take medicine is perhaps the greatest feature which distinguishes man from animals.

— Sir William Osler, MD (1849–1919)

Mood-altering drugs numb emotions. Painkillers/alcohol/antidepressants all mask the unmet need underlying the purpose for the drug. Antidepressants can be viewed as Band-Aids that stop emotional bleeding. But as Dr. Sarno has observed, taking away symptoms by artificial means (drugs, surgery, etc.) often forces TMS somewhere else, triggering sustained pain, anxiety, or depression. The drugs force TMS into another type of symptom; they don't stop the problems.

Switching back and forth between smoking, drinking, analgesics, and antidepressants is merely swapping one addiction for another. There's no net gain. The absence of purpose—a spiritual yearning—underlies the addiction to numbing agents, and usually presents itself in the form of pain or anxiety-related disorders. Do not use drugs to try to rid TMS pain. It can make the pain stay in the long run.

Drugs are **all poisons** to the mindbody. There is always a future price to pay for feeling better now, as apparent relief is simply borrowed with interest. When desperation decreases your ability to handle life's problems, drugs may be necessary short-term, but they are never a long-term solution. Drugs don't take care of the problem, they shift it. The problem remains and the sufferer then needs more drugs (as with back surgeries) to keep from attending to strong emotions. The net gain, once again, is nothing.

One of the first duties of the physician is to educate the masses not to take medicine.
— Sir William Osler, MD, *Aphorisms from his Bedside Teachings* (1849-1919)

America has become a nation of hypochondriacs. If you have constant heartburn you're under stress. You aren't suffering from acid reflux disea$e. Look for the reason behind the symptom and remove the reason, don't cover it up. If you suffer from migraines, look for the reason; don't begin routinely adding medications every time you have a symptom. The dependency creates codependency, as the drugs themselves become prescription-fulfilling prophecies.

This is what the **pharmo-medical machine** desperately desires. The book, *Selling Sickness: How the World's Biggest Pharmaceutical Companies Are Turning Us All into Patients*, by Ray Moynihan and Alan Cassels, describes the business well. Many of the physicians responsible for setting health standards also sit on the board of directors of the major drug companies.

> Eight of the nine experts who wrote the latest cholesterol guidelines also served as paid speakers, consultants or researchers to the world's major drug companies—Pfizer, Merck, Bristol-Myers-Squibb, Novartis, Bayer, Abbott, AstraZeneca, and GlaxoSmithKline.
> — Ray Moynihan and Alan Cassels, *Selling Sickness*[226]

Moynihan and Cassels reveal that cholesterol guidelines are only one example, and that approximately 90 percent of the physicians who set the guidelines for other physicians have conflicts of interest or financial ties with the pharmaceutical industry. It does lead us to wonder why they want to drop the guidelines for cholesterol so often. If they can convince people they need to drop 20 more cholesterol points, to say, 180 or 160, how many more millions of people can they pull into the circle of fear? How much more profit is generated? Moynihan and Cassels remind the readers of former Merck CEO, Henry Gadsen's, interview with Fortune Magazine in which he restated his frustration that his firm was only selling drugs to sick people, and that his "dream" was to be able to sell drugs to healthy people; they could then "sell to everyone."[227]

Having read this, don't think that you can suddenly stop taking your medication, because the reason for your need may still be present.

Mehmet Oz, MD, vice chair of surgery and professor of cardiothoracic surgery at Columbia University, has written that some older people with high levels of arterial blockage have no heart problems, and yet younger people with the same level of blockage have chest pain. Oz writes in *Healing from the Heart* that the reason two different people react differently to the same scenario is unknown,* and that, "It all depends on how pliable—how spasm-prone—a patient's vessel walls are." But Dr. Oz adds that much-needed nexus that reveals that heart attacks are more often tensionalgia events, by stating at a conference on the Mind-Body Connection, in 2000, that "it is his [Oz'] observation that many heart attacks can be traced back to a very stressful life event that occurred about four to seven days prior." This is after-storm, or Phase 4 TMS tensionalgia… beyond the battlefield.

The Hunter Becomes the Hunted, Turning the Tables on Health Myths

> My life is in the hands of any rascal who chooses to annoy and tease me.
> — John Hunter, anatomist, admitted Type A, father of modern surgery

As Hunter knew, until his abrupt end (a heart attack during an argument, in his mid 60s), our egos account for many of our infirmities, and as Dr. Oz knows, high cholesterol isn't the primary cause of heart attacks. Anger, frustration, and resentment

---

* The majority of physical symptoms where the etiology is described as "unknown" is normally TMS.

are, as well as the ever-present predisposition as to where people store anger in their bodies.

Paul Rosch, MD, clinical professor of medicine and psychiatry at New York Medical College and president of the American Institute of Stress, stated at a conference on cholesterol, "Anyone who questions cholesterol usually finds his funding cut off.... Stress has more deleterious effects on the heart than cholesterol."[228] At the same conference, Danish physician, Uffe Ravnskov, MD, showed reports on the ineffectiveness of lowering cholesterol in the attempt to decrease heart attacks, stating, "The reduced rates of cardiovascular mortality were small for men and nonexistent for women."[229] Ravnskov believes the problem began with the 1950s Framingham Heart Study's spurious correlation between high cholesterol and heart attacks—since cholesterol was only one factor out of over 200 other risk factors that could predict a heart attack. They could have chosen any one of the 240+ indicators that lead to heart problems, but they latched on to cholesterol—and here it remains—an enormous fear. This is similar to the nonexistent correlation between disc bulging and back pain.

Hidden anger induces the autonomic system to constrict important blood vessels when the individual feels overwhelmed. Here the message is no longer a warning—but a strike. If her cholesterol is high it merely exacerbates the problem, it doesn't create it. If the cholesterol is high, it doesn't take as much anger to damage the heart. So it's important to watch these levels—to a certain point. More than half of the people who die from heart attacks do not have the major predictors of heart disease, such as high cholesterol or blood pressure. As Deepak Chopra, MD, stated, the #1 predictor for heart attacks is job dissatisfaction, and the most common day and time for having a heart attack is Monday at 9 A.M.: the new day of the new conflict.

Rosenman and Friedman's earlier attempts to understand the metabolism of cholesterol and its links to coronary disease quickly focused toward personality characteristics as they began talking with their patients—much like Dr. Sarno did with back pain. These patients rarely felt that cholesterol was the reason behind their heart attacks, and "ranked job stress right at the top"[230] of the list. Their studies also corroborated their own suspicions regarding the missing linkages between cholesterol levels, high blood pressure, and heart attacks.

It became increasingly clear that these risk factors were merely markers that might predict coronary events, but did not cause them.

— Ray H. Rosenman, MD[231]

Heart attacks, high cholesterol, and high blood pressure result from unconscious rage (and stress and dietary considerations). The attacks in the heart are mindbody reactions to overwhelming stress and anger. If you don't have the tools (understanding or desire) to heal, then you will need medication.

I never had an ounce of pain relief from any type of anti-inflammatory medications such as the Cox-2 inhibitors—Vioxx, Celebrex, and Bextra, or any of the NSAIDs, among others. On 9/30/04, Vioxx was wisely pulled from the market, and its intended replacement, Prexige, has been pulled from many foreign markets and hasn't yet met approval for release by the FDA because of its potential for serious side effects. Hailed as **super aspirins**, the effects from Cox-2 inhibitors are often deadlier than the ailments they are prescribed for. This is true for many modern super drugs, as they become more dangerous than being married to Ben Cartwright. Bextra has been cited as a possible cause of Stevens-Johnson Syndrome (a severe reaction to chemicals). At the time of this writing, there are significant challenges to the use of these super drugs, since they are proven to do harm, and rarely do good. While researching, I met one person who told me that Celebrex always helped him. He said, "Steve, it does work for me." I told him that I truly believed it did work for him, but not for the reason he thought it did. It's only effective because he believed it would work for him, and so it did (or did it?). Placebos can be powerful healing forces.

Deep Belief in Anything Is the Master Key

This returns us to the very same question that Georg Groddeck, MD, had posed in the early 1900s as to why one drug worked for one person but not another, even though they shared the same symptoms, disease, and prognosis. It may well be because one sufferer had his confidence built up regarding the drug, and/or just happened to be having a good day when he took it, or from any other possible unconscious forces. Once it works, it tends to work repeatedly, as conditioning takes hold immediately.

The depth of the belief being a key component was confirmed in a University of Michigan study.[232] This is especially so if the symptom is or isn't relieved the very first time the drug (or surgery) was utilized. That first cut will always be the most influential because it creates a new experience, leaving the deepest scar.

Some would argue that the anti-inflammatories don't stop TMS pain because TMS pain has no swelling. But this is not always true. I had swelling from tension, Dr. Sopher tells me he has had it, and many others have as well. There can be swelling in TMS, and if symptom-relief is the question, then drugs may be a short-term answer—sometimes necessary.

Hemorrhoids are an inflammatory process, most often stress-induced. Tension can produce swelling in various forms. Many times I would exit a stressful meeting, my gums swollen from tension. Even though gums and hemorrhoids are on opposite ends of the body (depending on where your head is), the concept remains the same. There's a reason for the symptom and the drug doesn't alleviate the reason. Only the soporific effects of potent painkillers helped me during times of intense pain, and their effects wore off after a while, as my mindbody acclimated to their biochemical effects. Then the price had to always be paid for borrowed relief, as the withdrawal from painkillers became as painful as the pain itself.

People are in pain and depressed for a reason. Why would an individual rather pop a pill than find the core of his problem? John Lee answers: "Chemical addiction renders the mind incompetent." To confront and defeat anger takes "both halves of our bodymind."[233] The anger remains in the body, and the drug binds the anger to the body. Oftentimes, as long as the pain medication is taken, the pain remains, as the medication perpetuates an **association-pain response**. There are several people who have had multiple surgeries who have decided to cease taking pain medication postoperatively, and their pain abruptly ended. The drug had bound them to their pain—acting as a trigger for their pain. Stopping pain medication may stop the pain by not allowing the drug to trigger the pain through association.

Alter My Mood—Someone or Something Please Make Me Happy

What do mood-altering drugs such as antidepressants do physiologically within the brain? Their overall effect comes from increasing the flow of **neurotransmitters**. Some drugs can sync into the neurons and have a magnifying effect by releasing large quantities of neurotransmitters. Other drugs like the SSRIs, which block the reabsorption rate of neurotransmitters, can dramatically flood the system with them. Other drugs, which produce feelings of pleasure, enable the limbic system to release the neurotransmitter dopamine, further increasing the sensation of pleasure (aaahh, id does love pleasure). So drugs can either flush out certain transmitters, or slow the reabsorption of neurotransmitters, which magnifies their effect. We feel our best when we have a wide variety of available neurotransmitters available in our brain, and so drugs can make us feel good without having had any actual life experience. *The easy way out.* And—as former Ohio State University football coach Woody Hayes often said, "Anything that comes easy aint worth a damn."

Sidney Wolfe, MD, Acting Director of Public Citizen, states, "A lot of problems have been medicalized, like insomnia. There are a lot of reasons people can't go to sleep, but they should deal with those reasons instead of popping a sleeping pill." People are leaning heavily on the new super drugs for the same old problems when often "the answer is no drug at all." Antidepressant medication also inhibits the integration of TMS and should be stopped when possible. But the industry keeps pushing people to make them feel they need to be medicated to be well—and so the people keep wanting.

We are the people that can find, whatever you may need
If you got the money, we got your disease.

— Guns N' Roses, "Welcome to the Jungle"

Alternatively Speaking....

A 2006 Lindsey Tanner AP article on the 20-billion-dollar per year alternative drug industry cites a study funded by the National Institutes of Health on the effectiveness of glucosamine and chondroitin. One article, "Despite Tests, Many Consumers Swear by Remedies," reveals that glucosamine and chondroitin did "no better than dummy pills at relieving mild arthritis pain."[234] Recent studies have shown similar non-benefits over placebo for echinacea, St. John's wort, saw palmetto, and powdered shark cartilage.

One arthritis sufferer who naïvely believed he was getting benefit from glucosamine and chondroitin was quoted as saying, "I'll wrestle anybody who says it's no good." The study's co-author, Stephen Straus, MD, former Director of the National Institutes of Health National Center of Complementary and Alternative Medicine (I would hate to see the size of this guy's business card) had already studied the changes in the brain functioning of placebo users. Straus writes, "Their wishful thinking that they're going to get better, is harnessing the body's own mechanism for relieving pain." Their belief generates and ignites self-healing, since the mechanisms needed for healing are already within each individual.

But Oz never did give nothing to the Tin Man, That he didn't, didn't already have.
                                                    — "Tin Man", America

Pain sufferers have confided to me that they feel better as soon as the doctor has filled out their pain prescription form. I've had many people tell me that they feel better just knowing the medication is inside their home. Martin Rossman, MD, co-founder, The Academy for Guided Imagery, writes, "...many times people began to feel better as soon as I wrote their prescriptions!"[235] Emmett Miller, MD, has also stated that the hand that gives the pill is often a more powerful force than the pill itself. Drugs to these people are emotional safety nets. They don't fear falling once the drugs are in their possession, because the drugs give them a sense of confidence in themselves to cope through another day. Possession is nine-tenths of the law, of confidence.

Healing begins with belief, and that very belief is magnified when the individual takes the drug and just happens to have a good day, that day, or if the prescriber verbally sells it to the needer. They then associate the drug with the new feeling of wellness—immediate conditioning. After all, Pavlov didn't just ring the bell and the dogs came running. He had to feed them first.

Finally, the only reason to take a drug, either legal or illegal, mainstream or alternative, is to feel better, to fill the gap of isolation. But it should be understood always that the drug didn't make you feel better, it was your initial belief in the drug that did. You did it yourself! You just needed a jump-start and the drug was the jumper cable that extended from the manufacturer to your brain.

Full belief, or "positive expectant faith"[236] in the drug or procedure, is the force behind healing. What should be said when entering the doctor's office is, "I need something to alleviate my symptoms until I get through this emotionally tough time I'm going through." Drugs alleviate symptoms, not causes. A few people have told me, "I don't want to know what my problem is, Steve, I just want the drugs." God Bless America (national anthem begins here).

Yin and Yang

When this is, that is.
From the arising of this, comes the arising of that.
When this isn't, that isn't.
From the cessation of this, comes the cessation of that.
— The Noble Truth of the Cessation, discernment of dukkha

This is a good time to unravel the mystery of what yin chases yang means (since I couldn't figure where else to put it in the book). It simply means that the very same thing taken to its own extreme becomes itself once again as life folds over into itself to maintain balance. Every life experience and all creativity come from the clash of opposing forces—the collision of the energy of polar opposites. It's healthy to laugh and it's healthy to cry—the brightest stars eventually become black holes—the good person without accountability becomes the evil one.* Steroids take away skin redness, but if used too long, they redden the skin. The germaphobe cleans her hands to avoid germs, but cleaning too much destroys antibodies, allowing for infection. Lying down for a headache helps, but if you stay down too long it gives you a headache. The desire of total control results in the loss of all control. The greater the love you feel the deeper the pain of loss. If you help your child, she learns; if you do everything for her, she never learns… everything becomes itself—every opposite, its own opposite.

---

* *"Power tends to corrupt, absolute power corrupts absolutely—great men are almost always bad men."*
[John Emerich Edward Dalberg Acton (Lord Acton), Letter to Bishop Mandell Creighton, 1887]

25

Passus (Latin: "having suffered")

People who seem to be moving to greater levels of enlightenment and light actually experience darkness in more dramatic ways, and often times more tragic ways than people who live in the safe middle, people who are comfortably nice. Greek drama called this the tragic flaw... it said that every great person always had a tragic side, a tragic story, a secret wound that became the hole in the soul... the really great people I've met, when they (late at night) start telling you their story, there is always a big wound there or a big mistake or a dark side that they've never talked to anybody about... and you can't help but think that that very boxing ring they live in is part of what's made them great.
— Richard Rohr, OFM, *Quest for the Grail*

The aphorism states: *Experience is what we get when things don't go as planned.* When things do not go as planned, deeper understanding takes place and transformation begins. Will Rogers said, "Good judgment comes from experience, and a lot of that comes from bad judgment." Whether it is a huge mistake, or a traumatic experience, deeper understanding often comes through suffering, as ego dissolves into the light of consciousness. Knowledge can be purchased at any corner bookstore, but you can't buy understanding. Understanding comes through experience, and through relating knowledge to that experience. It is the valleys that make the mountains so towering; suffering that yields to compassion; death that makes life so precious.

It's Dark Inside This Whale's Belly.... Anybody Gotta Light?

Every problem, therefore, brings the possibility of a widening of consciousness, but also the necessity of saying goodbye to childlike unconsciousness....
— Carl Jung, *The Stages of Life*[237]

History has shown a pattern of malignant narcissism in people who have never been down-n-out. The only path to spiritual expansion is to experience life in many ways—the more dramatic, the deeper the understanding. How can there be high vibrational energy if there is no low vibrational energy? Where is the reference point? Enlightenment is only enlightenment because there first exists darkness—each relying on the other's existence. Even the beautiful flower needs dirt in which to grow.

Actor Michael J. Fox understands the concept well. Over a decade ago, Michael began experiencing Parkinson's disease (PD), a progressive and degenerative neurological ailment. This would destroy many people. But through his open heart

268

and mind, and the help of his family and a Jungian analyst, Michael found light where isolation and despair would normally thrive.

If you were to rush into this room right now and announce that you had struck a deal—with God, Allah, Buddha, Christ, Krishna, Bill Gates, whomever—in which the ten years since my diagnosis could be magically taken away, traded in for ten more years as the person I was before—I would, without a moment's hesitation, tell you to take a hike... I would no longer want to go back to that life—a sheltered narrow existence fueled by fear and made livable by insulation, isolation, and self-indulgence. It was a life lived in a bubble....

— Michael J. Fox, *Lucky Man*[238]

Michael recognizes his disease has been an enlightening blessing. He appears to be unconsciously punishing himself in order to assuage the pleasure of having had so much, overlain with deeper issues from his past. Michael is a rare breed—seeing light where many would perceive darkness. He is reconnecting by moving outside of his personal bubble and back into life's boxing ring with purpose in his corner, helping others through increased PD awareness.

TMS pain can be a blessing, since it provides the catalyst for needed change. Suffering also uncovers the deep desire for spiritual balance because it unveils to the individual that he isn't happy—not on his own path—out of balance. Worrying, trying too hard, and complaining, do not solve problems. Growth occurs not by solving problems, but by rising above them. Suffering is not the goal in life; it is an integral part of life that gives opportunity for creativity and growth as it insists upon needed change. When we don't change, we don't grow—we are stuck in suffering—heading for more suffering.

If you continue on the path you are on, you will get where you are headed.

— Chinese Proverb

Suffering Has A Purpose: Although It May Be Unknown

In their book, *Getting Well Again*, O. Carl Simonton, along with his wife Stephanie Simonton and his colleague James Creighton, asked their cancer patients to list the benefits they had received from getting cancer. The five benefits are consolidated:

1. Receiving permission to get out of dealing with a troublesome problem or situation.

2. Getting attention, care, nurturing from people around them.

3. Having an opportunity to regroup their psychological energy to deal with a problem or to gain a new perspective.

4. Gaining an incentive for personal growth or for modifying undesirable habits.

5. Not having to meet their own or others' high expectations.

— L. Creighton and O. Simonton and S. Simonton-Matthews,
Getting Well Again[239]

If a person desires to understand why he is in chronic pain, he could read *Getting Well Again*, and substitute the word pain for cancer. The mindbody is in the state it is—precisely as a result of the information it holds in shadowy places within the cells of the body. We tell our bodies what to do and when to do it—unconsciously—to run away from or reconnect with others.

> *A cell is like a computer chip. A chip is a bit of information and so is a cell... Bruce Lipton scoffs at the assumption that "cancer runs in the family." There is no cancer gene, he insists. Cells go cancerous when they are told to do so.*
> — Anna Spencer, PhD, *"Cell Consciousness—Proves Mind Over Matter"*[240]

TMS remains a tutor, as life can become a tough teacher that gives the test first, and the lesson later. Carl Jung wrote, "There is no coming to consciousness without pain,"[241] and through suffering, the unconscious rises toward consciousness. We learn, or grow, from suffering, most likely because we aren't yet evolved enough to have the ability to grow without suffering.

Martin Rossman, MD, writes of the benefits of his own suffering while studying to become a physician. One day while sitting at a conference table after rounds with other physicians from the pediatric ward, the chief resident of pediatrics broke down in what Rossman described as "deep sobbing." As he put his face in his hands he blurted out, "I can't stand it anymore.... I can't stand to see one more kid die."[242] The next day the chief resident quit. The day after, Rossman became ill with nausea, fever, and severe weakness. As I have previously written, we share grief and pain, often triggered by others' grief and pain. Rossman's lab results showed abnormal liver enzymes as well as an enlarged liver with signs of fatigue. His liver enzymes remained elevated for months until, as he writes, "I had my first normal lab panel the weekend my pediatrics rotation ended."[243] Rossman knows that it's often difficult to see the benefits of suffering during the suffering, writing, "Looking back, I have no doubt that this illness served an important function in me[244]. ... I can see that it relieved me from my responsibility I didn't want to have, and it gave me time to think a great deal about whether or not I wanted to continue in medicine."[245]

That hellfire that people roll through can burst their bubbles and often saves their lives through reflection, and then—rebuilding.

The Law of Attraction holds that we get back what we feel. All the labels in the world mean nothing; the only thing that matters is how we are vibrating. If we truly aren't where we want to be—we bring to us something that gets us to our destination, although not in the way we had planned. Like cancer—pain is not the enemy—we can create it if we need it. Illness is feedback regarding our deepest unmet needs.

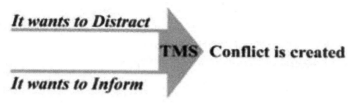

It wants to Distract

TMS **Conflict is created**

It wants to Inform

We suffer when we feel isolated, unappreciated, alone—unconnected. Suffering pushes us toward growth until we reach a certain level of awareness and then are suddenly pulled toward our predetermined path—toward our ultimate Self—the Truth. It is an intrinsic part of the human condition. The Four Noble Truths of Buddha refer to suffering, its role in life, and the way out.

Revered monk, Thich Nhat Hanh, describes the First Noble Truth: "The First Truth is the truth about suffering, and no one can see the path unless he or she sees suffering."[246] The Fourth Noble Truth is the path that leads out of suffering. No one can understand how to get out of suffering, until they realize how they got into suffering. The cocoon is the suffering; the butterfly born from suffering is happiness, the transformation process is life.

If we are not in contact with pain, we cannot know what real happiness is.
— Thich Nhat Hanh, Anger, Wisdom for Cooling the Flames[247]

Suffering opens the door to varying levels of consciousness. The human condition of suffering is an essential part of life, as Siddhārtha Gautama Buddha had been enlightened to, and Christ personified in His Passion. Without suffering, there is no compassion for the suffering of others because, like Parzival, you cannot know what questions to ask in order to relieve others from their own suffering. Wounds create experience from potential and reconnect humanity.

It seems that it's only the world of darkness, failure, disappointment, that teaches us the essential things: patience, letting go, surrender, compassion. You don't learn these in a world full of light. You don't have to feel the pain of others, or the pain of yourself, and so when the wounded ones come into your life you have no patience with them because you think it's all light.

— Richard Rohr, OFM, Quest for the Grail

We are born knowing the Truth—which exists inside everyone. The Truth also stands outside, in dimensions unknown. Only the body stands in the way. The body is a wall of fear and doubt that separates both halves of truth that desire to be whole and unified—as the deeper self knows exactly what it desires to be connected to. Pain is pushing us toward an inner truth—more content and aware.

Suffering has a noble purpose: the evolution of consciousness and the burning up of the ego. The man on the cross is an archetypal image. He is every man and every woman. As long as you resist suffering, it is a slow process because the resistance creates more ego to burn up. When you accept suffering, however, there is an acceleration of that process which is brought about by the fact that you suffer consciously... In the midst of conscious suffering there is already the transmutation. The fire of suffering becomes the light of consciousness.
— Eckhart Tolle, *A New Earth: Awakening to Your Life's Purpose*[248]

Tommy and Abe

In his life, Thomas Jefferson lost all of his children but one—he also lost his wife. He lost almost everyone that he loved and yet he helped found a free nation. Abraham Lincoln lost all of his children except one, and yet he helped ratify or unify that nation. Greatness can come from tragedy—yet there are the silent heroes, who, only late at night, speak of their great losses. The experience of darkness yields compassion, and through compassion comes forgiveness—and through forgiveness conflict fades into light. With each new scar comes a new birth, and the more scars the more rebirths. There is no death without birth—no birth without suffering—no life without death.

You know you got to go through hell before you get to heaven.
— Steve Miller Band, "Jet Airliner", 1977

26

Holding Onto Anger

You are like a man who wants to harm another and picks up a burning ember—he only burns himself.

— Buddhaghosa, Visuddhimagga, *The Path of Purification*

The final piece of the healing puzzle for me was the understanding of anger's role in pain. It wasn't that I didn't understand anger; I never knew it existed in me. I simply never felt it. Ego had sold out to superego. This final roadblock to healing rivals the understanding that herniated discs don't cause back or neck pain, and that shoulders and knees rarely need "surgically-scoped" for pain relief.

Many people in pain tell me they aren't angry. They often appear smiling, mild-mannered, polite, responsible, controlled, and cool-acting. This outward image hides a hellfire inferno lying just beneath their awareness—but deep within, they know it. It must be denied—OR, it has to be recognized—which ain't gonna happen because ego won't allow it. I believe the problem is in the fact that most people don't understand the concept of subconscious activity. It's difficult to believe what we can't see; skepticism is easier than seeking truth, as evidenced in atheism. It's easier to say something doesn't exist than to expel the energy and time needed to understand and to seek its essence.

Anger that is felt or recognized is acceptable anger. It is not part of the personal shadow, or the pain, because that anger is conscious. The unconscious anger is causing the symptoms and is of such unacceptable magnitude that it is relegated to the shadow. She has an anger problem—trouble feeling anger, trouble expressing anger, leading to bodily expressions of conflict.

The epiphany that led to my own healing was the understanding that I was furious inside, but never felt it, except through the multitude and severity of my symptoms. I had my light bulb moment when I bought a videotape by Dr. Sarno where he emphasized, "the rage that is causing your pain, you will never feel." Even though he wrote and wrote and wrote about repression, which I understood at an intellectual level, I didn't remember him saying those very words, that the rage is not felt. He stated, "Any anger you're aware of has nothing to do with TMS." And so, I truly didn't understand repression at an elemental level. Repression means you have paralyzed your feeling of that emotion associated with that event. My own thinking was—"well, okay, it's repressed, but I still don't feel it?" It was a DUH moment for me. But I don't feel so duh-mb as I talk with more and more pain sufferers who don't get it either. Nothing irritates me more than while trying to help people I hear them say things such as, "Weeelll, gotta disagree with you on that one SteveO, I'm a very calm person,"… as they suck on their asthma inhaler—OR—"Naw, you're waaaay off man, I'm a laid-back person, gotta give you a big fat NO on that one SteveO,"… as they have pain screaming down their legs, or anxiety attacks. They are livid inside; they just don't know it because they don't understand how the unconscious works in silence. I didn't get it at first, and neither do they. Repression works outside of awareness.

The notion of a structural cause of chronic pain is outdated. If a person can't get past the point that their on-again-off-again pain is not from those darn discs, or small rotator cuff tears, they will always be in pain… on again, and off again. Or, if they find a surgeon, perhaps farther away, who tells them that he can repair their problem—one who they believe in deeply—the placebo effect may take hold. When told they have a problem that can be physically repaired, their self-image can remain intact. Now—if the individual is insightful enough to understand that they themselves are generating their own symptoms, for a reason that only their shadow knows, then it comes down to understanding the role of anger—rage—vile energy.

The persona is like the tip of an iceberg. The tip is that part of the individual that he allows the world to see—while the bulk of his emotional self is buried beneath the surface of his unconscious waters. If the tip of the iceberg is very small, then he shows little of himself and there can be much anger hiding beneath. So, if he smiles a lot or is very quiet, polite, non-confrontational, a goodist—extremely isolated—then beware. Tragically, this was seen in the Virginia Tech massacre of 2007. Seung Hui Cho's roommates, to the person, stated that he never spoke and rarely acknowledged them. He continuously repressed everything, and everything that he didn't like—which was his life. Anger is only one letter from danger—if not properly released.

The reason that so many people withhold rage, is that as children, they learned that showing anger was a bad thing—sinful-like. And repression begins. This pattern becomes all that the individual knows—a part of his nature. He is conditioned to never let go, never cry, and never express his true feelings. Life becomes a baseball game, and everyone knows there's no crying in baseball.

People are angry that they are angry. And they are angry that the pain will not leave them, even though they believe the TMS process and understand it. This impatience leads to even more anger—a Ferris wheel that they can't get off. People then project their own anger onto others in order to place blame anywhere but on themselves. But the people they are angry with are the ones winning, because the ones they are angry with are controlling their behavior. The angriest people I talk with are those who were abandoned, molested, or ignored as children, or were forced into religious beliefs that they couldn't understand.

I'm often asked by pain sufferers how they can let go of their anger at a criticism directed at them. People bluntly tell me that they cannot release such a perceived rejection when someone stings their egos. They hold onto these criticisms forever. It's easy to say let it go, but it can be difficult to follow through when ego is dominating.

Anger guru, John Lee, contends that anger must be felt (brought to consciousness) before it can be released. As long as pain is present, there has been no purging of the specific memories of rejection, isolation, or—specifically, abandonment. Lee cautions us to be wary of abandonment addiction: erroneously associating being treated like garbage as good for us, or as a form of love that we somehow deserve. This, he writes, is because "We become accustomed to people not being there for us to the point that we feel it is right. Leaving looks like loving."[249] Lee continues, "Nine out of ten times, those of us who had a cold mother or distant father choose a cold wife or distant husband."[250] A very small number of former chronic pain sufferers have told me that their parents were very warm and loving; however, many still had fear of parental separation.

Many, as children, were forced into religious rituals before they were able to understand in life (Latin, religare, "to bind strongly"); they were made to feel guilty and told that they were sinners for enjoying, even contemplating, pleasure. They then feel forever flawed and think they must be perfect or they will find hellfire suddenly upon them. They are extremely angry at life—as well as religion. TMS then serves as a tool for self-punishment for things they unconsciously think that they have done wrong, or thought were wrong in the eyes of their culture. Murder, wounding others, lying, infidelity, stealing, suicide, and lack of compassion are culturally taboo—ineffable thoughts; but everyone has these darkside shadow images in what Jung called "positively demonic dynamism"*—and when they begin to surface, we must either act on them, or punish ourselves for thinking them. With TMS we punish ourselves—sometimes severely. The more unthinkable and reprehensible the thought, the more self-punishment must be imposed to assuage the guilt that society has instilled in us for possessing such condemnable images. For example, deep down inside, you really don't want to take care of your ailing parents. You are not as good as you imagine yourself to be. You seem to care outwardly—or you like to think you do—but deep within your shadow, you don't care that much, because your shadow has other interests that continually change. So when a loved one falls ill, we often find our own health failing because of the tyranny of the should—dividing our minds in conflict between the "I should" and the "I don't give a damn."

> ...it [pain and illness] has to punish a sin against a commandment.
> — Georg Groddeck, MD, *The Book of the It*[251]

---

* Jung also referred to our darker aspect as "a raging monster" in *On the Psychology of the Unconscious,* (1912). [CW 7: *Two Essays on Analytical Psychology,* p. 35]

All parents, including myself, damage their children in some form. Most do not purposely do so, but it still occurs as a natural part of life. Those who feel their parents did no harm to them are in denial; as Lee writes, "Denial saves them from having to go through the grief and rage that always follow embracing the truth. Denial protects them from losing their idealized childhood and mourning the self they didn't become, and from having to hate their parents and then learn to love them in a new, sadder, but authentic and adult way."[252] Lee continues his example with a client that he told, "If you're not happy with your life… then you were abandoned as a child."[253] I also found that well-meaning parents can lead their children to guilt and perfectionism by telling them that they are soooo good, that they never make mistakes—praising them to others, setting up the fear of failure, relying on others' approval to feel good about themselves.

Is this to say that all pain in life is because of parents? No—of course not. Parents often unintentionally, through criticisms or kindness, create problematic behavioral patterns in children. These children often grow up to become parents who pass those same patterns on to their children. I don't advocate blaming parents. My parents were good people, they loved me and my brothers—they persevered, tried to do what was right with what they had and knew—and they did. As free-willed adults, the choice is up to the adult to learn and to heal any unintended harm handed down to them.

There are of course the purposefully abusive parents. These pain sufferers harbor great amounts of rage from being abandoned, and tend to have more health issues. The abandonment in these cases, although painful, can be handled in the same manner suggested in the third trinity below, by dealing, feeling, and letting go of what was.

In my chronic pain program I found that the common denominator was child abuse—in all of these people—it was absolutely predictable.

— Robert Scaer, MD

A Trinity for Dealing With Anger—The First Step of Admittance

Sometimes, I guess there's just not enough rocks.

— Forrest Gump, *Forrest Gump*

Once the individual understands that the source of his physical manifestation is unfelt rage, and not a body defect, the question is always, "How do I stop being angry?" The answer is not always simple, as anger is a fiery behavior that sometimes needs to be discharged through appropriate expression. If we can take the energy of anger and turn it into motivation for change, we can divert the energy toward purpose and creativity and away from self-destruction. I've listed three broad-based categories for dealing with anger.*

Burn It—This is a temporary fix but in a day-to-day world it is a valuable and healthy tool to use in the short term. It can be thought of as a physical catharsis. Jogging, walking, table tennis, swimming, and many other forms of **continuous physical movement** temporarily discharge tension. However—the root problem remains and the seeds of discontent grow back.

Face It—Counseling or analytical introspection or any host of other insight-oriented therapies, including emotional release work, can cut through the heart of conflict. To feel and talk away anger may be two of the best ways to purge unexpressed energy, but it bypasses forgiveness. Understanding why someone did what they did to us does not necessarily mean we forgive them.

Stop Stress, a French company, once offered people use of an auto junkyard, for 40 Euros, to smash old cars in order to rid stress and anger. This is considered a form of emotional release. However, the revered Buddhist monk, Thich Nhat Hanh would understandably disagree with this methodology for dealing with anger. This leads us into the third and more spiritual method of dealing with anger.

Transform It—In his book, *Anger: Wisdom for Cooling the Flames*, Hanh writes that anger is a poison in the heart—and if it remains, there can be no happiness because happiness is a freedom that holding anger will never allow. Hanh advocates the practice of **compassionate listening** to dissolve anger. His premise is that we ingest anger every day. We eat anger because that which we eat must be killed. We watch anger on TV and read about anger in the papers and the Internet. Anger is inside all of us in what he calls the **seeds of anger** (e.g., two dogs in every man, yin and yang, Eros and Thanatos, creative instincts and destructive instincts—the divided mind). If the seeds of anger are watered, they grow and permeate the body, since anger is not psychological but organic in nature: that is, we feel and hold anger in our bodies.

Hanh's experience has shown that the best way to handle anger is to transform the energy of anger into compassionate and positive energy by embracing it. Anger, like pain, is not the enemy; it's a part of you that needs to be recognized and attended to. Who hasn't been angry with someone, gotten up the nerve to go talk, worked it out, and felt the burden lifted? Afterwards, the uplifting feeling is indescribable as the burden is rolled away. However, you must understand why the anger exists in yourself first—and only then, can you deal with anger in others.

This correlates with Dr. Weil's experience that his cancer patients did much better when they treated their cancer as a part of themselves rather than as a foreign invader. In *Spontaneous Healing*, Weil questions whether the notion of "I'm going to fight this

---

* Anger behind TMS comes, as Dr. Sarno described, from three possible sources or combinations thereof: id-superego conflict, residual rage from childhood, and daily stressors. The illness or pain merely exacerbates existing rage.

thing" is a good ideology regarding healing from pain and illness. *Sic vis pacem para bellum.* A man divided against himself cannot stand, and is merely two men in eternal conflict.

Anger can only be transformed through mindfulness. Mindfulness is the practice of being present, and aware of what is going on, without any judgment, simply observing what is: "Body and mind united."[254] With **presence**, you cannot suppress your anger or deny it. By taking care of your anger you transform it from negative to positive energy. Taking care of it means to not battle it, but rather, understand why it exists, and then use the energy of anger to transform it into something positive or useful. Hanh states that denying anger is due to pride. This is why so many people in pain claim they aren't angry. Their pride will not allow them to admit to such a cultural weakness. But anger is a seed born inside everyone—not only are we born with it, we also consume it daily, and need to attend to it with compassion.

As mentioned earlier, James Pennebaker, PhD, has shown that confiding and listening are major factors in healing and in dealing with anger. Along with forgiving herself, and showing compassion and kindness toward others, she desperately needs to know that someone understands her.

Compassion quells anger and protects us, since we are all part of potential higher streams of consciousness—One heart, One mind. When one person suffers—we all suffer. When you suffer, others suffer: when I suffer, I'm going to make certain you suffer.

Through conscious breathing, we connect ourselves to ourselves and feel and release our anger. It is impossible to be angry and to be calmly breathing at the same time. Anger shortens breathing as the body reacts to the tension. This is why TMSers are breath-holders—they are constantly angry.

Hanh doesn't advocate hitting pillows, or screaming at photos, or anything that is called venting. Multiple studies today show this is not helpful in the long run and is in fact dangerous because it strengthens the roots of anger. Venting is merely replaying or rehearsing your anger. Throwing things and hitting things only exhausts you and fools you into believing your anger is gone, but in fact, it just leaves you too exhausted to be angry. The roots of the anger remain buried. Venting can often make you angrier, and the next time you see the person you are angry at, you may practice what you have rehearsed by hitting him or screaming at him. **Venting is conditioning.** Hanh does not contend that compassion and understanding means that you let people walk all over you. If they try, walk away—breathe—and try to understand why they are suffering.

Most of our suffering is born from our lack of understanding and insight that there is no separate self. The other person is you, you are the other person.
                        — Thich Nhat Hanh, *Anger, Wisdom for Cooling the Flames*[255]

So the answer to cooling the flames, as Hanh has experienced, is to recognize that you are angry, and then "take good care of it." Also, recognize that when others get mad at you, they are suffering. Make peace with yourself first, and then you can make peace with others. Hanh would advocate that when you feel the pain in your back—send it your love.

A Philosophy on Life:
Acting on New Knowledge
and Healing

27

Physician Heal Thyself— How To Free Yourself From Pain

The man who insists upon seeing with perfect clearness before he decides, never decides. Accept life, and you must accept regret.

— Henri-Frederic Amiel, *Journal in Time*

Get a Physical Exam (uh—from a doctor… did I need to clarify that?)

Even though a vast majority of disorders are the effect of an emotional repression (barring the involvement of any overwhelming external factors, e.g., prolonged exposure to UV rays or years of smoking), you may first need external help (science) to rebalance. **Seek professional help first in order to rule out the need for further outside help.** If the diagnosis comes back as normal aging of the spine and joints (or whatever), rejoice in the fact that your life is in your hands and you are healable. If you fit the profile of what has been described in this book, then you are in a TMS-healable state and there is no further need for medical help. This is the good news proclaimed by the good doctor(s). Beware of professionals demanding unnecessary tests, exams, joint replacements, pseudo-therapies, medications, and surgeries.

If you are reading this and in great or chronic pain, or have any pain-equivalent symptoms—the healing can begin today with a fuller and deeper understanding of what comprises good health. The latter portion of this book is about life and living—practical and philosophical, immediate and concise—a viewpoint on healing as seen through the eyes of many who have healed, including moi. Become more aware of how **you** react to life and how your darker side motivates you to do good deeds—and bad, and you will discover a new path. There is no one direction. Healing is all about understanding **yourself**—your behavioral characteristics (the way in which you respond to stimulation), and your biography.

You may think it would be easier to follow my path where the weeds have already been trampled—an easier path laid down before you. But you won't learn anything new about yourself—your strengths and abilities, by following me. But I can guide you. If you desire to heal, then you need to walk over to the window, open it, and throw out everything you currently believe is true regarding pain. You also need to reach farther and expect less, it's not about lowering standards—everyone has the right to accomplish and to achieve. It's about understanding, and then believing.

Talk Through Your Current Issues—Not About Health

Confiding in others who care can be more healing than journaling, which is a great healer itself. As mentioned in chapters one and fourteen, James W. Pennebaker proved that denying mental pain causes physical pain, and illness. Finding the right person or confidant can have tremendous healing effects. While working on this section of this book, I received this voicemail from a friend (reproduced with her permission).

> *Hey SteveO… my neck was killing me, oh pain pain pain. It was because mom and I were on a disagreement, so I thought ok, I'm gonna call her tonight, and (um) it melted like butter. The pain is gone, isn't that amazing? I mean within five minutes of talking to mom, everything's fine, everything's ok… it's gone, the pain is gone, isn't that weird?*
> — Mrs. Olda Na'bohr

Pennebaker maintains that the key to good confiding is in choosing the confidant, and that the most important factor is **trust**. Beyond that, is finding someone nonjudgmental who will not criticize you, or who is a safe or anonymous listener. Talking with others who understand through their own experiences is a deeply healing mechanism. I found this to be true when I confided in pain forums toward the end of my healing. People will open up to virtual listeners and say things that they won't normally tell their family members because the family can be judgmental and defensive. People across the Internet are anonymous and therefore generally safe. Pennebaker also states that "self-disclosure will change the nature of your friendship."[256] As I became closer friends with others through healing, helping, and communicating, we eventually stopped talking about pain and only talked about life. It was here that I began to learn the deeper aspects of why TMS occurs.

Another valuable method is to find the professional listener. Or—if you don't want to offend someone in particular—write down all the things that worry and anger you, and then throw them away. Writing is self-talk, which is good, but confiding to another individual is a deeper healing. Pennebaker himself is somewhat ambivalent on whether you need another person to talk to in healing. He suggests that talking into a tape recorder may be as effective, especially if an individual doesn't open up easily or is racked with inhibitions. He asserts that writing is also invaluable in healing and the topic doesn't always need to be from the past.

> *It is not necessary to write about the most traumatic experience of your life. It is more important to focus on the issues that you are currently living with.*
> — James Pennebaker, PhD, *Opening Up:*
> *The Healing Power of Confiding in Others*[257]

Learn a New Language

First, stop placating your pain—become more confident. Throw away all aids and support devices. Get rid of pillows, back braces, canes, arch supports, crutches, comfy chairs, therapy, creams, drugs, shoe lifts, magnets, special mattresses, and self-pity. It's time to get tough now and to take your life back. You can do this!! I wasn't sure I could ever do it, and yet I did. I healed after nearly 30 years of pain, and as my internal language changed—so did my beliefs.

Change your internal language from can't... to am.... Tomorrow is not the day to heal, today am the day. Putting off the effort is what psychiatrists call **resistance,** and holds back healing. However, the desperation for immediate change is also expecting too much—just keep trying*—TMS-healing works! The subtlety is in the degree of expectation. One says "I am healing" and the other says "I must heal." Must-type thinking slows healing because it adds stressors, "Am healing" is relaxing confidence.

When pain strikes, talk to your **self** or think psychologically—in deep reflection; never look physically for the reason. What this means is to run back through your mind all the events that have occurred recently leading up to the onslaught of your pain (refer to Chapter 13). One or a few of these events is the cause of your symptoms—but may have been silently cast into your body by ego, bypassing your awareness. It has been estimated that we are only aware of about 5 percent of our surroundings. So it's important to look deeper, transforming the other 95 percent with dogged determination.

A new language of confidence shortens time in each of the **stages of TMS healing.** You must not think that you have TMS, you will KNOW it! The first stage is hoping you have TMS, the next stage is wanting to believe you do, the next stage is hoping that you are hoping for the right thing, the next stage is thinking you might, the next stage is thinking you do, the next stage is thinking you made a mistake when you first thought you had it, the next stage is worrying about the next stage, the next stage is being positive that you have TMS, the next stage, when the pain increases, is not being so sure anymore, the next stage is certainty that you have TMS, and the final stage is **knowing** you have it. There will be a point where you know it—doubt will be erased and the pain will suddenly... be... gone.

Self-Talk: Washing Your Brain Out with Soap

So it's vital to pay close attention to the internal language that you use when referring to yourself. Even those people who have healed completely, after reading Sarno, will inadvertently say to me, "Steve, my back never goes out anymore." The back never "went out;" that type of language needs to, though. Change your internal dialogue to the **language of improvement** because if you say something long enough, often enough, it begins to reinforce idle deeper beliefs in a manner similar to priming a pump. Is your language always negative? I once asked a former chronic pain sufferer if he would count how many negative thoughts he had per day. He wrote back and said he was astounded

---

* "There will be relapses into disbelief but the relapses will be shorter and shorter. Once you empower yourself, take control of your life, everything starts to go faster until ultimately you become your own healer." [Bruce Lipton, PhD]

at how negative he was. He spoke only one language to himself and it wasn't English—it was Neglish. Years and years of beating yourself up over every detail leads to a chronically negative atmosphere conducive to suffering. The negative must be switched for positive, even if the positive is not yet fully believed. The new language will eventually seep into the depths of the unconscious. It's hard to find the positive in everything—but it is possible to find center ground. You're never as good as you think you are, and you're never as bad as you think you are. Internal language is the filter by which we take action. TMSers are truly not as bad as they think they are, but they have convinced themselves that they are, and they continuously agree with themselves through negative reinforcement. A woman in chronic pain I communicated with sent me the following impromptu note of how she felt about herself:

You are lazy
You are out of shape
You look like your mother and a frumpy housewife
Oooh, the tears are rolling now....
You are broken
You are not good for anything
You don't do enough to be a good mother
You are a terrible homemaker
You never challenge yourself socially or intellectually
You don't deserve what you have, the house not having to work
You don't appreciate what you have
You never worked hard for anything in your life.
You are sloppy
You are pathetic
You are weak
You are useless
You are a disappointment
You never finish what you start
You aren't productive
You're a procrastinator

— Melanie Cawlie [Reprinted with permission]

Dr. Sarno refers to this overall view of self as the "beleaguered self." Many people feel they don't deserve to be happy and pain-free. I think most people in chronic pain could find many of these same self-descriptions in themselves. Sufferers tend to see the bad side, but only emit the good side, thus the conflict. Self-help stud, Tony Robbins, has stated that people could get whatever they want from life if they would just stop focusing on everything that can go wrong and only focus on the goal. It MUST be noted that "thinking positive" is not a healing solution. Positive thinking is only within a step of reversal, a change of direction that allows for the genesis of new beliefs to develop. TMS healing does not come from a positive attitude—only from full **belief**.

Joy and Sickness—Sides of the Same Vibrating Coin

The thought, "I think I am sick; therefore, I am sick," sends low vibrational energy out and pulls that which we don't want toward us. It tells the cells they are sick. Bruce Lipton, PhD, has learned through his extensive work on cell function that "Organisms always match their environment and as the environments change the organisms change to adapt to those environments (your genes adapt to your beliefs)."[258] By viewing yourself as broken, old, sick, and incapable—not in control of your health—your body responds physiologically to adapt to those beliefs—to "make it so," as Captain Jean-Luc Picard would say. How you perceive yourself is who you become. Modern medicine, in its fervent desire to mechanically alter the body, tells you that you are in dire need of this or that. Your beliefs control your health, and if those beliefs are based on false perceptions such as bad knees, feet, shoulders, skin, digestive tracts, and backs, your anatomy will crumble—adapt—and match your perception. We are right back to the archetypal influence of physicians once again—and the power of belief. If your doctor tells you Dr. Sarno is wrong, that's it—your belief in a process that has been repeatedly proven to work, has abruptly ended. Your misguided belief has failed you.

With regard to TMS, there should be a shift in vibrational energy toward higher energy frequencies. Seek happiness in more of life's outcomes, scenarios and opportunities. A change in thinking is the precursor to action, and action is the precursor to physical change, and change is the answer to healing. Thoughts such as **can't** or **never** must be replaced with **will** and **am**. I will be ok, therefore I am ok—altering cell structure and physiology.

One of the most common affirmations people use to increase vibration in healing is the Couéism from Émile Coué, "Every day, in every way, I am getting better and better." Also very common is, "I deserve to be happy." These are all good measures and may spark what is already within to vibrate with new life. However, Dr. Weil is correct when he says that experience has shown positive thinking does little if anything. It is far more important to connect with someone who has experienced healing—to read about or communicate with someone who has healed from the same malady you currently have. The unconscious is more susceptible to altering its belief if it witnesses healing—as opposed to trying to convince itself of something it can't comprehend. Affirmations, at times, can be as useless as bead counting or banging your head against a wall or the chanting of phrases—if the ritual is not fully believed, but rather done for ritual's sake. If the individual continuously affirms something he does not believe with all of his Being, he continuously reaffirms the negative—more deeply ingraining failure. **Affirmations often mask negativism.** This is why prayers don't always work. The person doesn't fully believe it will happen. She must believe in her new words eventually or the words are useless. "Managing pain" is affirming a negative—confirming that something is unfixable.

Build Some Fences

Yes people become weighed down, feel torn, trapped, or taken advantage of, and as a result are unhappy or annoyed with themselves.

— Susan Newman, PhD, *The Book of NO*[259]

You need to define personal boundaries that others understand and respect—or as Dr. Newman said, you will become angry at yourself! This is readily accomplished by telling them how you truly feel. I know people who get migraines whenever they go with their friends because they are unconsciously angered at themselves because they don't want to go, but they cannot say no. Susan Newman lays out the basics for Stepping into No:

- *Make a list of your yeses over the period of a week*
- *Pay attention to how you parcel out your time*
- *Get your priorities straight*
- *Know your limits—start to define them if you don't know what they are*
- *Give control to others to ease your responsibilities.*

— Susan Newman, PhD, *The Book of NO*[260]

Newman then goes on to give scenario after scenario on how to set boundaries— how to say no. What does pain have to do with saying no? Only those in pain "no". When someone asks you to do something, they are asking you for a part of your life— stealing your privacy, energy, and time. Be careful when you ask someone to do something for you because you may be asking more than you think.

In a 2008 television interview, Randy Owen, lead singer for the country rock band, Alabama, responded to a question regarding his "dark period" of anxiety and deep depression that he had suffered through by exclaiming, "Yeah—that was from trying to solve everyone's problems!" Know how to say no.

Exercise and Fitness

Citius, Altius, Fortius (faster, higher, stronger)

— The Olympic motto

One of pain's purposes is to keep individuals fearful of moving, and they shouldn't begin moving until they have gained confidence in the TMS diagnosis. Activity begins to reverse the false notions of structuralism.* After so many decades of believing falsehoods about back nerves somehow being pinched, it can be very frightening to think of pushing the physical envelope. The more fear that accompanies the pain, the more power will be given to it by avoiding movement. This is why **activity is the single most important aspect in healing**. However, the fear of the pain should be

---

* Structuralism is a term I have used for the notion that we have no control over our health—a helplessness— that our bodies simply fail "because they do" and not for any underlying reason or purpose.

drawn down gradually. People often fear becoming active, and I don't blame them. The seeds of doubt have sprouted over time that increasing physical activity is causing further damage to the spine or joints. This is not the case.

> *...the advice to resume normal physical activity, including the most vigorous, has been given to a large number of patients over the past seventeen years. I cannot recall one person who has subsequently said that this advice caused him or her to have further back trouble.*
> — John E. Sarno, MD, *Healing Back Pain*[261]

On the other end of the physical spectrum, I have seen people get much worse through inactivity and rest. One man told me he rested his so-called tennis elbow for months but it didn't get any better until he started using it again. Others have told me that their tennis elbows got worse when they rested them. I empathized as my own back and elbow pain got worse with continued rest.

The body, bones, muscles, heart muscle all need to be under some physical stress. The entire vascular and neurological systems need to be stimulated through healthy and fun movement. The body cries out to be used. Decrease the mind's activity and increase the body's ...**find balance....**

Becoming even a little more active can be difficult if an individual has been inactive for prolonged periods; coordination problems may occur as clumsiness stumbles in— a state of proprioception deficiency. This often occurs after a person is injured and has been in recovery for extended lengths of time. Proprioception (defined as "one's own") is the ability of the mind and body to work together. A protracted period of rest has diminishing returns and ultimately becomes incongruous with healing. With proprioception the inner workings of the mindbody aren't shaking hands as well, and the mindbody doesn't quite know where each body part should be when the body is in motion. This dormancy resulting in mindbody atrophy occurs rapidly when motion ceases. We are beings intended to be in almost constant motion, vibrating a full life, driven by purpose.

Proprioceptive sensory loss creates anxiety in individuals but it can be easily reversed. Common methods of regaining control of motion are to run or walk figure eight patterns. Another method is to walk heel-to-toe—retraining the mind and body to work together again as a unit.

The next step after belief change and initial movement is to get into the best physical shape that you can be in for your age and your health status. Include **both** aerobic and anaerobic activities, as well as a healthy diet.

Your pain may increase as you become more active. The increase is frightening and immediately depletes confidence in the TMS diagnosis. Over time, I began to appreciate the increases in pain because I knew it indicated that my brain was resisting the changes—becoming more desperate for a distraction as I dismissed through movement a structural cause for the symptoms. I began to see victory as the pain intensified. I was beginning to understand the concept of the **liminal threshold**—the time and space where all change occurs. Bore tension out of your system by physically and redundantly moving through physical activity until your brain gives up its weapon of obsessive fear. Why is this important for treating chronic pain? By redundantly challenging the body, the fear of hurting herself diminishes as she realizes day after day, week after week, month after month, that her pain is not going to worsen. In fact, it will begin to recede. If the pain begins to move around she has won the battle. And since the mindbody is a process to be maintained, it's paramount to give it what it needs and wants. The body cries out to be pushed, and the mind agrees.

> *Perhaps the most important (but most difficult) thing that patients must do, is to resume all physical activity, including the most vigorous.*
> — John E. Sarno, MD, *Healing Back Pain*[262]

When I first attempted increasing activity, the pain would cut through me. I couldn't even bend enough to touch my knees—the pain was just too intense. So in order to change the manner in which my mind interpreted the pain, I would scramble my thinking pattern by forcing my mind off the pain. I often tried to spell the word Titleist backwards (and that isn't easy 'cause I always giggled at the last three letters). This is the same process I used early on while running, where I forcefully thought of an area on my back that felt great—redirecting my mind's eye from the pain to a feel-great area. I thought of this process as a cognitive transversal but it was simply rearranging my molecules of emotion by changing awareness, perception, reasoning, and judgment to another point where the mind intersects another body area. The breaking of the focus is vital because the obsessive mind latches on tightly to suggestion.

Dr. Sarno concluded that you don't necessarily need to do anything at all to heal except to deeply integrate that the pain is from unconscious rage. But this doesn't always sink in for people and so I included physical fitness. Dr. Sarno also suggests resuming physical activity, the more aggressive the better. Exercise and train as if the pain was not there. Do not think about how the pain will be before going to exercise. Do not purposefully exercise the area in pain. If you do this it becomes physical therapy again, which hinders healing. Train for good health and a sense of well-being. If a particular exercise really hurts the painful area, keep doing the exercise (assuming there has been a doctor's clearance to train). Push through the pain and focus on the exercise or another body area, or someone else's body area—never the pain itself. Continue the movement until the fear and pain vanish. I have seen the pain move quickly when confronted with increased activity and by ignoring it. The area in pain may also need strengthening, not because there is injury there, but it may be weakened due to a lack of bloodflow for prolonged periods. If the spasm is severe enough, the nerve or tissue can be oxygen-deprived, leading to weakened muscles. Increasing strength and aerobic endurance happens quickly, and is one highly effective healing tool. Change takes courage. Take your life back. It's worth it!

Tension has trouble hiding in a body that is balanced and running healthily and efficiently. Exercise also decreases those lingering and harmful cortisol levels.

Stay Somewhat Socially Engaged

Chronic pain, anxiety, and depression can be signs that the individual has either lost the desire for social activity, isn't socially active enough, or maybe never was. The first instinct is to fade into the woodwork, which falls right into the teeth of pain and depression. Stay socially engaged or depression may creep in. Social activity enables us to share our problems, reminds us that we are never alone, and also adds competing stimuli to the pain. Many people have written to me that when their pain strikes, they head over to a good friend's house for a good conversation and a glass of wine (btw, wine is a depressant but also a relaxer) *...as the sober yin chases the drunken yang....* They invariably report that they felt better afterward because social banter draws the focus away from the pain and problems—for the moment. It is imperative to live in the moment.

Praising the Almighty… Dollar That Is

How much does money mean to you? Is it worth your li$e? Healing from pain often means stopping worrying about how much you own. Find a slower more satisfying career, a slower, more relaxed life. It's difficult to spend money when you're dead (although banks will still accept your checks). Some jobs are not meant for all people because some personalities tend to care too much for their own good. I became acquainted with a man who was a doctor and was in severe TMS pain. He eventually left his practice and found a more under-stimulated life and career and is pain-free after reading Dr. Sarno's books. Perfectionists can take a mediocre job and turn it into a stressful job through self-imposed pressure. People often get into careers to please their parents and in the process they become disenchanted and depressed. Lose your dreaded job before you lose your precious life.

Relationship

The healthiest people among us seem to be those generous souls who laugh easily, forget unpleasant events quickly, and are quick to forgive even the gravest offenses. This kind of childlikeness keeps a person unencumbered emotionally and spiritually, and in the end, unencumbered physically.

— Don Colbert, MD, *Deadly Emotions*[263]

From the beginning, TMSing is the resultant effect of conflict in unresolved interpersonal relationships, including the relationship with self, the emotional loss of which has never been expressed away, and by which the fear of abandonment remains as an ever-present memory. Recently I received an invitation to the Chopra Center for Wellbeing. The Newsletter/invitation began with the following: "As humans, we share a common set of emotions; we can all relate to feelings of anger, sorrow, pride, and joy. Our ability to feel these emotions and empathize with others as they experience them keeps us connected with the universe and ourselves." Full—healthy—and for-giving relationships are another set of keys to a healthy pain-free vessel. We feel safe and alive when connected with others.

Brennen

[Reprinted with permission]

> Hello All…. I have suffered from TMS since childhood. A little background info:
>
> My parents divorced when I was five and I had terrible thoughts of being left alone. I had horrible leg pain (growing pains) when I was a pre-teen and occasionally during my teen years. Acne was VERY bad despite medication. Acne got a little better during my twenties, varying in intensity.
>
> About three years ago while unemployed with a new mortgage, we were leaving for our vacation we had already paid for. In helping my mother complete a project before I left, I noticed a pretty good backache starting. Never really had one before so I took Advil and went on vacation. I couldn't move the next day and the rest of the vaca was spent on my back. My sciatica was so bad I wanted my leg cut off. I did 14 months of chiro, pain meds, muscle relaxers, massage, stretching, etc…. You know you've probably all been there.
>
> Second vacation nursing a backache came and went. Doctor said surgery needed, even though he hadn't ordered an MRI yet. Chiro said the same thing. I wasn't going to do surgery, so I started searching and came across Dr. Sarno's book. Read it and it helped show me I was the classic perfectionist and worst critic of myself. It was like reading my biography. So I applied that knowledge and my pain lessened. Not really finding a good course of action I bought Fred's book and made a complete recovery in around 3-4 months.

I'm happy to report that Brennen recently wrote to me, "I have no symptoms and am completely pain-free." His story is somewhat typical of pain sufferers—extremely well phrased and succinct. He had essentially summarized this book. I asked him if I could reprint his biographical synopsis because it contains many of the life-triggers and subsequent effects. His was, in essence, **a perfect TMS storm**. As is typical, he had a first-cut of parental divorce and fears of abandonment that planted the seeds of perfectionism. Then began the cycle of the sciatic leg pains, skin eruptions, unemployment, obvious vacation syndrome (leisure sickness), searching for external cures, depression, finding of Sarno, searching the psychologicals, standing against the pain, success as the pain moves around, financial worries, and finally full circle to the resurfacing of reduced bloodflow when new tension reaches new heights. Brennen is further proof that we all can heal no matter what our biography tries to hold us to. He also tells me that he, too, has met with resistance to TMS. The thing that stood out most with me was that his doctor(s) told him surgery was "needed" before the MRI was tak$n.

Healing Connections—Touch Is One Letter from Ouch

In *Body, Mind & Soul*, Deepak Chopra, MD, describes the Ohio State University study performed on rabbits to test their metabolization of cholesterol. All the groups of rabbits were given a diet extremely high in cholesterol. But to the amazement of the researchers—one group of rabbits had 60 percent less incidence of hyperlipidemia (elevated fat molecules in the blood), even though their diets remained identical. This was a mystery to the researchers until it was discovered that one of the technicians was holding and petting that particular group of rabbits. The connectivity and ease of fear of abandonment had, as Chopra described, "transformed the cholesterol into a completely different metabolic pathway." Touch heals the body because it reverses the sense of isolation and keeps us connected to life. As I mentioned in Chapter 9, several people have told me their pain immediately stops when someone touches them (similar to the chiropractic phenomenon).

Easing the fear of isolation reduces the level of stress hormones in the body, and releases all sorts of good chemicals, profoundly affecting the body's ability to heal from pain and disease. This is reiterated by Stanford University professor of biology and neurology, Robert Sapolsky. During his lecture at Ohio University's Memorial Auditorium, and from his book, *Why Zebra's Don't Get Ulcers: Stress, Disease and Coping*, Sapolsky examined how stunted growth, or more precisely psychogenic dwarfism, is caused by stress. He explains that having the stress hormone constantly ON damages the body by taking energy away "from other important processes, such as digestion, growth, tissue repair, reproduction, and the immune response." Psychogenic dwarfism is caused by "extreme emotional deprivation" and involves an overactive sympathetic nervous system.[264] Emotional deprivation leads to physical deprivation through the same sympathetic nervous system dysregulation involved in chronic pain.

Everyone (even rabbits) needs nurturing attention and touch—to be heard—and in this hearing, each heart is reconnected with another as metabolic functions are stabilized and restored. These physical symptoms represent the emotional distance we maintain between us. We suffer because of the pressures we place on ourselves to succeed, to go it alone—to be independent—and in the process forget that we need to stay connected, loved, and secure. Dr. Weil has said that he has seen several people's back pain disappear after falling in love—no longer feeling alone.

Why is this concept so important to healing from pain? Healing is not about getting rid of the pain; it's about getting rid of the tension build-up from the guilt and fear that is born from isolation and abandonment. Pain is a symptom of a deeper need to feel connected and understood. Anger is the knife that separates hearts, and ego the wall that prevents hearts from reconciling.

Daddy's Influence

Nothing exerts a stronger psychic effect upon the human environment, and especially upon children, than the life which the parents have not lived.

— Carl Jung, on *Paracelsus*

In the February 2004 issue of *Reader's Digest*, comedian Ray Romano stated, "I used to say that if my father had hugged me once, I would be an accountant, I wouldn't need to do comedy. He loved us but couldn't show affection in any way."[265] Ray needed to know if he and his dad were okay relationship-wise, he needed some type of non-tacit approval and acceptance from his dad—just once—but in its absence, he sought attention in others' eyes—larger arenas. Fathers have much trouble showing affection to sons because their own fathers were absent or unaffectionate. Non-praise then follows non-praise until **the man** has the courage to break the cycle.

In 2003, W. Singleton wrote in his dissertation, "The Father Archetype and the Myth of the Fatherless Son" that, "Nature abhors a vacuum. Father-absence or emotional abandonment by the father leaves such a vacancy."[266] The problem is that the vacancy is either filled by external rage (breaking laws), or by internal rage (chronic illness). The direction of the rage depends on the personality type and the first method of fight/flight utilized for survival.

A man I know well had a contentious relationship with his own father. When his father suddenly died he didn't shed a single tear. During the funeral he was being touted as "the strong one" because he appeared to be holding up so well—even smiling. It was a paragon of repression. A few years after his father's death he developed multiple sclerosis. Holding back tears and emotions prevents the freeze response from being discharged, because it never allows for the completion of the state of helplessness and trauma. Those father-son bonds that are broken often manifest in the physical and psychological realm.

Carl Jung described the story of a 20-year-old banker's son from Hungary. The son had become ill shortly after his own father became ill. From his illness, the father lost the use of his right side and shortly afterward the son also lost the use of his right side. So the son was sent to Zurich where Jung put him through intense psychoanalysis. During analysis it was discovered that the son had a strong father-son complex. The son revealed a dream to Jung where he was lying in a coffin beside his father in a vain attempt to open the coffin's lid. Jung explained to the boy that he had too strongly identified with his father and the father's invalidism was becoming his own. Once explained to him (knowledge therapy? ... yes!), the son became better after a few weeks and was sent home. Jung noted that the key to the boy's healing was in his expressing his feelings to Jung, and by the fact that "his heavy burden has been rolled away."[267] The son had taken on the father's symptoms due to his love and strong need to tracordify with his father.

If a son or daughter becomes ill, or suffers severe chronic pain, one of the first relationships to look at would be the type of relationship with either father or mother—the other being the spousal relationship. Are these relationships lacking affection—or stifled with praise?*

> If you love your children, be happy, share your happiness with them, and value their opinions. Children want their parents to be happy and to know that they are a part of that happiness. If you're negative and judgmental and tense and arguing or missing—so will they be—eventually.

---

* "Our ability to nurture children is strongly influenced by our own conception, birth, childhood, and life experiences. When we are not aware of unmet needs of our own childhood, we can easily hurt children in their care, often without realizing it. When we understand and address the unmet emotional and physical needs of our own early years, we are better able to meet the needs of our children, even when the child's behavior is challenging or provoking—and we break the cycle of abuse otherwise handed from generation to generation," *Blueprint for Transforming the Lives of Children.* [aTLC.org]

28

Breathe In....
and Don't Forget the Out Part

The Lord God formed the man from the dust of the ground and breathed into his nostrils the breath of life and man became a living being.

— Genesis, 2:7

There is no life without breath. Tensionalgia sufferers need to breathe with conscious awareness. The goal should be breathing toward a state of alpha brainwave activity. We can approach this state of peace and awareness through deep, relaxed breathing. As stated before—the Type Ts are short breath-takers, breathing from the top of the lungs and ignoring the all-important bottom. The "bottom drop" in the breathing process not only allows for air to be released but also for tension to be released.

As Andrew Weil's breathing CD title, *Breathing: The Master Key to Self Healing*, suggests, conscious breathing is key to living healthily. Dr. Weil has also called breathing, "The doorway to control of the autonomic nervous system." Pain sufferers have on occasion commented to me that as they exhale, they stop at a certain point before fully releasing the breath. But the last amount of air that needs to be breathed out is important. It is this last small portion of the exhale that takes the autonomic nervous system overactivity with it. It brings down tension as the lungs fall empty and the body acquiesces—in rhythm.

When I jog I don't consider it simply running. I think of it as an oxygenation of my mindbody. Like Dr. Sarno, Majid Ali, MD, founder and professor of medicine at the former Capital University of Integrative Medicine, discovered that pain results from oxygen deprivation, a product of "dysfunctional oxygen metabolism"[268] in intracellular activity.

Our natural breathing pattern is most likely set at birth. The first conditioned response in life is breathing. Robert Fulford, DO, felt that many health problems were the result of the lack of fullness of the **first breath** at birth. The second conditioned response is crying, as the baby quickly discovers that crying brings others to him to fill his needs, and id is born. Later in life—when people need others deeply—they may simply and unconsciously give themselves symptoms (as acceptable substitutes for crying) to fulfill those same primal needs.

Dr. Fulford felt that the first-breath trauma was one of the main reasons that people became ill and suffered pain. If the first breath taken at birth was not full, "the cranial rhythms are restricted from the start."[269] Dysoxygenosis* is Dr. Ali's term for the failure of cellular oxygen metabolism due to damage to the enzymes of oxygen metabolism. Whatever the reason(s), abnormal oxygen metabolism, oxidosis and dysoxygenosis are the physiological instigators behind pain and fatigue—factors that directly result from the emotional responses that initiated them. When tragedy or trauma occurs, when stress accumulates, the breathing mechanism is disrupted.

Short breathing signifies an unwillingness to relent, relax, to let go and move forward—to free the spirit to soar where it may—and heal. The Latin word for spirit, *spirare*, means "to breathe."

Consider Counseling

Anyone who needs psychiatry is sick in the head.

— Major Frank Burns, *M*A*S*H*

Personal counseling is highly recommended before the pain becomes intolerable. Pain would never get to the point of intolerance if counseling was sought early on. Women are far more likely than men to turn to others for emotional support—a Western cultural meme. To many men, the need for another's listening ear is a sign of weakness, but this is an outdated fallacy sustained by the presence of the cultural male ego. Men instinctively know if they begin to let some of their emotions out, they may fall apart altogether, which is an emasculating no-no in their minds. Counseling sheds healing light on the shadow—the blacker, denser aspect of the individual—holding all the answers necessary for healing. But people fear the painful truth, so counseling can be a frightening prospect. Effective counseling enables the individual to slowly peel their mask (persona) away. Most people can't recognize the masks they wear because they've never looked in the mirror with objective eyes—so they see only a reflection of what they want to see.

No matter which counseling method is chosen, counseling will most likely fail to heal if the nexus between the psychological and the physical is never made. Digging deeper into your past may well be very helpful and satisfying, but it won't take your pain away unless you understand how your mental process is creating the physical problem.

---

* "Oxidosis leads to dysfunctional oxygen metabolism, which is the basis of all symptoms of fibromyalgia and chronic fatigue syndrome. It is the molecular basis of pain, fatigue, and brain fog in those syndromes. 'Dysoxygenosis' (dys-oxy-gen-o-sis) is my term for dysfunctional oxygen metabolism." Majid Ali, MD.

29

Set Goals—The Big Picture with the Fine Print

...people who continually ignore their emotional needs pay the price physically. Good health in contrast, is the result of paying attention to your needs—mental, physical, and emotional—and then translating this awareness into action... The most effective tool we have found for getting our patients to take specific, positive action is to ask them to set new life goals.

— O. Carl Simonton, MD, et. al., *Getting Well Again*[270]

Healing from pain often requires setting new goals or redefining old ones. There are two types of goals, the long-term new-life goals and the short-term **physical goals**. Long-term goals require an individual to reflect deeply and come up with a new future vision where she envisions herself at peace. Where does she want to be in life, and how does she want to feel? What does she want to do with her life?

Short-term goals are more readily tackled. They are simple—intended to get the individual up and moving around. Short-term goals described here are movement goals, not mental or life goals. Almost everyone I have met who has healed has set short-term goals for themselves in order to overcome their debilitating pain. A friend crippled with TMS pain so badly that he could not climb steps, found Dr. Sarno's book, and then found *Rapid Recovery* by Fred Amir. After taking Amir's advice on goal setting, he began setting goals of climbing, by first climbing one step and then another, and was eventually able to climb all the steps. From being essentially crippled on the ground floor, he climbed his way up to pain-free which all began with a first step. He's currently 84 years old, so healing knows no age limit. It doesn't matter the age or how many surgeries you've had, the pain can go, if you want it to. By setting goals, you make the rebellious child listen to you and not the other way around. Movement and goal setting tells the id that the "matured self" is in control, and that crying (pain) no longer brings people to him. Soon the child will begin to listen and change **but** he will not commit easily unless you reward him for his acquiescence. If the child understands that movement will be rewarded, he is more likely to stop throwing fits (symptoms). This is soothing, which counteracts the rage, altering behavioral and conditioning responses. In *Rapid Recovery from Neck and Back Pain*, Amir accurately describes how it is necessary to "associate the reward with the goal" and to "Make sure to reward yourself as soon as your goals are achieved."[271] The brain needs to create the nexus between movement and reward—if not immediately rewarded after movement, **delayed reinforcement** occurs; the association may not be as strong and change may not occur.

While accepting your pleasure-reward, continuously visualize yourself moving pain-free and easily. This reminds the brain to associate pleasure with moving—thereby reversing the current conditioning that associates pain with moving. The process may take some time, but it works! The brain's behavior is now being altered which may or may not lead to a permanent cure, but it will certainly ease the pain and put the individual back on a confident path—beyond the physicophobia.

> Make certain not to make pain reduction the goal. This is yet another example of monitoring progress. What we are looking for with goal setting is rewarding activity—nothing more. The pain will eventually leave as a byproduct of increased activity, and confidence. Finish the goal whether the pain is present or not. Just do it!

If still possessed by fears of structural damage, build yourself up through incremental movement. If your feet hurt and you can't stand without pain—sit down! Then slowly push your feet into the ground, day after day, a little bit more, a little bit harder. Then begin to stand while supporting yourself with something: day by day. Then try to stand up for thirty seconds, then forty, fifty, and finally alone with no support. Then begin taking small steps, traveling farther every day, always rewarding yourself with something that makes you feel good, something that soothes your id-self. Eventually, you should be walking or running without pain, all beginning with a goal; a single first step. I have yet to see anyone who has set goals and **stuck to them**, who has failed to heal. People who don't heal, do set goals, start them, but don't stick with them. They don't follow through with the repatterning, or reconditioning. They're not yet ready to heal; they still need the physical distraction. Consciously they are determined, but unconsciously they resist.

If the bottom of your feet hurt and you are afraid to walk, the goal should be to walk or to run. Let's say you choose walking, starting with a few yards a day. Do this daily until you no longer think of the walking part, or the stepping, until it becomes secondary mechanically. Force your mind to a non-pain area, and as always, immediately reward your mindbody for the activity while reflecting on the activity. At the end of the walk, have a pleasurable reward ready. Some people use food, others sex as their reward, others choose long hot baths with candlelight (mostly females), and yet others choose just listening to healing relaxation tapes and music.

You can also develop a personal ritual in which you take yourself into your own heart. Do something enjoyable or appreciative each day for yourself. Use meditation tapes, soft music, yoga, or massage to assist you in feeling tranquil so that a sense of harmony can penetrate into your spirit and your physical body.
            — Caroline Myss PhD, *Why People Don't Heal, And How They Can*[272]

I believe that people who cannot stay the course long enough to achieve even short-term goals (the Jeffersonian phobia of resolution) are afraid that they may just accomplish their goals—destroying all excuses for healing. This I believe, is frightening to their child-primitive because they still need their pain for unconscious reasons—unconsciously sabotaging the goal. These are the **trouble healers.**

So you can approach healing from the physical end, or the psychological end, or better yet from both ends simultaneously. There are also the fortunate 20 percent or more who heal as soon as they are told what is happening within their mindbodies, without having to do anything! These are the people who annoy the trouble healers.

30

Visualize! Imagine Being Healed— and Heal

Imagery gives the silent right brain a chance to bring its needs to light and to contribute its special qualities to the healing process.
— Martin Rossman, MD, *Guided Imagery for Self-Healing*[273]

Perhaps there is no more significant mechanism for healing than visualization or **guided imagery**, as it proves that we have great control over our health. The mystery is in how to allow the healing answers to surface—how to entice what is in the shadows to consciousness.

Imagine the brain as having two separate functions; I say "two" for example's sake only because the mind is incredibly complex. But for now, think of the "first" part of the brain as having that part that controls conscious activities like raising your arm, standing up, turning your head, or talking. The mysteries with pain and illness are that they stem from a "second" part of the brain that does not appear to be within direct conscious control. The problem is that there are no direct synaptic routes to the unconscious world, and so we must find an alternative pathway. The inroad into this autonomic/unconscious arena is through the use of guided imagery—or imagining.

Martin Rossman, MD, calls this inroad the Inner Adviser. It knows the cause of the problem but is reticent in un-repressing what it doesn't want made known. It doesn't communicate well verbally, it only feels and exists in real time, and only expresses itself physically. Like a mute that cannot directly tell you why he is angered, the Inner Advisor reveals discontent by "signing" pain and illness through the body. To find out what made the child throw its fit, you must learn how to look, or how to ask. The techniques can be easily learned if they are practiced. This is exactly what the psychic and healer, Edgar Cayce, did. Cayce could also peer into the other person's Inner Adviser (subconscious). Cayce said that anyone could do it if they practiced. Learning this art of finding the source of unhappiness and imbalance by simply asking has saved many lives. The more advanced the individual becomes in the art, the more able he becomes in gaining control over his immune system, autonomic functions, and overall health.

All of the body is in the mind, but not all of the mind is in the body.
— Swami Rama[274]

You may wonder why I chose this quote by Swami Rama. It is for the same reason I mentioned Edward Cayce, Paracelsus, Peggy Kessler, Jesus of Nazareth, and Reverend Henry Melvill. We are connected by forces inside and outside of us—by mind—stretching beyond the physical arena. This is why, if your physician doesn't believe you will heal, you often won't heal. When she says you are damaged—helpless—she has created a condemnation that your unconscious instantly integrates and accepts. It has to do with mirror neurons—metaphysically connecting our emotions, thoughts, and feelings with those people near us.

In 1969, during a visit to the Menninger Foundation in Topeka, Kansas, and under "laboratory controlled testing," Swami Rama demonstrated that he could consciously raise the temperature on various parts of the palm of his hand 11 degrees. He also slowed his heart rate from 74 beats per minute to 52 in less than a minute—even stopping his heart from beating altogether. He also generated specific brain wave patterns on demand—deliberately and consistently producing theta and/or delta waves. With his entire body wrapped to prevent movement and wearing a mask to prevent air from leaving his nose and mouth, Rama spun a 14-inch knitting needle from 5 feet away. He had proven the ability to voluntarily control what is considered to be an involuntary system—disproving that autonomic functions are entirely involuntary. Rama's demonstrations prove that we have control over our bodies, and also, that there is much more to our lives than we can see. We can heal if we communicate with our inner-world, and listen.

> Visualization Is the Virtual Language between
> the Conscious and Unconscious Mind
> **Pain Is the Physical Language of the Unconscious Mind**

Listening to the Mute

The first and most important step in guided imagery healing is **relaxation** to drown out mental chatter. Since relaxation is a foreign concept to the driven individual, initial attempts can be very unrelaxing. Nevertheless, without it, visualization is marginally effective—if at all. The mindbody must become extremely silent to hear a mute. To learn how to relax, I headed straight for the experts in the field—sought out their CDs, books, and videos. There are many relaxation techniques, and it is imperative to find one that works for you. The method of relaxation that is most popular and has persevered the longest is **progressive relaxation**, pioneered by psychologist Edmund Jacobson in the 1930s. This method takes you through the body parts, one at a time, relaxing each area until the entire body is relaxed.

The unconscious mind is more susceptible to suggestion when relaxed or sleep-deprived. The first step in interrogating prisoners is to sleep deprive them in order to persuade them. So it is important to at least perform guided imagery at night before sleep, as in **programming dreams** where the unconscious mind is more likely to be coerced—to "speak up" as the chatter of the day fades. Relaxation compensates for adrenal exhaustion by allowing for the natural healing capabilities of the body to take over, and increases serotonin for sleep while reducing cortisol levels. Once relaxation is achieved, and if the ailment hasn't been satisfactorily alleviated, it will be necessary to delve deeper into the right side of the brain. The entire concept of imagery healing is to increase self-awareness behind the physical problem—to listen to the inner you. The process works so elegantly that it is hard to believe that people will not try it. People more often seek outside help for answers because they feel others know more about them than they do. Once relaxed, images will begin to surface in the form of clues. Try to read them. Listen to yourself!

Go not abroad; retire into thyself, for truth dwells in the inner man.

— St. Augustine

How Imagery Works

Every time you focus on the image, it becomes stronger, and over a few weeks it becomes lodged in your unconscious mind.

— Martin Rossman, MD, *Guided Imagery for Self-Healing*[275]

Imagery helped me heal from 27 years of pain. As I finally understood that my herniated discs, arthritis, and stenosis were not the cause of my back pain—I knew that I needed to unravel almost 30 years of having the wrong visual image of my spine. I began imagining my spine as perfect, with anatomically perfect discs and huge openings for the nerve endings to float out through. I imagined my discs as perfectly cushioning my spine with each step I took. After weeks of practicing this, my pain would cease for a few seconds at a time. Eventually, the pain began bounding all over different areas such as my knees and the bottom of my feet. The foot pain was new to me and so I knew I needed to visualize something that would counter the images of my feet pounding the pavement when I ran. The idea that jogging is damaging to the feet and knees is an elderly wife's tale, but it was deeply ingrained in my mind. My breakthrough came on a snowy day when a soft powder of snow covered the ground about two inches deep. I took this image and ran with it. I imagined that I was running on cotton and that the cotton was cushioning my knee and ankles, and feet and back. Within seconds my foot pain disappeared as my unconscious mind actually began believing my visual image that I was running on cotton. In that moment I realized the power of belief—and have never looked back. I also never stopped imagining that the blood was pouring heavily into the painful area of my back like a large waterfall. I "heard" the sound of the falls as the blood cascaded over my now inconsistent pain, pouring blood and oxygen everywhere. Over months it actually began to work. The pain would start as I began to run, but when I actively imagined, the pain would cease. Eventually, I was running pain-free and to this day I never have any pain when I run. I successfully reconditioned my brain from all the insane admonitions about running and lifting and exercising. Never listen to people who tell you that running is bad for your knees or back or feet. We are not that fragile (I believe this is the third time I've stated this, and that it will be the third time many people won't believe it). We become our persistent thoughts, and if those thoughts are intended to keep people down, they will. People who really don't want to expend the energy to run will always come up with the old excuse that running or walking is bad for their knees and feet—but it isn't true. Running dramatically strengthens joints, bones, and muscles.

Guided Imagery Is Nothing to Sneeze At

A Swiss research team led by psychotherapist Wolf Langewitz, PhD, conducted a study on the effects of visualization and pollen allergies—covering two consecutive pollen seasons which included tree and grass pollen sufferers. Volunteers were asked to visualize a place where they felt free of their allergies. The purpose was to see if the sufferers could induce themselves into a hypnotic state where their brains could reduce the symptoms just by imagining a symptom-free state. Using outcome data of "nasal flow under hypnosis, pollinosis symptoms from diaries and retrospective assessments, restrictions in wellbeing and use of anti-allergic medication," the study concluded that symptoms were reduced by approximately 33 percent.[276] It should be noted that visualization and self-hypnosis have no side effects. Several former pain sufferers have stated that their lifelong allergies have disappeared after TMS healing. Allergies are the immune system's overreaction to a pollen trigger or foreign substance.

Whatever we can visualize, our bodies can feel and react to, as the appropriate neuropeptide chain for that emotion is sent into the blood stream toward the matching receptor cells—creating that particular experience or re-experience. By imagining, we create or recreate prior physiologic responses, enabling the body to match the experience. The most common example is the lemon or orange experience. By closing the eyes and imagining eating a freshly cut, juicy, dripping orange, the salivary glands release saliva. Even though the orange was never real, the mindbody process doesn't know the difference.

Imagine a picture of your mother. Do you see her? That image came from every cell in your body that holds her memory. If you had never seen or heard your mother, you would have no experience to draw her picture from. Did her image make you tense or happy? Whatever experience you had with her is the emotional state you have unconsciously assigned to her memory. Now imagine a crumbling spine, scoliosis, ankylosis, arthritic diseased knees, stenosis, degenerating joints and bones, pinched nerves with bulging painful red swollen herniations. Having been told that these are bad things—and cause pain—the frightening sensory experience is held within each cell of the body, as bad memory experiences, such as victimization, disease, or fear.

These images now become your new reality, and the body re-experiences these painful states with every trigger. Visualizing a healthy body reverses, or interrupts, prior false experiences by breaking the long-term neural relationships. It works—and has worked for thousands of years, and is an invaluable tool in healing. You can't heal until you can imagine yourself as "okay" and as being healthy and happy and pain-free. If you can't imagine right away, fake it until you make it. Push your imagination to its limitless potential until you finally become what you visualize.

Imagination is everything. It is the preview of life's coming attractions.

— Albert Einstein

> The idea in guided imagery healing is to relax and to allow symbols and images to rise to some form of awareness—especially before sleep—to ameliorate the reason for the pain by implanting healthier images. You may have a dream that night or an image that your body, or a higher source, reveals as an answer. These images and symbols are the reasons behind the symptom. Guided imagery also has another equally important direction and that is to send good imagery into the mindbody to alter prior experiences: imagery is a two-way street.

A Super Man's Power of Visualization

In 1997, actor Christopher D'Olier Reeve developed an ankle infection as a result of complications from his quadriplegia. His infection was so severe that it became an open wound that Chris described as going "all the way to the bone." His doctors tried powerful antibiotics on him but he was allergic to them and had to stop. The physicians finally told Chris that they would need to amputate his leg to save his life.

I remember spending most of that summer, sitting on the deck of our house in the country looking at the mountains and just picturing my ankle the way it used to be, and remembering that the body wants to be whole. And sure enough, after six months, it started to close up, and after eight months it has healed, and today you wouldn't even know there had ever been a wound there—I pictured my ankle the way it used to be, the normal ankle—that's what it wants to be. It doesn't want to be this open wound where you can literally see the bone, it doesn't want to be that way.

— Christopher Reeve, PBS[277]

This is precisely what I mean by tracordifying… "the way it used to be"—dyad from monad, wanting to be as—**One**—again. Christopher went on to state that it was so easy that he couldn't understand why people wouldn't try visualization. Here's why. Many people only believe what they can see. But there is much more, as Max Planck, the father of quantum theory, understood when he stated, "There are realities apart from our sense perceptions," or as Bruce H. Lipton, PhD, might say, Chris sent a signal to his cells to heal.

Fear of health, and of symptoms, are also guided images. Persistent images of crumbling spines, joints, digestive systems, ulcerations, cysts, etc. will bring symptoms as the image becomes organic reality. Dr. Rossman states, "The most common form of imagery that affects our health is worry."[278]

Top athletes routinely use visualization techniques for improved performance. All great athletes and successful people do this naturally—it's one of the reasons they are great. When I first began visualization to rid my back pain I felt foolish. It just didn't seem practical. But Olympic athletes were doing it, so I decided to give it a try. It took some time but there were ever-increasing reductions of pain, along with all of my symptoms.

> Pain is a message with its own language, asking questions, and hiding answers. By sending and looking for images, the body can be altered, since every cell in the body has receptor sites for neuropeptides. The correct neuropeptide is the key, and the cell is the lock that needs to be opened. Emotions alter the cells when the neuropeptide chain is attached to it. So visualization can change the body's state of existence by merely imagining. A friend who had a constantly reoccurring cyst on the same spot on his body— each surgically removed—tried guided imagery healing, and has never had a cyst since.

31

Communicate

Whatever you condemn, you have done yourself.

— Georg Groddeck, MD (1866-1934)

The previous chapter on visualization explained the importance of the healing communication with the self. This chapter concerns healing through communication with others—knowing there is no difference between the two. There is a universal consciousness shared by all people and life everywhere, at varying times, and has been shown by such people as Edgar Cayce, Swami Rama, and Jill Bolte Taylor. The actions and thoughts of one affect the actions and thoughts of others at levels unseen. The closer the relationship, the more is shared. The net of life catches everyone together, as good open-hearted communication is vital to good health because it affects everyone's lives, through their health.

> *Ye cannot live for yourselves; a thousand fibres connect you with your fellowmen, and along those fibres, as along sympathetic threads, run your actions as causes, and return to you as effects.*

— Reverend Henry Melvill, sermon,
St. Margaret's Church, Lothbury, England (1798–1871)

In his book, *Opening Up: The Healing Power of Confiding in Others*, Pennebaker describes a study he conducted on the healing power of expression catharsis. Students were asked to write down their deep thoughts about any trauma they had experienced. Pennebaker admitted that he and the other study designers were both "stunned and depressed by the stories."[279] One student had written that as a 9-year-old boy, his father walked him to their backyard and nonchalantly told him that he and his mother were getting divorced. The boy describes his father's explanation for the divorce, "Son, the problem with me and your mother was having kids in the first place. Things haven't been the same since you and your sister's birth." The child often blames himself when there is any type of relationship problem between mother and father. But this father didn't leave anything to chance, telling the boy that it was basically his fault—for being born. Another student wrote that when she was 10, her mother asked her to pick up her toys because her grandmother was coming to visit. She didn't pick up the toys—her grandmother visited that night—tripped over the toys, broke her hip, and died after hip surgery a week later. Pennebaker writes, "Now eight years later, the woman [girl] still blames herself every day."[280] Adults need to forgive themselves for their past—it's gone.

The mass of men lead lives of quiet desperation.

— Henry David Thoreau

Daily there are people living with stories of deep relationship guilt. This often leads to firing salvos at people because we see in them characteristics that we don't like in ourselves, projecting our faults onto them. The woman who criticizes another woman for the risqué clothing she is wearing, does so because she, too, deep down, would like to dress that same way, and so it provokes an image of herself that she both likes (id) and cannot like (superego). She must condemn the other's actions because they jeopardize her own self-perceptions. People criticize because they, too, hate being criticized. People hate bigots because they hate that same bigotry they see within themselves, and are afraid it may surface. Groddeck's Proposition holds true—we condemn in others what we already know is within ourselves. Effective communication begins with understanding that the things you hate in others are traits that you despise within yourself. The closer to your own nerve, the deeper the pain you engender onto others **...and the vicious cycle continues... to hide the self... by pointing toward them....** This is precisely why people get angry when they are told that their pain is coming from hidden emotions. At some level of consciousness— they know it is true and so they must condemn it and find a physical cause to bury an unwanted image of themselves. The more fiercely they condemn TMS, the more they know it to be true.

It's not the message delivered that is important, but the message that is received. If the two aren't the same, either the communication of the message was poor or someone wasn't listening. It takes two to lingo.

Connecting With Others—Healing Communication

Rapid Recovery from Neck and Back Pain was an important tool in my recovery. More than anything else, it communicated to me that I wasn't dying, but it also connected me to another person by hearing Fred's woes, which were almost exactly what I was experiencing. A portion of *Rapid Recovery* was dedicated to good communication—a necessary component in the healing process because it is almost always relationship issues behind our maladies. Healing is an awakening; it can occur instantly and is always here and now—but life is a journey, and communication the road we travel while in search of good relationship. When I speak of new relationship, it doesn't necessarily mean new people, but more likely a new relationship with the same people, and of course, the self. Sufferers must find words here and words there to construct their own temple of healing... built on diminishing ego. Healing will never be lasting without great communication. *...and the yin chases the yang... as they become you....*

Advertisements for cancer-fighting drugs begin with statements such as, "I'm ready to fight this cancer." Fighting anything—either mentally or physically—gives power to the object of resistance. Cancer cells recruit other cancer cells to fight with them when they are attacked by chemotherapy. The idea in healing is to begin to understand why the imbalance has occurred, and to begin accepting disorders as a product of self-expression, that has gone unexpressed. My customized healing routine began when I read the words from Dr. Sarno, "one must confront TMS, fight it." But I missed the message on a more subtle level. I now see his statement as, "you must not let it get you down" and that "you must stay persistent!" I misunderstood the communiqué and attacked it like an outside invader, which prolonged my re-balancing act toward healing. Even having misunderstood it, it was **the most important point** I took from Dr. Sarno's work. Self needs to be heard—connected—to keep unwanted emotions from being relegated to the body. With heart-to-heart communication comes a sense of peace that purges the body of guilt, and guilt is the primary source of conflict that generates pain.

In 2005 I read the following posting on the topic of TMS:

"In a follow-up this morning to my previous post, last night I spent some time talking with my wife about our finances. Just before I went to bed, I noticed that my back pain was virtually gone."

This man's relief from tensionalgia comes from expressing his feelings from his heart to his wife, and assumingly he also listened to her heartbeat. It was not merely the dread of facing their finances that was causing his tension, but also his need to communicate his concerns, and to listen to hers. Communication eases tension. Which broken relationships are the primary culprits behind chronic pain and illness? They are the ones closest to the heart, of course—family members or close friends. When disease or pain suddenly occurs, these ties are most likely the knots behind the tension. Rarely does conflict result from anything other than the family dynamic—both past and present.

All family relationships are emotionally loaded. It is one of the first things to be considered when someone has an attack of TMS that seems to come out of nowhere.
— John E. Sarno, MD, *Healing Back Pain*[281]

Nana I Ke Kumu

The ancient civilizations knew the healing value of family communication, but the concept got lost in modern-day healing as techno-medicine made its debut from European culture. It's widely held by many historians that at one time—thousands of years ago—there was one healing method in the world. Only remnants of it remain today, in Hawaiian cultural practices, most likely protected until recently by their relative isolation. These practices are traced directly back to the ancient Hawaiians—the Huna. In 1972, the ancient concept was re-introduced to the public in a book called *Nana I Ke Kumu*, by kumu (defined as "teacher") Mary Kawena Pukui. *Nana I Ke Kumu* means "look to the source." Since this source is almost always family or extended family, the ancients utilized a process called **ho'oponopono**, which roughly translates as "to set things right," or "to set right." Succinctly, ho'oponopono is pulling the family or extended family together in order to discover what went wrong, to find the source of the illness (psychic disharmony) and to bring back into harmony the intertwined forces of "God, nature, and man."[282] Where there's a problem, look to the source for healing—not at the ends (symptoms) for cures.

The ho'oponopono process is designed to restore harmony and is quite intuitive and varied. Generally, the **highly formal** process follows:

- All the members of the family that are believed to be involved in the disharmony are called together. E. Victoria Shook writes in her book, *Ho'oponopono,* that *"The family is a complex net of relationships, and any disturbance in one part of the net will pull other parts. This metaphor reinforces the Hawaiian philosophy of the interrelatedness of all things."*[283]

- Then a prayer, or **pule** is offered to bring in Divine guidance and also to add strength to "the emotional commitment."[284] This entire process can be led by a respected senior member of the family or by an outside healer or kahuna (this is where the term, Big Kahuna, comes from).

- The problem is then identified. Following the identification of the problem, each individual has an opportunity to speak their grievances, and during this time, no one else is allowed to speak, except for the kahuna. Each individual present is asked to be honest, open, and fair in expressing true feelings, but they are warned not to place blame or become angry.

- Once the grievances are stated, each individual is asked to forgive, to sincerely admit any wrongdoings. If restitution is required, the individual(s) must make a promise to try to resolve the actions that created any imbalance.

- The most important part of the process is the "mutual release" where all individuals must agree on the problem, its source(s) and those who have confessed must be truly forgiven, and those who have wronged must have truly confessed. Without the entire family unit in harmony, the process is not complete. This can take 20 minutes, or it can take days if the "clearing of the air" is laborious, or if there has been no complete agreement of forgiveness, or if total confession hasn't occurred.

One can only imagine how much pain and disease could be avoided if family units still rode the ho'oponopono-pony today. There would be many tears shed and many hearts healed if families could be this open and honest. Pain would most likely fade from memory as deep, open, and honest family communication brings deep healing. But the family unit, as we know it, is largely fragmented, exclusionary, recalcitrant, proud, isolated, and increasingly disappearing in a secular, impersonal, self-centered world.

Once you tell somebody, the way that you feel, you can feel it beginning to ease.
— James Taylor, "Shower the People You Love with Love"

Relationship clashes, however, show us a side of ourselves that we would not otherwise see. We must be and have opposites, a polarizing other. From the book, *Jung on Evil*: "without the experience of the opposites, there is no experience of wholeness."[285] These others can be observed best through family. If it weren't for family, people would largely avoid anyone they didn't agree with; so family forces together people who would otherwise avoid each other. This is the **soul purpose** of a family unit, to see yourself through forced proximity, to live, struggle and grow together in spiritual expansion. Eventually, however, she must learn to live alone (differentiate) before she can once again live with others, moving from the natural phase to the cultural phase, and finally returning home again. The family is the foundation of relationship that gives birth to all other relationships. The family is the answer; it is both stressor and healer.

What does communication have to do with pain? Everything. If we could sit and talk with those who left us, or hurt us, and purge all the past pain, there would be less suffering. But—ego, time, and circumstance don't always allow for open communication to occur and so we are given the gift of forgiveness to fill the voids of rejection—as well as—the gift of understanding.

32

Power Therapies

The "power therapies" are alternatives to standard behavioral psychological techniques. They aim to interrupt the attention of the debilitating effects of stress and trauma—by reducing fear through reconditioning habits. Si, in Inglís now, por favor? Power therapies are techniques used to heal broken hearts, where psychology has failed, or isn't available. They often deal with meridian points, or the chi, or energy fields, and are aimed at working through or redirecting pain from the mind. They are labeled power therapies because of the speed and effect they supposedly have on reducing or diffusing the fear and anger from past trauma.

Common Power Therapies:
ISTDP Intensive Short-Term Dynamic Psychotherapy
NLP Neuro-Linguistic Programming
TIR Traumatic Incident Reduction
EFT Emotional Freedom Technique
EMDR Eye Movement Desensitization and Reprocessing
TFT Thought Field Therapy
V/KD Visio/Kinesthetic Dissociation

Programmed Dreams

> *The programmed dream can out-do even the power therapies. It can find the source and the cure for any problem in a single night.*
> — Clancy McKenzie, MD, author of *Babies Need Mothers*

Interestingly, deep healing can also be found through programming dreams—which Freud stated were "The royal road to the unconscious." In a related email, psychiatrist Clancy McKenzie relayed the following experience to me:

"I treated a woman who had severe chronic pain and multiple operations. When she mentioned her mother—who had died 10 years earlier, she would burst out in tears. I had her program [herself] to have a dream about her mother, which would not be upsetting, and programming the dream itself would resolve all the upset feelings. The next month I asked her about her mother. For the first time in 10 years she did not cry. She matter-of-factly reported that the dream was about shopping together, and the upset feelings are all gone. The next month the chronic pain and even the medical and surgical problems were resolving. All had related to the unconscious guilt about the mother's death."

The key words here are "unconscious guilt" and the key concept is self-blame when separation occurs or any ambiguity remains following the loss of a significant love.

With Dr. McKenzie's above quote, we come full circle from separation, to guilt, to self-punishment, and suffering. So if all the answers are ever-present in the unconscious mind, then programmed dreams would be the roadmap for the journey, speeding past psychoanalysis and beyond the unconscious process. The programmed dream goes far beyond the unconscious mind. It is the same technique that Daniel used to interpret King Nebuchadnezzar's dreams. Dr. McKenzie tells me that he has not known one person to get a wrong answer with a programmed dream, which can be likened to a prayer. The programming—or asking before sleep—may provoke a "visit from the highest source" during the night with the answers at will.

> *Your subjective (unconscious) mind performs its highest functions when your objective (conscious) senses are not functioning. In other words, it is that intelligence that makes itself known when the objective mind is suspended (sleeping) or in a sleepy, drowsy state.*
> — Joseph Murphy, PhD, DD, *The Power of Your Subconscious Mind*[286]

The stories of Dr. McKenzie's patients' healings are astounding, as healing emanates from enticing the mind to work through "altered states of consciousness" to allow answers to rise to awareness. The lady who dreamt of a winding highway, turning left and then right, back and forth, was subsequently diagnosed with an intestinal obstruction and scheduled for surgery. McKenzie then had her program a dream to rid the obstruction, and it was suddenly gone. People with Raynaud's syndrome had dreamt the answers behind the cutting-off of the blood supply to their hands, which McKenzie had described as the "extreme need on one part of the mind to control an extremely objectionable impulse belonging to another part of the mind." This confirms Dr. Sarno's work that when the mind is conflicted, the blood supply is reduced to create a symptom.

Enough people told me they received good relief from pain using power therapies that it was important to mention them here. I list the more popular therapies for possible help in alleviating pain, even if through placebo result.

33

Laugh Dammit!—Seriously

Life would be tragic if it weren't funny.

— Stephen Hawking, PhD, astrophysicist

There would be no need for therapies if genuine laughter won the day. Power therapies walk the individual through the trauma to discharge a freeze response that was never released. People get so caught up in trying to do right or be good, held in self-pity and victimization, that they forget to look at the absurdity of life—the funny side—the side they cannot control. The angriest and most controlling and critical people have the worst senses of humor—most dominating superegos. You won't find people in critical TMS laughing either. Yet humor heals.

Laughter dramatically increases the denominator of the rage/soothe ratio—aiding in healing. At one point during the darkest days of his presidency during the Civil War, Lincoln asked his cabinet to laugh, telling them, "Gentlemen, why don't you laugh? With the fearful strain that is upon me day and night, if I did not laugh, I should die. You need this medicine as much as I do."

Laughter suppresses the release of the stress hormone and immune system suppresser, cortisol—boosting the immune system's power. Laughter also releases endorphins and natural painkillers into the spinal canal. The endorphins generate a sense of peace and happiness and pleasure—an analgesic effect that alters mood—relieving depression and boosting disease fighters. All good stuff. Laughter is the antithesis of anger and worry. Worry demands control, laughter is losing control. You cannot be both in control and out of control at the same time—laughter unites our extremes, pulling out of us paradoxes of thinking and feeling, hero and thief, sadness and happiness. Something is only funny if we understand its opposite side, that's what makes it so funny. So in his quest for perfection and his need for control, he forgets how to laugh in order to fill the gaps of the opposites.

The **International Society for Humor Studies** (ISHS) holds conferences and workshops on the effects of humor and health. Much of the research is on the effect of humor on biological sciences and the human anatomy. Therapeutic humor is used as a complementary treatment for treating pain and illness. Once again, Norman Cousins becomes a paragon in the effectiveness of this type of treatment, as his work became synonymous with laughter as a healing tool. Professor Sven Svebak's study on svhumor and its svhealing sveffects on kidney disease, concluded that people recovered from kidney disease much more rapidly when in the playful state of laughter.

Learning how to laugh is as simple as seeing the absurdity in the circumstance, and relating it to your own experience. The TMS sufferer understands that she needs to laugh, she just can't figure out the details because she's too busy analyzing. Jerry Seinfeld has said that you cannot explain that something is funny to someone—it either makes you laugh or it doesn't. In the explanation it loses its appeal due to intellectualizing, along with its spontaneity. People forget how to laugh because they get caught up in the adult world; they forget how to be a kid. As the great sage Homer Simpson said, speaking of a little boy, "he reminds me of me, before the weight of the world crushed my shoulders."

> *We begin naïve, now that's the true fool, we really don't know anything, but the end of the journey is what I like to call second naïveté, returning back to another kind of innocence, maybe we weren't wrong when we spoke of second childhood, a kind of non-need to impress people, a kind of non-need to be important, a freedom to say almost silly things, because there's no competition anymore—that's a great freedom.*
> — Richard Rohr, OFM, *Quest for the Grail*

When laughter stops, pain starts. When was the last time you laughed freely with milk coming out of your nose? A controlling superego on constant watch will not allow for silliness. If you are suffering from TMS, seizures, constant infections, fibromyalgia, chronic fatigue, psoriatic arthritis, etc., you must stop your vehicle, see the flowers and breathe. Live with more silliness. Laughter lives in the moment and breaks tension. It is the most honest expression of a free individual, and expression heals.

Some Homerisms to Break the Tension of Intellect:

- How is education supposed to make me feel smarter? Besides, every time I learn something new, it pushes some old stuff out of my brain. Remember when I took that home winemaking course, and I forgot how to drive?
- Oh, everything looks bad if you remember it.
- It's not easy to juggle a pregnant wife and a troubled child, but somehow I managed to fit in eight hours of TV a day.

Homer: *Son, I just want you to know I have total faith in you.*
Bart: *Since when?*
Homer: *Since your mother yelled at me.*

Comedy writers are most adept at seeing causes and effects in life—not burdened by medical degrees, they are free to simply observe life and report on it. It didn't surprise me when I heard Homer say the following in the episode, "Pokey Mom"—on my birthday.

Oh, God, my back! It hurts so much! And my job is so unfulfilling!
> — *The Simpsons*, "Pokey Mom," January 14, 2001

Why is this important to healing from pain? Laughter unhinges the neuron's long-term relationships with one another. Self-pity, guilt, anger and victimization strengthen the neural-set—forming **nerve cell identity**. Laughter breaks these hardwired neural-sets and begins rewiring new neural relationships with happier, more fun, and pleasurable small peptide chains. Laughter changes the biochemistry from bad to good. Find humor all around you, and heal.

34

Giving Aid and Comfort to the Enemy

I have seen the enemy, and they are us.

— Walt Kelly, *Pogo Possum*

Once again—the pain is not really an enemy. It is a message from you to yourself. Accepting pain does not mean accommodating it, which is giving it aid and comfort. You can welcome a guest into your home and talk with him, but you don't have to let him sleep in your bed or use your ATM card. Bending more slowly, sitting or walking sideways, favoring one side over the other, are physical accommodations. Walking robotic-like in protective fashion is a form of accommodation. Throw away the pillows (not just the throw pillows) and aids and ingenious gadgets designed for making money from fear. Start walking straight, tall, and proud. Do not fear any range or type of movement. Become relentless!!

But What About Bob?

In an article in *Health Magazine,* March, 2004, Linda Marsa writes the story of a woman named Kim Chester who had hurt her back in the summer of 1999. It reads:

"For the next several months, physical therapists treated Chester with heat packs, electrical stimulation, and light exercise-special stretches, 'nonimpact' water aerobics, easy walking. But the pain never went away completely. And Chester feared it might get worse, so she constantly babied her back. She even quit her software sales job because the travel was too hard on her…. She lived this way for three long years. Then out of desperation, Chester enrolled in a special back-pain program at New England Baptist Hospital's Spine Center in Boston. At first she couldn't believe it when the doctors told her to do everything the physical therapists had cautioned her not to, like running on a treadmill or riding a stationary bike. But three months later, Chester felt better than she had in years."[287]

Renewed aggressive activity is what Dr. Sarno has been recommending for decades, with **one major exception**—he has found that attacking the back specifically does not work in the healing process as quickly or permanently as does simply stopping all back pain treatments. The action of specifically attacking the back in a bootcamp manner is still accommodating—more deeply integrating the structural beliefs by erroneously attacking the symptom. DO NOT do back stretches and exercises for the back! Stretch because it feels good—exercise to burn tension and for bettering your health—never for pain release.

Conceptually, prescribing physical therapy contradicts what we have found to be the only rational way to treat the problem; that is, by teaching, and thereby invalidating, the process where it begins—in the mind.

— John E. Sarno, MD, *Healing Back Pain*[288]

Now—by attacking the back or shoulder or knee, or whatever hurts—you may get good results because there will be less fear of hurting yourself. There will also be more blood sent to the afflicted area as well as moving toxins out of the area and gaining range of motion. These all give much needed confidence to an individual in fear of pain, but it is only a **baby step** in the right direction.

35

Repetition Repetition Repetition...

Insanity is doing the same thing over and over and expecting different results.

— Anonymous

Elephants captured in the wild in Asia (particularly India and Thailand) are tied to large chains that are attached to heavy metal posts. After a few days of the elephant attempting unsuccessfully to get free, the heavy containment system is replaced with a light rope or string and a tiny stick. With his mighty strength, the elephant could easily pull free now, but it gives up challenging, as its memory imprisons it forever. Even though it could easily overpower the stick, it will no longer challenge the containment system because its mind has been imprisoned by its first experience. It has been limited by the chains of its current knowledge because it tried several times to get free and couldn't—so it gave up trying—imprisoning itself without the help of others. It is imperative to let go of all that you have learned about the back, the body, and chronic pain. Let go of those things that do not serve you, or you will end up serving them. The direction needs to be changed in thinking from backwards to forward.

It often takes much repetition to break old behavioral patterns and it cannot be accomplished by sticking to a closed mind. Deep inside people still believe the old ways and fear the new ones since change is frightening, often more frightening than pain. The unconscious mind is very slow to respond to certain changes—which is a good thing or we would be those "highly unstable animals" that Dr. Sarno spoke of.

The Brain's Prefrontal Cortex Contains Our Self-Conscious

The precise healing mechanism behind knowledge therapy is unknown—but it works! People can heal in a few minutes, or take much longer, if the new information isn't accepted by the deeper primal brain. Healing may take much repetition or rereading of the TMS material—a deeper acceptance and confidence, with the reduction of fear. Although the exact mechanism is not understood, healing begins in the prefrontal cortex of the brain, also known as the "frontal association," and its specific influence over the amygdala.* So many people had asked me how knowledge

---

* The amygdala fires signals to the hypothalamus (mentioned in Chapter 2) to ignite the sympathetic nervous system—the system causing all the health problems if chronically strained with tension, from obsessive thinking. This is why Dr. Sarno called the hypothalamus "an essential way station in the (TMS)

therapy worked that I decided to research it more deeply by contacting Robert Sapolsky, PhD, a MacArthur Foundation Genius Fellowship Award winner, and sent him my Neanderthal explanation to get his feedback. His response to my explanation of knowledge therapy-healing was, that although the field is light years ahead of the type of brain regulatory issues I was trying to explain, he did say, "I think the scenario you outline [regarding the prefrontal cortex's interaction with the amygdala and knowledge therapy healing] is probably the best informed guess one could come up with." So we don't know precisely why knowledge therapy works, we only observe that it does. The one thing we know for certain is that healing finally occurs when the brain loses its grip on fear.

The amygdala is responsible for emotional processing and the expression of emotions. It regulates our rage, fear, and pleasure—components of id. When we fear something, such as fearing our bodies are flawed and failing—our health deteriorating, or death, that fear is stored in the amygdala. Each time we think of these body areas or systems being worn out or crumbling, the amygdala reacts in fear because of the **stored emotional memories** of fear already within it.

> *The amygdala probably functions to alter autonomic activity during responses to threatening or anxiety provoking stimuli.*
> — *Biological Psychiatry*, Volume 1[289]

Anger is governed by the amygdala. When removed from the brains of animals, they lose their anger response along with their sexual response—becoming indifferent to external stimuli.

TMS repetition-healing reverses fear by training the amygdala that "you are safe"—you're okay, don't fear, you will be fine, your symptom is from a harmless source—replacing fear with feelings of safety. Once it feels "all is safe"—the amygdala then eases up on the autonomic nervous system, and in turn, the ANS begins to re-balance and settle down—it stops overreacting as strongly, and symptoms ease.

So we import healing symbols and new mental imagery through the prefrontal cortex, which causes the conditioned and unconditioned responses in the physical body. What we imagine, our bodies adapt to. When told our bodies are flawed—through faulty medical advice—our mindbodies adapt to that image. The new TMS information, or knowledge therapy, is a mental rescripting.

The prefrontal cortex is the center of conscious action and activity that is responsible for thinking, planning, self-control, empathy, reasoning, judgment, personality expression, and social control. More specifically, the left prefrontal cortex

---

process." It is responsive to the autonomic nervous system inputs: sleep, thirst, fatigue, hunger, stress, body temperature, circadian rhythms, and blood pressure. You can view the hypothalamus simply as sticking its toes into "life's waters" to see how hot or cold the water is and adjusting the ANS levels accordingly.

generates positive feelings, and the left cortex also inhibits negative emotions from the amygdala (so it is very important in healing).

The prefrontal cortex also helps us focus on the task at hand—what we are doing right now—and it is a major player in pain and health. We pour new healing knowledge into this conscious prefrontal cortex—a portal if you will, into the entire self. This 5 percent "conscious section" of the brain is the doorway into the 95 percent unconscious where we ultimately heal—by reducing fear. In people who are happier there is higher activity in the prefrontal cortex, and in people severely depressed the cortex is diminished in size and activity. It's not surprising that the cortex has its greatest growth during the first three years—as psychiatrist Clancy McKenzie, MD, has shown, the first three years are the most critical in determining our mental development, for better or worse.

Dr. Sapolsky, a neuroendocrinologist has said, "The frontal cortex is the closest thing we have to a neural basis for the superego." It delays our gratification if it feels it is warranted. It has been described as the conductor of our deepest goals and desires—a regulator of our emotions responsible for cognitive control of our emotions. In other words, the frontal cortex keeps our deepest darkest impulses and desires at bay and in check—and also sends messages into the deeper part of the brain "to be good." Trying to be good is enraging to us if we don't want to be good, if we HAVE to be good.

Here is where the change begins in TMS healing. Repeating the truth into this frontal cortex slowly seeps into the deeper self—the limbic center—where there are no inhibitions, and where our impulsivity resides. Scientists can observe when a breakdown occurs in this prefrontal cortex because the people become more aggressive and primal, more outward, less concerned about the public eye. It can no longer screen deep dark thoughts as well—no longer contain primal impulses.

The most important point here is that this deeper portion of the brain doesn't see in maybes, it only sees yes or no. The prefrontal cortex is the planner—weighing all possibilities, sometimes confusing and gridlocking the individual. If the correct information, in this case, TMS, gets filtered through the prefrontal cortex into the deeper portion of the brain where emotions reside, it will alter the deeper brain from a no to a yes, or yes to a no, depending on what information is being delivered, and what information is being held. Once the deeper portion accepts the new information, the body relaxes and alters its physiology. In the end the truth sets you free—but sometimes you have to fight to free yourself, and the weapon is persistence.

The conscious mind allows itself to be trained like a parrot, but the unconscious does not— which is why St. Augustine thanked God for not making him responsible for his dreams.
— Carl Jung, Psychology and Alchemy[290]

There are some sufferers who heal quite quickly. Many have reported losing their pain after one or two meetings with Dr. Sarno. But from what I have seen, it takes much repetitiveness or reversal of old thinking and ingrained patterns. I **intentionally repeated** many important topics in this book. This is oftentimes necessary to integrate or reintroduce light into the mindbody. People regularly report that it was in the rereading of the material that caused the light bulb to click ON inside their heads. Don't be held back by a stick and string; keep testing your own ability until you finally break free. Destroy benchmarks with hope and persistence—you can do it! Persistently imitating what you desire will ultimately bring about that state of existence.

There are many different light bulb moments for many people with different light bulb heads. I found a few major things in each one of Dr. Sarno's first three books that I used to escape from my personal self-containment system. When I finally "got it," the light bulb over my head was so bright that my electric bill went up. The following are the primary connections that he made with me that helped me heal. Maybe one or a few will resonate with you.

From Dr. Sarno's first book, *Mind Over Back Pain*:
- the pain is due to mild oxygen deprivation
- tyranny of the should
- knowledge therapy

From Dr. Sarno's second book, *Healing Back Pain*:
- one must confront TMS, fight it, or the symptoms will continue
- you cannot hurt yourself
- the idea that a nerve is being pinched is fantasy
- stop all therapy
- emotional barometer

From Dr. Sarno's third book, *The Mindbody Prescription*:
- rage to soothe ratio

If the unconscious still doubts and fears (hanging on to tiny sticks of misinformation), the change and reintegration of the truth can be painstakingly s l o w. It may be that the wounds are so deep, the fear so great, that she really needs to move slowly for the psychological health of her entire self. Flood your life with appreciation and fearless thinking, and you will heal, in your time, not according to anyone or anything else. Trying to heal quickly is tying yourself to someone else's stick. Everyone's emotional biography is different. Know that you will be okay—stop putting so much pressure on yourself to follow someone else's method and timeframe. Relax and good luck! With the information in this book you have the tools to heal.

Different Learning Styles—Left- or Right-Brained?

Healing may come from simple knowledge, but it may not if you're in your right mind. It may have to come from an incessant pounding into the right brain as to what is occurring until the "whole picture" suddenly comes into focus, and then, ah-ha, the brain finally gets it and the pain leaves. I am reminded of my friend, Georgina, who read, and read, and read, all of the TMS material out there. She asked and asked questions of me and of those who had healed. She couldn't get enough information fast enough as her impatience led her right past the answers and back into her own questions. Then one moment—while in a jet plane, she was rereading Dr. Sopher's book, and... her back pain suddenly left her. Sometimes it's meant to be, or not to be, it all depends on which reality you choose to accept, and by the way in which you have learned to learn.

From communicating with hundreds of chronic pain sufferers over the years, I'm inclined to believe that they heal according to how they learn. This makes sense. Since it is knowledge that heals, how you acquire that knowledge must be an important factor in how you heal. I now realize that this was another reason that I healed more slowly. I happen to be a right-minded individual: right-brain dominant.

The left hemisphere of the brain thinks sequentially, line by line. Left-brainers can read books and understand it in its order, line after line, and they may just be the faster healers—healing soon after reading the books. The right hemisphere of the brain thinks holistically. Right-brainers see the book as a whole, and they may be slower healers for reasons explained below. However—we function best when we are using both "halves" in counterbalance... *yin and yang together in balance.*

Martin Rossman, MD, examines the revolutionary breakthroughs by Nobel Prize winner, Roger Sperry, PhD, and his colleagues regarding the brain, its two halves and how they are "simultaneously capable of independent thought."[291] We also saw the experience of Jill Bolte Taylor when her left brain lost communication with her right brain—illustrating Sperry's assertion. Rossman describes the two halves:

> **The left brain: sequential**
> Logical
> Analytical
> Takes things apart
> Concerned with outer world, business, and time
> **The right brain: simultaneous**
> Emotional
> Thoughtful
> Synthesizes, puts things together
> Concerned with inner world, perception, physiology, and form[292]

Dr. Rossman uses this example: the left brain sees a train coming down the tracks, one by one, as each car passes. "He can see just a little bit of the cars ahead of and behind the one he is watching."[293] This is left-side **sequential integration**.

The right brain, however, sees the train as if in a hot-air balloon overhead. It sees the train, its direction, the track, and the town it has just departed from and the town it is heading toward. When I read this, it immediately clicked with me. I've always been able to see the big picture, which makes for good humor, but I often struggled with the succession of events. Sequential learning was difficult for me because I wanted to know the purpose before I drudged through the details; why, where, how long, how much, howz come? My strengths are to be able to pull large amounts of information together, large picture perception, and understanding inner workings. The details are ancillary necessities to me. I tend to think in terms of images and sensations, and so my own healing took its own course because I needed to repetitively challenge the larger picture; but I erroneously challenged the details in futility.

> *This ability of the right hemisphere to grasp the larger context of events is one of the specialized functions that make it invaluable to us in healing.*
> — Martin Rossman, MD, *Guided Imagery for Self-Healing*[294]

As a right-brainer, or visual spatial learner (VSL), I needed to pull back from all the information that I had accumulated—to find a way to engage my learning strength.

> *Visual-spatial learners who experience learning problems have heightened sensory awareness to stimuli, such as extreme sensitivity to smells, acute hearing, and intense reactions to loud noises. They are constantly bombarded by stimuli; they get so much information that they have trouble filtering it out.... These children are highly perfectionistic, which means that they cannot handle failure.*
> — Linda Silverman, PhD, Jeffrey N. Freed, MAT[295]

At Least He's In His Right Mind? (a matter of opinion I spose)

The VSL has been described as perfectionistic. Other characteristics as described by VSL authoritarians Silverman and Freed are:

- Holistic learners.
- Multitasking learners, see the big picture, nonlinear learners.
- Extremely sensitive to external stimuli.
- All-or-nothing learning style, "they either immediately see the correct solution to a problem or they don't get it at all, in which case they may watch quietly (while pretending not to watch) or avoid the situation completely because it is too ego threatening."
- Visual-spatial learners have amazing abilities to "read" people, since they can't rely on audition for information.

- So adept at reading cues and observing people that they can tell what a person is thinking almost verbatim. Oftentimes, in school, they sense a teacher's anxieties and ambivalent feeling towards them and react with statements such as, "that teacher hates me."

- Systems thinkers—they need to see the whole picture before they can understand the parts.

- Highly aware of space, but pay little attention to time.

- Inventiveness and ability to see the relationships of large numbers of variables.[296]

If you happen to be a VSL—once you have the overall concept of TMS, then repetition may no longer be necessary; it may be time to stand on Dr. Sarno's second pillar, and act on that knowledge. Stop going over the same information, expecting different results. If your healing strategy isn't working, change the strategy to fit your nature.

36

Trouble Healers:
Unconscious Resistance to Change

It has become apparent to me that assuming that everyone wants to heal is both misleading and potentially dangerous.... Because change is among the most frightening aspects of life, you may fear change more intensely than illness and enter into a pattern of postponing the changes you need to make.
— Caroline Myss, PhD, *Why People Don't Heal, And How They Can*[297]

CS Lewis once said, "You have to sneak past the watchful dragons of self-consciousness." If you are thinking about healing—then you are no longer healing—you are only thinking about healing. A small percentage of people don't heal or they heal more slowly from mindbody disorders. The most obvious reason is **early extreme emotional separation trauma**—intense anxiety—which cannot be overcome through mere knowledge—requiring intense counseling, shadow-work, or programmed dreams. Here I want to address trouble healers—an interesting and frustrated group.

When Jesus saw him lying there and learned that he had been in this condition for a long time, He asked him, Do you want to get well?
— *John* 5:6, NIV

I vividly remember thinking as a young kid when I had first heard the above statement, "why would this Jesus ask someone if he wanted to get better?" What kind of silly question was that? Everyone wants to get better! It would take me 40 more years to understand the expanding depth of that question. Deep down inside—some people still need their pain, although they don't consciously want it.

I was reminded of that Biblical verse while watching a movie called *The Singing Detective* with Robert Downey, Jr. and Mel Gibson. The story's main character, Dan Dark, played by Downey, was a deeply disturbed writer suffering from psoriatic arthropathy, a serious type of painful psoriasis* that can affect the joints—his case

---

* As Dr. Sarno writes in, *The Mindbody Prescription*, "Not everyone agrees that these are mindbody disorders (psoriasis, et. al.) but I have found them to be so in my clinical practice." Sarno's findings are supported by studies at the Department of Dermatology of the University of Pennsylvania School of Medicine, which linked brain factors to a "cellular inflammatory response seen in a variety of skin disorders" which includes eczema, acne, and psoriasis. "Such a link could have clinical significance in the commonly observed exacerbation of many dermatoses, such as psoriasis and atopic disease, by emotional stress." Other studies also support the findings of psoriasis having an emotional cause. In 1994, *The*

324

emanating from unresolved childhood trauma. *The Singing Detective* dramatizes how trauma from childhood can lurk and grow into generalized anger at the world, and how disease is chosen and harvested when the time is ripe—although not always at logical times.

Mel Gibson played the psychoanalyst, Dr. Gibbon, who was working with the angry and extremely bitter Dan Dark. Dark had been told by the medical staff to "reassemble yourself," and that "the poisons of the mind have somehow erupted onto the surface of the skin"—that he would not get on top of his condition until he dealt with his "bitterness." A conversation from the movie:

Dr. Gibbon: Mr. Dark, do you plan to get better?

Dan Dark: Hmmm? (sarcastically uttered, not wanting to heal)

Dr. Gibbon: Chronic illness is a shelter. Yeah, a cave in the rocks into which a wounded spirit can safely crawl.

I have learned through personal experience and many conversations with other TMS sufferers that there are a multitude of reasons that some people heal more slowly than others, and indeed that a very rare few don't heal much at all. Pain and illness can enable people to opt out of situations that they don't want to be in because they are unconsciously feeling trapped by outside observers, or they simply cannot say "no." Sickness allows people to ask for help where they normally wouldn't ask because they unconsciously feel guilty knowing that other people have their own problems and needs as well. Pain and illness can also give them a stage to be heard—a means by which they can express themselves where their egos wouldn't normally permit them to do so.

> *True healing is one of the most frightening journeys anyone can undertake. For some people, illness can provide a feeling of physical safety that sometimes allows them to slow down the speed at which their lives are moving or changing. Illness can also offer the safety of not having to confront your inner issues or change yourself... when you become seriously ill, you may experience a level of concern and attention from others that you might not otherwise receive.*
>
> — Caroline Myss, PhD, *Why People Don't Heal, And How They Can*[298]

The acceptance of crumbling body parts as sources of pain can be a face-saving mechanism when conflict becomes insoluble. There are people who unconsciously do not want to heal because they may be forced back into that personal arena to face more rejection, back into that unwanted responsibility, or job, or significant other. These self-sabotagers are by far the angriest—often very polite and quiet—sometimes loud and obnoxious. Consciously they do want to get better—BUT—unconsciously

---

British Journal of Dermatology published a study entitled, "The Relationship Between Stress and the Onset and Exacerbation of Psoriasis and Other Skin Conditions" that linked stress to the onset and exacerbation of psoriasis. Thus, stress not only exacerbates psoriasis, it can initiate it.

they resist. They make up excuses as to why they aren't healing; cling to old beliefs for security; constantly talk about their symptoms, and routinely identify "other" causes behind their pain and fatigue, beyond TMS. This is the TMS process working as the brain designed it, to keep them hunting for "real" physical problems—when they don't have any. Some have such low self-esteem that they actually feel they deserve suffering. Multiple abandonments, or fear of abandonment, or memories of abandonment fears have made them collectors of pain. They have been beaten down since childhood leaving them feeling that they are less than they truly are, and have more than they truly deserve.

> *Finally, I have also met some people who have refused to relinquish their pain because they believe it is a justified punishment for something they have done.*
> — David E. Bresler, PhD, *Free Yourself From Pain*[299]

A small percentage of people prevent healing through repeatedly and unconsciously resisting treatment. A common example is overeating. The conscious-self attempts dieting but suddenly one day she gorges herself on desserts. She has unconsciously rejected the notion of weight loss. Her current self-image is comforting because it's known to her. She may fear becoming her true self for fear of succeeding. If she succeeds she is now in the spotlight. Once in the light her shadow is more likely to get caught and her weaknesses revealed—her inability to restrain her inferior vulnerable self, frightens her. So, internal conflict rages onward because her motivations are instinctively at war.

Jessica

Jessica had TMS foot pain so intense that she had difficulty walking. Through encouragement and self-determination, she went from painful walking to a short jog. Not long after, she sent me this note regarding a dream she had (reprinted with her permission). "I was late so I ran back home as fast as I could. I had such determination on my face and was running so fast and I was using my arms to help me run faster. All of a sudden I saw my mother hanging out some washing and I stopped abruptly, thinking, I can't let mother see that I can run and that was when I woke up... I can still remember that the running felt good and normal until I saw Mom. I panicked, but why? Perhaps it suggests that I am still holding back from allowing myself to be and act normally. My body wants to run and be normal but something is stopping me—still wanting to be looked at by my mother?"

Jessica knows her pain is emotional and somatized. She understood and implemented the concept of TMS very quickly—yet her pain lingered. She was unconsciously fearful of the changes necessary to heal and she fully understood it. To her credit, she made a full commitment to herself that she would change, which is not easy, since people don't always desire to become who they truly are; in fact, it may be "the most difficult thing one can do" as Richard Rohr has stated. Jessica's unconscious motivation for change may not have outweighed the attention that her pain brought her at the time.

The road to recovery can have many potholes, and people sometimes fear twisting an ankle in one, so they avoid the road to recovery all together. Most sufferers I have spoken to have indeed felt that TMS is a message that change is needed. In his book, *The Purpose Driven Life*, Rick Warren writes, "Growth is often painful and scary. There is no growth without change.... You must let go of the old ways in order to experience the new." Growth takes unparalleled courage—and ultimately only you can free yourself.

Migraine Momma

A tremendous obstacle in my own healing was that my back pain had become a part of who I was—who I identified myself as. Hi, I'm Steve, I have a bad back, it's nice to meet you. I had become like Kerry the Cripple, or Migraine Mary, or Harry Hemorrhoid. But I was more than my pain. I was limiting myself because of the unconscious acceptance of early false meme. It's plain and simple: people begin to see themselves as they feel that others see them, and so that perception malfunction eventually becomes them. The crutch becomes part of the man's arm—the hacking cough part of his speaking language, the limp a part of his own self-pity, as he holds his traumas, fears, and separations in his body. The individual with the old hip or knee injury doesn't realize that he healed years ago—but continues to limp. But due to the bombardment of false information by the medical industrial complex, family folklore, and his resistance to becoming whole again, he keeps recreating the same victimization neurotransmitters. He feels he is forever disabled, but he isn't. He has chosen to accept the notion that he is flawed, and so he is.

> *As soon as you start to tell yourself in your perception that you can't do something anymore, then your biologic system will adjust to prove you right... you will not do what you think you can't do.*
>
> — Bruce Lipton, PhD, cell biologist[300]

Finally, I have discovered that many people do not heal because of sheer and utter pretentious, pompous, ego-arrogance. No one will ever tell them what to do. Good luck with that one.

Sticking Points in Healing

Caroline Myss, PhD, has observed a fine line between those who heal and those who don't. Dr. Myss writes in her book, *Why People Don't Heal: And How They Can*, "...because we fear change, most of us remain in the old and familiar places, clinging to situations and relationships that have essentially ended."[301] She continues—"The fear of quitting a job or facing up to a deteriorating marriage is actually fear of taking charge of your own life."[302] The end result, she writes, is that "your spiritual and life potential [go] unrealized."[303]

This isn't to say that every time you get back pain—or any disorder—you should get a divorce or quit your job. But when healing doesn't come, and doesn't come, you must look more deeply into your situation and current relationships, and at the severity of the symptom—such as cancer. A minor back pain doesn't warrant a divorce or separation, but a crippling pain or illness may require intense shadow-work— perhaps permanent relationship change. Having written that—it is important to add that statistics show divorce is more dangerous to health than is working through the problems, so feel your way through the process. Balance is always at the center of healing through good communication, as well as knowing when to allow for change. Caroline Myss poses the following questions for self-examination in slow-healing individuals:

- Are you afraid that if you heal, your support group will abandon you?
- Do you see emotional wounds as a means of bonding with another person, and does healing mean having to separate from that person?[304]

These are very important questions. Does your pain give you a sense that you won't be taken care of if it fades? Or that you won't have any way to be heard, or be recognized? As a wise man once said, "Life is relationship," so will any relationships change if you heal? Will you have to face a failed relationship? Would healing require that you face a new life or redefine your position in a relationship with someone close to you? Will your private nest, or the bubble that isolates you from the world collapse if you heal? Will you have to finally face the world and do things for yourself?

Purple Hearts

> *At times he regarded the wounded soldiers in an envious way. He conceived persons with torn bodies to be peculiarly happy. He wished that he, too, had a wound, a red badge of courage.*
>
> — *The Red Badge of Courage*

Wounds of honor lead us to Dr. Myss' concept of **woundology**. This is when someone not only has an unconscious reason not to heal, but capitalizes on the circumstance by using the "street" value or social currency of their wound—that is, the manipulative value of the wound."[305] Woundology is Myss' warning of getting trapped with regard to healing. This is similar to John Stossel's notion of **jurosomatic illness**. If people can be compensated either emotionally or financially, they tend to have more ailments and complaints. If a health system is set in place to handle a certain disorder—people are unconsciously drawn to that disorder. This is why people who don't have health insurance tend to be healthier people—comparatively. Badges of honor also have social value—giving individuals their stage not only to be heard, but honored.

Myss describes the sharing of a wound as a possible "shortcut to developing trust and understanding."[306] People can use pain or illness to manipulate others, gain trust, and to compete with other sufferers for attention—attention they never received or were once showered with and deeply "myss" today. In a conversation with a sufferer, Myss asked the woman how long she anticipated the level of support that she was currently receiving from her support group. The woman replied, "It may take years, and if it does, I expect my support system to give me that amount of time."[307]

I went it alone when I was down in critical pain—routinely criticized for having pain, as it was a nuisance to those around me. Most people, however, who I have spoken with, had someone or a support system in place that helped them work through the integration of the TMS concept. Paradoxically, however, this "being taken care of" can also inhibit healing by stealing motivation to heal from the painee *a yin chases yang thingy…* **right?**

A man once wrote into a mindbody help group, "I find myself wanting to talk to people about the pain." Sometimes we need to itemize our infirmities to others to ease fear—to be heard—because we don't feel like others are listening, or even care. If the support system is there, and the stage is set, turn up the lights and let the show begin. However, I discovered that talking about my pain only prolonged it. It is better to talk about frustrations, disappointments, and fears, never the body. So with pain, there can be camaraderie and comparison and manipulation all under the banner of **shadowy needs.**

Shadow-Work and Sheltered Needs

Understanding shadow work and how the shadow-self can "emerge in self-sabotaging, uncontrollable behavior,"[308] is important to understand for trouble healers—in the chronicity of pain and illness—because shadow-work establishes a conscious relationship with hidden unconscious forces. Connie Zweig, PhD, and Steve Wolf, PhD, write in *Romancing the Shadow*, regarding establishing this conscious relationship, "In this way,* eventually we can accomplish directly what the shadow tries to accomplish indirectly."[309] Healing expands by tracing the root of the problems back to the deeper needs by enticing the shadow to reveal what it already knows. Andrew Weil stated in the *Frontline* interview, "The Alternative Fix: Pros and Cons of Integrative Medicine," that when people are not healing he pauses and asks himself—"Okay, what's preventing healing? What's blocking it? What can I do as a physician to facilitate healing?" The roadblocks lie in the sheltered self, and it should be noted that psychiatrists specializing in Jungian shadow-work believe, as Dr. Sarno does, that behavioral therapy does not necessarily solve problems. It is necessary to

---

* "In this way" refers to **shadow-work** which includes attempting to try to "identify shadow figures," and "bodily and emotional cues," all with the purpose of "uncovering their deeper needs." [*Romancing The Shadow*, p. 12]

look inside and to find reasons, not to try to alter behavior and symptoms, since symptoms and behavior are only effects.

A final caveat: if someone you are in relationship with is in pain or in a state of chronic illness, take a close look at yourself. You may be the one who is the source of their extreme tension and physical problems. You may be the triggering mechanism by which they repress their emotions. Are you listening to them at all, or are you contrarily babying them too much? By telling the sufferer "no wait, I'll pick that up, I don't want you to hurt your back," you more deeply reinforce that they are broken. Are you fulfilling their emotional needs, or stifling them by doing too much or too little for them?

37

Is it Gone Yet? Uh—You Still Here?

Attention to health is life's greatest hindrance.

— Plato (427-347) BC

She gets up in the morning anxious to see how her pain is going to be today. Will it be better? It's best that she rise and focus on how thankful she is for the things she can do that day, and also that she has things to do. I still cannot remember the exact day my pain left. It was sorta like, "Hey, I haven't had pain in a few weeks." I had given up checking on my progress altogether. A watched pot never boils, as a watched body never heals. In the end—time ends up framing you. In the words of a former sufferer, "I think that as a TMSer in the stages of still having pain or in decreasing pain, we frequently do the 'systems check.'" Yes—and it must stop.

Don't Pay Attention to Your Healing Progress—Go Live!

Understand waves of possibilities and how your watching something alters it.* Through **quantum healing** we can see how consciously observing health can alter desired healing outcomes. When you fully understand that pain is coming from a hidden, unfelt, unknown, unrecognized emotional process, do nothing about it, relax in the knowledge, have fun, become physically active, imagine a healthy vessel, and allow healing to simply happen. Don't attempt to push faster than the light allows.

Any shadow of doubt in the TMS process and the pain will linger or return. All the will in the world cannot overcome one shadow of doubt. From the Law of Attraction, "If you have a strong desire but lots of doubt, your desire will never come to you."[310]

If you are thinking about healing, then you are no longer healing, and are only thinking about healing (CS Lewis' Watchful Dragons of self-consciousness). The conscious watchful eye is a thief of the present, because it demands energy and intellect for anticipation and away from feeling, healing, and enjoying.

In my healing, I learned toward the end to simply **allow** pain. When you feel a muscle cramp coming on, do you tense-up and squeeze it—fight it—or relax and allow it through breathing (by the way, a muscle cramp is TMS)? I eventually let the pain do what it would, and lived and moved normally, making it irrelevant, as my

---

* Watch this 5-minute Dr. Quantum—Double Slit Experiment video on how observing something changes it, just as with healing: youtube.com/watch?v=DfPeprQ7oGc

virtual friend and rapper, Tractor-D, wrote about her pain, "let it wash over me." It also helped me to stop feeling the pain as a pinched nerve—which it wasn't. I began to visualize the pain as a sucking or pulling sensation, a different way of viewing and understanding the information the pain was sending me. Pain is a cramp from hell. If the sufferer cannot stop thinking that structural problems are the reasons behind his chronic (and often acute) pain, then he is unconsciously resisting the changes necessary for healing.

The Paradox of Trying Too Hard

When you cease to try to understand, then you will know, without understanding.
— Kwai Chang Caine, "A Praying Mantis Kills"

All beings perform more efficiently when not overloaded and pressured. Former Ohio State University football coach, Jim Tressel, was once asked about his laid-back coaching style—why he didn't yell at and berate his players like some coaches. He said that he didn't want them to have to worry about him yelling at them on top of all the other things they had to think about. Added pressure makes simple tasks more difficult and muddles the interpretation of subtle messages. Change occurs much more rapidly when relaxed and at ease, and with confidence. So making healing fun is an important decision—it expedited my recovery. People heal faster when they "let life's problems resolve themselves." Go do something you've always wanted to do, with excitement—and ease up on you.

Worsening Pain—The Edges of Truths

Be advised—pain may worsen during various healing stages, for no obvious reason. As the emotion rises to the surface—and it will if you're healing—the pain must increase in order to prevent the expression or recognition of the unwanted. Pain tells us that we are on the verge of change—coming face to face with what we know to be true deep within, yet won't admit to. Faith is then necessary to move forward when the other side can't be seen—and isn't fully known. TMS is a **liminal effect** (Latin, limina defined as "threshold"). Liminal space is that space where the first door has been opened but the second has not yet been entered. It is the space in between knowing and not knowing—the threshold of understanding... *the space between the yin and yang....*

Anthropologist Victor Turner first introduced the term liminal space, which has been described as "neither this nor that." Limina is used to describe the transformation from one state to another: the dissolving edge of one state, but not yet the beginning of another. **All transformation takes place within the limina.** Indian post-colonial theorist, Homi K. Bhabha, has described the limina as being "interstitial," deriving from the word interstice (in-TUR-stiss). This term is used to describe a very small opening, or a gap in something in nature that appears to be continuous. It can also refer to a pause in an event, or in time. Suffering is indeed a pause or space in the life of the person. Illness and pain knock her down so that she CAN pause. The step through the next doorway is a rebirth—enlightenment, or as the Buddha referred to it, "crossing to the other shore."

Oliver Wendell Holmes wrote, "Every now and then a man's mind is stretched by a new idea or sensation, and never shrinks back to its former." After TMS healing, you cannot go back through the first TMS door. You may want to turn the previous knob a few times, as old ways die hard, but you can't reverse understanding gained. Pain itself stands at the edge of transformation. People invariably come through their pain a changed person.

> *The patient who has recovered from TMS grows into a happier, more comfortable, more peaceful person who sees new paths toward greater personal fulfillment.*
> — Andrea Leonard-Segal, MD, *The Divided Mind*[311]

Groddeck—das Es—The It-Force That Controls All Disease?

> *…man creates his own illnesses for a definite purpose, using the outer world merely as an instrument, finding there an inexhaustible supply of material which he can use for this purpose, today a piece of orange peel, tomorrow the spirochete of syphilis, the day after, a draft of cold air, or anything else that will help him pile up his woes. And always to gain pleasure, no matter how unlikely that may seem, for every human being experiences something of pleasure in suffering; every human being has the feeling of guilt and tries to get rid of it by self-punishment.*
> — Georg Groddeck, MD, *The Book of the It*[312]

Groddeck's assertion brings us to the pinnacle—and reaffirms my earlier notions that our next in-vogue form of suffering will be whatever the guy next to you has, and that today our backs and feet and hands are collectively failing. "…today a piece of orange peel, tomorrow the spirochete of syphilis, the day after, a draft of cold air." What is currently popular in suffering, is what people will catch or use at an unconscious level for self-punishment against **darker pleasure**.

Georg Walther Groddeck, MD, was one of the most prolific healers of modern time. You may not have heard of him—that's simply because he didn't care about his reputation in posterity; he simply healed people, lots of them, mainly the chronically ill. Although he considered Freud a genius (and vice versa), for Freud's discoveries of ego, transcendence, and resistance, etc., he parted ways with Freud on the philosophy of disease, health, and healing. Groddeck felt there was something much greater—a force happening with the human organism that could not be defined within the human psyche, as Freud attempted to do. Groddeck called this unknowable force that animates humankind—**the It** (Groddeck spoke German, so the "foreignclature" would be—**das Es**). This is where the id stems from, das es = the it = the id. Groddeck claimed Freud stole the term id from him and Freud claimed Groddeck stole the term id from

Nietzsche. No one knows the real source because of all the various egos involved back then. No matter, Freud eventually gave Groddeck credit for id in his book, *The Ego and the Id.*

The **It hypothesis,** as Groddeck put forth, is "The sum total of an individual human being." **It** determines what we do and what we experience. Groddeck moved beyond ego as the component that defined us, by pointing out that ego doesn't determine our heartbeats per minute, our cell structure, our need for oxygen, or that we are even organic beings—something else determines that: our **It.** The fact that we live, Groddeck felt, was only a "superficial part of **It's** total experience."

> *I assume that man is animated by the It, which directs what he does and what he goes through... Man, then, is himself a function of this mysterious force which expresses itself through him, through his illness no less than his health.*
>
> — Georg Groddeck, MD, pioneer of psychosomatic medicine (1866-1934)[313]

Groddeck's experiences as a medical doctor led him to conclude that there was something beyond what we could comprehend occurring behind illness, since people with the same disease and prognosis often had different outcomes. He therefore concluded that the causes of disease were unknowable, that "disease as an entity did not exist, except inasmuch as it were an expression of a man's total personality, his **It,** experiencing itself through him"—disease then, Groddeck proclaimed, is a form of self-expression of the entire Self.

Through his understanding of **It,** Groddeck's healing methods drastically changed; he abandoned most of his medical training and experience and turned to psychoanalysis, which he thought could help in every disease—with every physical problem. To Groddeck, modern medicine was simply performing ritualistic practices—it didn't matter which one was used because the only thing that was important was how the sufferer's **It** perceived "the prescription." Therefore, the physician's medical-techno know-how did little for the patient; healing was determined by how **It** responded. The doctor could dress a wound, apply ointment, set a cast, or amputate—but the **It** controlled the final outcome.

Groddeck felt that the physician could influence the **It** through psychoanalysis—from there the **It** could learn from its mistakes and correct them. **It** caused the cancer and car accident, broke the leg in the fall, infected the lungs and blinded the eyes. **It** is the architect of mankind—metaphysical in nature—beyond Freudian causes and effects. The **It** is the cause that needs to be understood in healing. Groddeck knew that science was working fervently on effects alone—but to him, it wasn't possible to stop the effects (symptoms) of disease until the cause was more fully understood. Here is where Groddeck and Sarno collide in success because Groddeck felt that healing came through understanding. Groddeck didn't meddle with disease—he tried to understand what the **It** was trying to express through the disease by trying to influence the **It** through psychoanalysis, teaching **It** how to express itself in a less painful fashion.

Groddeck's **It** also confirms the notion that we will use whatever is within our means for self-punishment—any new symptom, cured through any new fad. Today it is those deadly soft mattresses, wrist-breaking computer keyboards, devastating $150 shoes, dreaded comfy chairs; and tomorrow, **It** may just be an orange peel— anything to keep the dark from becoming light. People will find what they need to punish themselves for desires of pleasure, by piling up their woes using an "inexhaustible supply of material" to hide their guilt and shame.

> *With Groddeck has gone one of the most remarkable men I have ever met. He is indeed the only man I have known who continually reminded me of Lao-Tzu; his non-action had just the same magical effect. He took the view that the doctor really knows nothing, and of himself can do nothing, that he should therefore interfere as little as possible, for his presence [alone] can invoke to action the patient's own powers of healing.... In this way Groddeck cured me in less than a week of a relapsing phlebitis, which other doctors had warned me would keep me an invalid for years, if not for the rest of my life.*
> — Hermann Graf Keyserling, philosopher (1880-1946)[314]

38

Letting Go

There is only one way to happiness, and that is to cease worrying about things which are beyond the power of our will.

— Epictetus, Stoic philosopher (55 AD-135 AD)

Eustress versus Distress

Life events do not cause tension—destructive emotions assigned to the events do, just as fear doesn't cause TMS—the reaction to overcoming the source of fear does. Tension is a psycho-physiological reaction to the interpretation of an event. The majority of people were understandably irate when OJ Simpson was found not guilty for double murder, while others with ego-vested interest happily cheered that he walked away freely. The same event—with two different behavioral responses, or emotional attachments: one of anger and one of joy. By not holding on to an overzealous interpretation of any event—medical imaging or prognosis—the body doesn't respond as strongly. The pain of TMS begins to wane when you no longer attach any meaning to the structural changes—or when you let go of those things that sting your ego.

In his book, *Deadly Emotions*, Dr. Colbert writes of a middle-aged patient that had developed rheumatoid arthritis from her inability to let go of an attachment. She had complained that her husband had left her for a younger woman and that her lifestyle had gone from one of luxury to just getting by. Her interpretation of the event was manifest as rage toward her ex-husband. She openly admitted to Dr. Colbert that she hated her ex-husband and she wished him dead. She not only wanted him dead, she wanted him to suffer agonizingly and painfully. Her condition worsened as her years rolled by. Colbert described her as being "once lovely, gentle, and gracious."[315] He had even asked her if she could ever forgive her ex-husband, to which she replied, "No. I plan to carry the way I feel to the grave."[316] Colbert wrote that through the years she became "bent over, twisted, and contorted."[317] She could never let go of her resentment toward her former husband—all the way up to her death. Her own inability to forgive only burned her by fueling the fire of her ego; it never hurt him.

Holding on to things that do not serve self can be a deadly course of action. People in general don't understand what cancer is. A cancer cell is a cell that will not die—will not live in harmony with its cell community. It is a cell—the ground of all consciousness—that refuses to change, to surrender, to let go. And in its refusal, it can kill the entire being. By holding steadfast to anything, to everything, we may be killing ourselves.

39

TMS Gives Hope
"Hope is the mainstay, hope is everything."

Thanks for the memories…. "I'm so old they've cancelled my blood type."

— Bob Hope

Five Golden Keys to Health and Happiness—Beginning with Hope

The iconic comedian, Bob Hope, was a shining example of how to live a good, fulfilled, productive, happy, healthy life. I believe Bob did five things right in order to live healthily and happily, right up until he died at age one hundred. The most important thing Bob did—was to do what he loved. He didn't do what others wanted him to do, he didn't do what he felt he should do, he did what fulfilled HIM. He became Self, which Jung felt was the goal of life—self-realization through individuation. Laughter heals, and Bob loved making people laugh. He enjoyed his career, generating laughter—a golden key to happiness, since it's impossible to experience anger and laughter simultaneously.

The second thing Bob did right was to take a long walk every day. His daughter Linda said that wherever he happened to be, you could find him with his golf club in hand taking a walk—widening his proxemic space. It is great meditation to go out alone and to quiet the chatter of the day. The physical health benefits of walking are as important as its meditative benefits. We are bipeds—meant to walk, walk, walk.

The third thing Bob did right was to get a daily massage. Massage is a tremendous way to soothe the sympathetic nervous system. Tension melts away and the reason for the anger often melts with it. Georg Groddeck—an MD and natural philosopher, abandoned most of his medical training and resorted to a combination of two things: **psychoanalysis** and **massage**.

The fourth thing Bob did right was to use his power and fame for benevolence. No single person has ever given more to those who fight for freedom than Bob Hope. He entertained millions of GIs for over 60 years. This no doubt would have helped assuage any guilt over living wealthy in a free land. Giving can assuage the deep guilt of having, where others don't.

The fifth thing Bob did right was to nurture a loving healthy relationship. Partners who support each other tend to be happier and healthier. He was married to Dolores for nearly 70 years. When she asked him where he wanted to be buried, he reportedly said, "Surprise me."

It's no mystery why Hope lived happily and healthily for an entire century. I read his golf book, *Confessions of a Hooker: My Lifelong Love Affair with Golf*, in which he stated that he had only been in the hospital once in his life. Bob gives us hope—a guide to happiness. Happiness is the feeling of connection, joy, love, and serenity. It is living free and with purpose; feeling self-worth by adding value to the world.

40

Beyond TMS

The most tragic events are a great benefit to mankind and therefore necessary.

— Chuang Tzu

What I Learned: My Road Home

I saw the angel in the marble and I just chiseled 'til I set him free.

— Michelangelo

- I learned that there was a part of me, hidden by me—from me—for reasons unknown to me—that makes me who I am, that I never knew existed—that causes all my physical effects.
- I learned to move from demanding perfection to the giving of and feeling natural compassion.
- I learned to forgive myself for things I felt I had done wrong, had left undone, or could have done better.
- I learned to focus on life instead of death—love instead of fear.
- I learned that love is immensely greater than the emotion that we feel as love.
- I learned that many of the false beliefs we accept today are based on the egocentric self-centered actions of others from the past.
- I learned that what I saw in myself as weaknesses were my greatest strengths—as nature intended me.
- I learned that intimacy is the greatest fear to those who love the deepest.
- I learned that life's hurdles strengthened my body and expanded my mind—to greater consciousness.

When my wife was handicapped, it cut my heart in two. My heart longed to beat again to the rhythm of One. Then began a great pain that held within it the potential for transformation—yet I filled my heart unknowingly with self-punishment. With time and grace, I began to see my error and from tragedy I awakened to a higher plane of awareness—moving beyond ego and inward toward my-Self.

Whether it is from Divine Providence, or from crossing to the other shore, the song remains the same. Learning came from a higher source, a more knowledgeable teacher, a Master's plan so infinitely intelligent that my only understanding is that I can never understand it—and yet I see its effects daily. Each set-back opens the mind wider because it forces introspection, creating ripples inward to be reflected upon as reconciliation with the unwanted unfolds. Through grief, we discover what sustains us—given the opportunity to search inward, to the beginning, uncovering truths and marveling at life's mysteries along the way.

The most beautiful experience we can have is the mysterious. It is the fundamental emotion which stands at the cradle of true art and true science. Whosoever does not know it and can no longer marvel, is as good as dead, and his eyes are dimmed.
                                                                              — Albert Einstein, 1931

The concept in healing behind all the ego and shadow-work—and self-introspection—is to experience wholeness through happiness. The real tragedy in tragedy is if nothing is learned and old patterns remain. Dr. Sarno's School offered a degree in the study of pain and unconscious behavior—I graduated with Honors. And I know—without a flicker of doubt—that you can, too.

Building Our Chain of Awareness—Beginning with Forgiveness

There are two things to aim for in life: first to get what you want, and, after that, to enjoy it. Only the wisest of mankind achieve the second.
                                                     — Logan Pearsall Smith, *Life and Human Nature*,
                                                                      literary perfectionist (1865-1946)

At early ages, we are hard-wired to certain realities—false images of ourselves built upon rejection. We see what we think we should see, act like we think we should act—burying any darker images of ourselves along with a portion of light—and our personality is born. Each self-built personality reacts to life in its own way. But if that personality's foundation is built on a demanding superego, true happiness is lost in the conflict of egos. The individual now gets trapped by her emotions—thinking she is those emotions—unable to move beyond them, unable to forgive herself, unable to push beyond her memories, unable to experience deep happiness.

Memories are stored within each cell of the mindbody. The mindbody is a storehouse for memories that react to the emotions attached to those memories. In *Anatomy of the Spirit*, Caroline Myss writes that, "Your biography becomes your biology." In the foreword to the book you are now reading, Dr. Sopher stated that your "psychology affects physiology," and I have written "your biology follows your belief." The concepts are the same. The physical body reveals the content of the psyche at any one time in the form of pain, illness, or good health.

We learn self-punishment during early separation trauma (trauma, as defined by Robert Scaer, MD, is "a state of helplessness under life-threat"). For survival, we then utilize either the flight (withdrawal/capitulation), fight (aggressive assertion), or freeze (avoidance of pain trauma) response—whichever originally worked for our survival will be our method for life. If freeze is chosen—the genesis of TMS begins. The physical symptoms that result from the freeze response are the TMS symptoms discussed throughout this book. These symptoms result from a lack of discharge of the energy pent up by a fight or flight response that never took place—expressions of conflict that desire to be known, and yet for personal reasons, cannot.

> People who wear masks seek to hide their faces. It takes energy to design and to build a mask. It takes energy to sell the mask. It takes energy to put that mask on. It takes energy to make sure that mask is on every day. It takes great courage to recognize it as a mask. It takes greater courage to peel the mask away... and to reveal the face beneath... as love replaces fear, and Self rises to Consciousness.

Emotional pain is culturally taboo, and so masks of physical pain are worn instead. This book is about revealing human misconceptions. If you believe you are failing, you will fail, through unconscious actions, as your shadow tries in desperation to hide a side of yourself that you fear. If you believe in hope, there isn't enough light to shine on all the possibilities in healing. With hope comes calm—and from calm, peace.

When I first began to read Dr. Sarno's work, I thought he was just a strange old Q-wacky guy trying to sell books. I made the great error of judging something beyond the realm of my current understanding. My physical pain was so sharp, so deep, and so life-altering, that I would not believe it could have been emotionally driven. I just would not believe it, and yet it was. I was wrong—the good doctor was correct.

Toward the end of this writing, I contacted psychiatrist Clancy McKenzie to verify a few things he had previously explained to me, and to clarify some of what he had written, since so much suffering begins with early separation, isolation, rejection, and perceived emotional abandonment. At that time I wasn't sure how to end this book. I needed to stop at some point or the manuscript was going to make *War and Peace* look like the menu at Denny's restaurant. I wasn't quite sure how to end—but I didn't tell Dr. McKenzie that. Then out of the blue, clear sky he wrote back to me these words of advice for my book, "Don't forget to mention forgiveness." That was it! He had given me the ending and the beginning that I had been searching for. Forgiveness is the beginning that ends self-induced suffering. I already knew that happiness was the antidote to TMS venom. You can't be happy if you fear. You can't be happy without hope or love. Fear is **darkness**—an interstice—a brief pause in the awareness of the continuity of love, where we must decide whether to give in and believe that this is all that there is, or to move to that next depth of consciousness. No love, no hope, no happiness can exist without first forgiving the Self. But how do you explain happiness to people who don't feel worthy of it? Indeed dozens have asked me how to become happier. It comes from letting go of fear—and becoming yourself—who nature intended you to be. Once fear is faced—anger from conflict fades. The only way to be truly happy is to love deeply, laugh freely—forgive genuinely.

Many years ago Gerald Jampolsky, MD, had figured it out, and so it didn't surprise me when I read this in his book in the spring of 2007.

> *For many years I had been bothered by chronic disabling back pain. Through those years I was not able to play tennis, garden, or do many of the things that I liked to do. I was hospitalized several times, and at one point the neurosurgeon wanted to perform surgery on what was called an organic back disease—a degenerative disc. I chose not to have the surgery... I thought I was upset because of the pain and the distress caused by it. Then one day there seemed to be a small voice inside which said that, even though I had an organic back syndrome, I was causing my own pain. It became clear to me that my back condition became worse when I was under emotional stress, particularly, when I was fearful and holding a grievance against someone. I was not upset for the reason I thought... As I learned to let go of my grievances through the practice of forgiveness, my pain disappeared. I now have no limitations on my activities... I was upset because of unhealed personal relationships.*
>
> — Gerald Jampolsky, MD, *Love Is Letting Go Of Fear*[318]

Dr. Jampolsky had seen the light in the 1970s. I went through this same process myself and have watched many others do the same. I would be hard-pressed to look back and to find someone who was in pain who hadn't recently had a major change, was experiencing overwhelming demands, or was holding a grudge—necessitating repression—leading to their symptoms.

Most felt that at some odd level, they were indeed punishing themselves by attaching themselves to disorders that didn't exist—or weren't in a position to even succumb to. They all knew deep under their turbulent conscious waters that they were somehow conflicted—and they also knew that they were hiding that conflict in their bodies. They weren't happy—and so their minds set upon their flesh. I made this book a comprehensive health book, rather than just focusing on pain itself. I meandered from the psychological to the physical—back and forth—knowing they could never be separated.

Pain is a part of life and the philosophy upon which that life is based, and so this book attempts to shed light on the larger life—which is the origins of pain, not merely the characteristics of it. This book isn't about what TMS is. It's mainly about "**why**" TMS is. My intention is to provide a map that shows the many roads leading out of conflict; it's up to the sufferer to decide which fork in the road to take on the journey to healing—persistently plodding toward truth, away from man-made problems.

Mortals obtain the harmony of health, only as they forsake discord, acknowledge the supremacy of divine Mind, and abandon their mortal beliefs. Eradicate the image of disease from perturbed thought before it has taken tangible shape in conscious thought... and you prevent the development of disease. This task becomes easy, if you understand that every disease is an error, and has no character or type, except what mortal mind assigns it. By lifting thought above error, or disease, and contending persistently for truth, you destroy error. When we remove disease by addressing the disturbed mind, giving no heed to the body, we prove that thought alone creates suffering.

— Mary Baker Eddy, *Science and Health*, 1875[319]

I'm often asked if I could sum up TMS in one word. Although tension results primarily from id-superego conflict, if I had to give the cause of pain an emotional label, it would be **guilt** (or shame—guilt is a personal reaction, and shame is a social reaction to embarrassment). We cannot fully concentrate on worrying about others and our own happiness simultaneously, and so we suffer from experiencing deep inside what we would like to be doing instead of caring about them. Guilt is the residual conflict from trying to be good and right, while simultaneously not wanting to be good or right. Lost in the conflict of trying to make everyone happy simultaneously is the ability to enjoy what already is—absent is presence—and guilt crowds out happiness if self-punishment is the mechanism for coping. Other people cannot make you happy—only you can: you own your life. The past must be forgiven, or released for the move forward.

Deep down inside, people know where they need to be, and what they need to see in order to become happy; they just lack the faith needed for the journey and so pain and illness are messengers that push them toward the wholeness of love and truth. Once happiness is chosen over fear and conflict, problems fade from memory—the body is no longer a prison for emotional wounds, and becomes a vessel for more spirited journeys.

Happiness first,
and good health will certainly follow....

Appendix A

TMS Equivalents—
Serving the Same Purpose as Pain

Your body does your feeling for you. Every feeling—from pleasure to pain and everything between—we feel in our bodies first and only secondarily through our minds.
— John Lee, *Facing the Fire*[320]

This section contains a simple list of common tension-induced mindbody symptoms—equivalents of TMS tensionalgia—physical manifestations of an emotional response. The following list is an array of tension-induced symptoms that either I defeated through TMS healing, or have read about, or have seen others heal from. The manifestations listed below could also be divided into TMS categories such as gastrointestinal disorders, skin disorders, genitourinary disorders, cardio-pulmonary disorders, autoimmune disorders, circulatory disorders, dysthymic disorders, and immune deficiencies, among others. The array is for easy reference. Have at it.

Acid reflux (gastroesophogeal reflux, or heartburn, or GERD)—It's frustrating to hear television commercials claiming this to be a "disease." Acid reflux is a symptom of stress, anxiety, and sometimes poor physical conditioning. It is not a disease. However, anything allowed to remain chronic can become dangerous. It has the potential for Barrett's Syndrome.* As with all symptoms, take the reason away.

Acne—Pimples are anger and anxiety, bursting eruptions through the skin. People are often astounded by the fact that right before their big date or their big event they get a pimple squarely in the middle of their forehead or on their face. What they don't realize is that it was the anxiety of the upcoming event that precipitated the burst of emotion through the skin—revealing the level of heightened anxiety and hormonal activity.

Acute pseudo-gout (false gout)—Forms of so-called gout are emotionally driven. This is Phase 2 TMS since it is often triggered by dehydration, stress, or a hit or twist of the joint, with no elevated uric acid.

---

* Barrett's Syndrome or Barrett's Esophagus occurs when the lining of the low end of the esophagus forms new types of cells like intestinal-type cells. GERD is a major suspect in the anomaly.

Addictions—Drug, alcohol, sex, gambling, video games, etc.: all are distractions that allow the mind to be focused elsewhere and away from the unwanted emotions and anxiety; the problems of the day.

Alcoholism—Alcohol numbs emotions—abused in an attempt to fill a separation void. Alcohol is a legalized drug that is consumed in place of attempting to satisfy a spiritual yearning and/or to alleviate the anger of earlier relationship separation.

Allergies—Several people I know have rid their lifetime allergies with TMS healing. These include both food and pollen allergies. An allergy is the immune system overreacting to external triggers.

Angina—This is chest pain caused by the heart not getting enough blood. Psychological factors play a heavy role but there can be an underlying physical reason. Find out why the heart isn't getting enough blood; get a heart check-up first before attempting tensionalgia healing. People can actually get TMS chest pains by the contraction of the chest muscles themselves, making them feel as though they are having a heart attack.

Ankylosing spondylitis—This disorder was brought to the public eye by Norman Cousins, who successfully defeated it through relaxation, laughter, and the intake of large amounts of ascorbic acid. It was ultimately his ability to take possession of his own health that cured the disorder.

Anxiety—Given the choice of anxiety or pain, people's brains often choose pain because of their superego. Thus, they suffer from chronic pain until they become aware of its purpose.

Arrhythmia—This describes an irregularity in the heart's natural rhythm. Get a heart check-up first before trying tensionalgia healing.

Asthma—People become so fearful that their next breath may not come that they panic. They push ahead of the light in faithless fear, not allowing it to simply happen. Exercise is one trigger for an asthma-panic and anger is another.

Atrial premature beats, APB, (heart in the throat feeling)—Get a heart check-up first before trying tensionalgia healing.

Back pain—Ouch (see the above book).

Bell's Palsy—As Dr. Sarno described, if the bloodflow is unconsciously reduced at the base of the skull, nerves do not regenerate and permanent damage can occur. Nerves encased in bone, as in the skull and spine are not regenerative. Oxygen loss to these types of nerves after 24 hours is permanently paralyzing.

Binge drinking—This is sudden sustained bursts of heavy drinking; it is also known as falling off the wagon (see Alcoholism).

Broken heart syndrome (stress cardiomyopathy)—This is often misdiagnosed as a massive heart attack but is a reversible state. It is caused by an emotional overload that "shocks" the heart into a state that mimics a heart attack. The loss of a loved one can literally "break" the heart.

Burning mouth syndrome (BMS)—The sensation of a burning tongue and oral mucous membranes, can be banished with TMS healing.

Bursitis—This is a term that is too loosely tossed around. Most cases of so-called bursitis are TMS. It alludes to swelling of the bursa but there is often no swelling. Many TMS pains that cannot be identified by physicians are erroneously labeled bursitis or tendonitis… or any host of "itises."

Calcium deposits—The presence of calcium deposits often leads to a misdiagnosis of the deposits being the cause of pain, followed by unnecessary surgery—but it often is TMS.

Carpal tunnel syndrome—With the advent of computers, we acquired this modern man-made delusionary social-replication phenomenon. When the medical industry introduced this term they planted the seeds for pain. Anyone who hits the emotional threshold now has a perfectly legitimate physical outlet—a new place to bury unwanted emotions.

Cholinergic urticaria—This is a case of hives that suddenly appears under extreme stress. They tend to itch and form a bump like a mosquito bite. This manifestation was made famous by the Chris Elliot character in the movie *There's Something About Mary.*

Chondromalacia patella (supposed wear under the kneecap)—This is TMS in the knee and is incorrectly associated with a wearing-out of the knee.

Chronic cough (bronchitis)—I had months of continuous chronic cough that I learned, years later, was due to repressed anger. Get a check-up first before trying tensionalgia healing. Coughing could be indicative of a later stage of lung disease.

Chronic fatigue syndrome, CFS, (benign myalgic encephalomyelitis)—Symptoms of this syndrome include muscle weakness, cognitive dysfunction (mental fogginess) often accompanied by muscle fatigue, joint pain, respiratory dysfunction and depression. Rest is non-beneficial. It often begins with a flu-like feeling or after periods of prolonged stress (Phase 4 TMS). It occurs more often in women and at midlife. Dr. Sarno has had much success treating CFS as TMS. They are one and the same.

Coccydynia—The location for this pain is deep in the tailbone, in the crease of the buttocks. It, too, leaves with TMS healing (the pain, that is—not the crease).

Cold sores—Induced by tension or anxiety, these viral skin eruptions are the wart's handsome half-cousin.

Constipation—Under severe stress and anxiety, some people can't go doo-doo. When the body goes into fight/flight, the digestive processes are triaged as an ancillary necessity.

Coronary artery disease—(See angina) From Type A to Type Z, the heart takes much of the brunt of repressed anger.

Cramps (spasms)—The TMSer often suffers leg and foot cramps at night when the bloodflow is further decreased at rest and unconscious activity increases. The unconscious and autonomic systems never sleep; if they did, you would sleep forever.

Dandruff—The flakes provide further evidence of autonomic involvement since skin secretion is a part of the thermoregulatory function of the ANS. During stressful periods, the ANS can increase sweating or reduce it—drying the skin.

Depression—There is rarely chronic pain without first mild to severe depression (acute pain may not be preceded by depression, but rather by overstimulation); it manifests as the loss of purpose.

Dizziness (lightheadedness, floating)—As anger tries to surface, the dizziness holds the anger down as conflict attempts to surface. The energy build-up of trying to hold down anxiety and anger swoons the person.

Drop foot—With TMS, when the muscles and nerves that control the foot aren't getting the needed blood (oxygen), the foot begins to drop with weakness.

Dry eyes—Dry eyes often serve the same distractionary purpose as pain, and this symptom can also be halted through gaining knowledge. As Andrea Leonard-Segal, MD, has written in *The Divided Mind*, dry eye is simply a distraction that the brain chooses and is TMS. She asked one of her patients if he had ever cried before, to which he replied "yes." She checked his tear ducts and they were open and functioning. She cured the man with TMS knowledge and has had success with others in showing that dry eye is simply a diversion from hidden emotional conflict.

Dry spot in throat—This may feel like a dry spot but it usually occurs when there is a tense situation, like when you need to communicate something difficult to say. The inner self does not want to talk and so id rebels.

Dyspepsia (indigestion)—The Civil War general, Stonewall Jackson, was famous for having this disorder. He also fit the Type T personality perfectly. He was anxious and restless and somewhat of a paranoid worrier. He was also an excellent planner.

Ear flutter (sudden sharp pain or thumping)—During overwhelming periods of stress, the brain often chooses the ears as an outlet for repressed anger. It sometimes sounds like a fluttering, and can be accompanied by sharp pain to hold one's attention. Loss of equilibrium can follow. Not wanting to (h)ear.

Eating disorders—

Anorexia Nervosa (AN)—This psychological-refusal to maintain a healthy weight for one's frame is a form of self-punishment combined with low self-esteem: not feeling good enough.

Bulimia Nervosa (BN)—Binge eating is followed by self-induced vomiting. Often this is compensatory behavior to prevent weight gain—the psychological self-destructive preoccupation to punish the self for perceived flaws, such as a failure to fit in and be accepted. It is a distractionary technique to keep the individual away from her emotional base through a preoccupation with her weight and body image. It is a TMS pain equivalent. **Binge-eating disorder (BED)**— This is compulsive over-eating to quell anxiety and thwart emotional pain, even when not hungry. Guilt then follows. The following is a quote from *Make the Connection* by Oprah Winfrey and Bob Greene (her personal trainer). Greene writes: "We all have different ways of coping with pain.... Food just happens to be the most socially acceptable coping mechanism.... Oprah clearly used food as her primary coping mechanism.... In the past, Oprah would simply go to the refrigerator and eat the stress and pain away. But when she no longer used eating as an outlet, she began to experience physical pain. Pain is a part of life. I'm happy to report Oprah now also experiences backaches, muscle spasms, and cramps.... The kind of emotional issues I'm referring to generally come from childhood experiences or traumatic events."[321] The key words here are, "socially acceptable coping mechanism." Food consumed, or food denied, to some people is their pain pill, their alcohol—their **distraction**.

Eczema (or dermatitis)—This includes skin rashes of various sorts. They, too, leave or get much better with TMS healing.

Emetophobia—This fear of vomiting is a common distraction.

Epicondylitis—Elbow pain. Lateral is **tennis elbow**, and medial is **golfer's elbow**.

Epstein-Barr Syndrome (EBS)—A virus, associated with CFS and benign myalgic encephalomyelitis. Fatigue with aches and pain, similar to CFS but with EBS, people have elevated antibody titers. Dr. Sarno points out in *The Mindbody Prescription* that these antibody titers can be reduced when people are given the opportunity to express or speak about their feelings.* People are fighting to get "fatigue" labeled as a disease. This would be a setback in recovery from it. Once something is labeled a disease, there will be lots of mon$y thrown at it, all in the wrong direction. Seek the answers inside first.

Facial tics—See fasciculation.

Fainting—Fainting can have numerous causes; however, fear, overstimulation and the battle for outer control (superego) are primary causes.

---

* "A paper published in the *Journal of Consulting and Clinical Psychology* in 1994 reported a decrease in antibody titers for the Epstein-Barr virus in people who were given the opportunity to write or speak about feelings that had been hitherto repressed.... The syndrome appears to be a combination of immune system malfunction (giving rise to the elevated antibody titers) and TMS symptoms, both of which can be attributed to the emotional process...." [*The Mindbody Prescription*, pp. 118-119]

Fasciculation—This is an involuntary muscle twitching or contraction under the skin that is not sufficient to move a limb but is visual to the eye. Most people can relate to the face twitches, triceps twitches, eyelid twitches, etc., as being stress related. The majority are benign mindbody tensionalgias. There are more serious afflictions that can be underlying these symptoms and as usual, get an exam, exam, exam (please don't get three exams, it's just a mantra borrowed from the realtors). For the most part, these minor nuisances are surfacing rage or hidden anxiety, pushed back into the depths until they burst onto the skin-scene. People have reported that they get fasciculations all over their bodies when under stress on vacations, before weddings, big events, etc.

Fibromyalgia (a.k.a. myofibrositis, fibrositis, or myofasciitis)—Here we have TMS on steroids. Fibromyalgia = TMS = subconscious rage. This is a common example of physicians getting together and establishing a disorder that didn't even exist (it happened in 1971). Females suffer this emotional effect over men at a ratio of approximately 10:1, resulting in about 90 percent of fibro sufferers being non-men. Currently, a TV ad is running for Lyrica, where the actress says her doctor tells her that her fibromyalgia is caused by "overactive nerves." This is not true. Pain always results from a lack of oxygen.

Floaters—Many tension sufferers have reported that they have an unusually high number of those distortions that are visible in the eye. They are shadows caused by degeneration of the gel-like vitreous in the eye. People in chronic pain appear to have many more of these. People have also written that they have reduced the number by relaxation and reduction in tension.

Frozen shoulder (a.k.a. adhesive capsulitis)—This is a very common TMS equivalent where the shoulder joint feels immovable or stiff and sometimes painful. Symptoms leave with TMS healing.

Gambling (chronic)—This takes the individual out of his mundane world and away from his life. It is fantasizing away current emotional and financial status.

Gas—Self-imposed pressure creates self-imposed pressures. Abdominal gas pains and cramping are tension-induced equivalents of pain as fight/flight pressure builds.

Gastritis—(inflammation of the stomach lining) This can lead to bleeding brought on by prolonged periods of extreme repressed stress and anger. It is an emotional response.

Gastroparasis (a.k.a. lazy stomach)—My father had this manifestation and it was quite frightening. The stomach simply stops digesting food. The more solid the food, the more uncomfortable and indigestible it is. I communicated with one other man who had this TMS equivalent, who had eventually read Sarno and had also healed. My father lost 54 lbs. as the symptom came out of nowhere and left just as mysteriously. TMS can wreak havoc in any system that the ANS controls and digestion is one of its primary functions.

Globus pharyngis—Broken down by word, we have Globus (ball), and pharyngis (throat): ball in the throat, or squeezing throat. It is the sensation of the need to cry but there are no external tears. It is a sign of depression and high tension. I developed this soon after my wife was handicapped: it, too, left with TMS healing and is a TMS pain equivalent. Studies on this symptom show its onset is related to not having a close confidant to which personal feelings can be expressed; aloneness.

Gout—I know people who get gout whenever they are under "stension," and as soon as the stress leaves, so does the gout, swelling and all. Something somehow alters the biochemistry under stress that produces inflamed joints. Often people will get red and swollen knees under tension that also leaves when the tension leaves.

Growing pains—There is no such thing as a growing pain. Growth heals pain, it does not cause it. To a child, the world is much larger and more frightening than to adults. A child's universe is overwhelming and this often becomes manifest in the form of extreme anxiety and TMS. Children often get leg and hip and ankle pain, or any other TMS symptom, such as stomachaches, rashes, etc., from overstimulation.

Gum swelling (gingivitis)—This is a good example of the existence of swelling in TMS. Gum swelling leaves when tension subsides.

Hair falling out (alopecia)—There are many reasons the hair can fall out, and tension is one of those reasons. Get an exam first before trying tensionalgia healing.

Hamstring pull—Though it feels like a pulled muscle, it is more often blood withdrawing to key muscles on the back of the leg—a cramp from tension.

Hay fever—This is also known as allergic rhinitis or allergies to pollen. For many people, allergies disappear when their pain subsides. As shown earlier in Chapter Thirty, in the Wolf Langewitz study, guided imagery and relaxation techniques significantly reduce hay fever symptoms.

Heart flutter—This is the feeling of the heart skipping beats. I always got this symptom when I was physically exhausted. It was always frightening and went away with relaxation. It felt as though it was taking my breath away. It stems from the energy demand imposed on the body, angerziety interfering with pacemaking.

Heel spurs or heel pain—As with calcium deposits, most heel spurs are blamed for heel pain. But as Drs. Sarno and Sopher have shown, the clever mind simply finds these sites to keep the mind's eye away from unconscious anger. The pain regularly leaves with TMS healing even with the spurs' existence.

Hemorrhoids—Think of this as varicose veins in the anus, or "vanus of the anus." Under stress, many people have tissue swelling around the anus. Life has literally become a pain in the arse and manifests itself in the form of its mental imagery.

Hiatus hernia—Part of the stomach pushes through the hiatus (opening in the diaphragm) and into the chest cavity, allowing gastric backflow into the esophagus, causing heartburn. Symptoms leave with TMS healing.

Hiccups—I have a cure for hiccups that has never failed to work yet. Give me a dollar and I'll show you how to rid them. Hiccups serve the same function as bronchitis and all the other TMS equivalents: distractions.

Hip pain—Both hip socket pain and trochanteric bursitis, which is outer hip pain, are symptoms that leave with TMS healing.

Hot flashes—This is a feeling of being flushed with wild autonomic swings. Wild swings in the thermoregulatory function are common with TMS overload and stress, in both men and women.

Hyperacusis—This sensitivity to sound leaves with TMS healing and relaxation.

Hypertension (chronically elevated blood pressure)—In its acute form it's referred to as transient high blood pressure and is a short-term occurrence as it rises and falls with stress and exertion, which is normal. In chronic form it's labeled as hypertension and is oftentimes a mindbody disorder. Read *The Divided Mind*, Chapter 5, Hypertension and the Mindbody Connection: A New Paradigm, with Samuel Mann, MD—an excellent explanation of TMS as a main cause of hypertension. According to Dr. Mann, approximately 20-25 percent of hypertension is due to TMS.

Impotence, sexual (not mental)—Stress can dramatically reduce the ability to perform sexually. So I'm told.

Infections (frequent)—The infections would include upper respiratory, urinary, genital (non-STD), bronchial, etc. Tension reduces the immune system's ability to protect against inside and outside invaders.

Interstitial cystitis: IC/PBS (painful bladder syndrome)—Interstitial cystitis is "claimed to be" an inflamed bladder. Approximately 15 percent of the people I have seen in TMS pain also experienced this form of bladder pain. Its etiology is unknown, and yet many surgeons rush in to remove the bla$$er (cystectomy). Later they find it was only TMS pain and they're left without a bladder, for no reason. Common cystitis, also known as a urinary tract infection, is caused by bacteria and is usually treated with antibiotics. Unlike common cystitis, IC is believed not to be caused by bacteria and does not respond to conventional antibiotic therapy. At the IC website, it specifically states that IC is not a psychosomatic disorder and is not caused by stress. But later in the self-help section on "what you can do" to help alleviate the symptoms of IC, it recommends, "stress reduction."[322] If stress can aggravate it, stress can cause it. There are enough former sufferers who have healed from IC who are living testimonials to the truth that IC is indeed a mindbody stress disorder.

Irritable bladder (IB)—This is an involuntary muscle contraction of the bladder with the uncontrollable need to urinate. Symptoms leave with TMS healing.

Irritable bowel syndrome (IBS, once commonly called colitis)—By any name, it is a sporadic mix of constipation and diarrhea that often is accompanied by pain and bloating. From the Johns Hopkins website, "Emotional stress may be a contributing factor... often possible to relieve symptoms with a combination of diet and stress management."

Knees (red and swollen)—(see stigmata) I see people with this symptom on occasion. Some also get red ears when tired. The body reveals the deep inner unresolved emotions through the knees, which are symbolic of support.

Lyme disease (LD)—Just because the LD antibody titer is in the blood doesn't mean the symptoms are coming from Lyme Disease. As Dr. Sarno has shown, so-called LD symptoms are mitigated through TMS healing.

Metatarsalgia—This pain and inflammation occurs at the ball of the foot. Symptoms leave with TMS healing.

Migraines—Most headaches have been proven to be psychosomatic, barring any disease process. They can fade with TMS knowledge and deep healing. Vasoconstriction creates deep pain within the head as a message and/or distraction. I experienced the pre-headache symptoms, pre-Sarno, but never the actual pain.

Mitral valve prolapse (MVP, click murmur syndrome)—I was not surprised to find out how many pain sufferers also had MVP, as I do. Two people I know have had their heart murmurs suddenly disappear with TMS healing. Dr. Sarno, a TMS sufferer himself, also has MVP. After 45 years of MVP, my friend Allan Masison's murmur disappeared when his TMS pain left him.

Nausea—Frequently this is a result of TMS, and a distraction.

Neck pain—A.k.a., pain in the neck, which is merely back pain: the "northern back."

Neuroma (metatarsal foot pain)—Most commonly found as bottom-of-the-foot-pain in the metatarsal region, it is tension-related and dissipates with TMS healing. For years I had this pain and it, too, left with the back pain and has not returned.

Non-gonococcal urethritis (NGU)—While often infectious (usually chlamydial), this urethral infection can stem from the guilt of sexual pleasure. Dr. Sopher wrote to me, "I have seen quite a few just like this" regarding sexual guilt and urethral infections. Symptoms leave with TMS healing.

Nose bleeds—Under tension people's noses often begin bleeding as the blood vessels vacillate and sometimes burst. Bleeding episodes can be stopped with TMS healing.

Nosophobia—This is a fear of becoming ill. On rare occasions people don't even need to have any symptoms in order to be TMSing. The simple fear of possibly falling ill can rivet attention and focus away from their problems.

Numbness (face, hands, feet, toes, etc.)—As always, more serious disorders must be ruled out first! Numbness may be serious and it may be harmless, as it was in my case.

OCD (obsessive compulsive disorder)—An anxiety disorder characterized by intrusive thoughts that produce uneasiness, apprehension, fear, or worry, the visible symptoms can include repetitive behaviors aimed at reducing anxiety; the disorder can also produce a combination of thoughts (obsessions) and behaviors (compulsions).

Palpitations—A racing and or pounding heartbeat are symptoms that leave with TMS healing.

Panic attack—Panic is strongly repressed rage breaking loose; outer control suppressing inner turmoil. Superego has id in a death grip.

Paresthesia—Tingling in the legs or extremities can be quite frightening and should be checked out. Leaves with TMS healing. This pins-and-needles feeling can occur anywhere, even the face and arms. It comes from a lack of oxygen to the nerve.

Periodic limb movement disorder (PLMD)—Flinching of arms and legs during non-REM sleep, once known as nocturnal myoclonus—I had never heard of this malady until a friend of mine with TMS and PLMD explained it to me. I went to a site on the subject and read about it that day. That very night my hands and arms began flinching as my body began integrating the thought. It woke me up for several nights in a row until I realized that I had become a host for the meme. I treated it like TMS and it immediately went away.

Peripheral neuropathy (a nerve condition that affects the extremities, particularly the feet)—This is attributed to various processes, but is clearly idiopathic. Many people whose feet hurt do not realize that it is an emotional response. A friend, Bart la Dose, used to call his the "rolled up socks syndrome." It leaves with TMS healing.

Phobias—These are irrational fears that run deep from early separation fear or trauma. People with phobias desire more control and are far more likely to experience TMS.

Piriformis syndrome—This symptom surfaces when TMS becomes more severe. At the height of my TMS, the oxygen deprivation was so bad that my hip piriformis muscle began to cramp as the bloodflow reduced in my hip. Tingling and pins-and-needles soon followed. These symptoms disappear with TMS therapy. This is clearly TMS muscle cramping and not a pinched nerve.

Plantar fasciitis—Pain occurs on the bottom of the foot along the arch. Symptoms leave with TMS healing.

Post-polio syndrome—Pain at the muscle sites that exhibited polio, but as Dr. Sarno points out in *The Divided Mind*, "there is no proof that this is the cause."*

Proctalgia fugax (levator ani syndrome)—A TMS disorder where people have severe rectal pain. It is not uncommon and is "curable" with TMS healing.

Promiscuity—One must heed the need to breed with speed because coping this way is meant to mislead.

Prostatitis (acute bacterial prostatitis, chronic bacterial prostatitis, nonbacterial prostatitis, and prostatodynia)—Of these four types, I've seen two people recover from nonbacterial. In *Healing Back Pain*, Dr. Sarno writes, "an academic urologist of my acquaintance has said that over 90 percent of his cases of prostatitis are due to tension."[323]

Psoriasis—This is a chronic skin condition where the cells multiply too quickly, resulting in red, or white, or silvery thick patches of skin. There is an extremely high correlation of psoriasis with back pain, further proof of autonomic involvement. From *Deadly Emotions*, "Psoriasis is like a volcano erupting from the pressure of unseen forces just below the surface of a person's life. The body is releasing fear, frustration, anger, and other toxic emotions."[324]

Pyloric spasms—This is the feeling of being kicked in the stomach and getting the wind "knocked out," as the hands and legs become weak and shaky. After a pyloric spasm I always felt as if I had just had a seizure: exhausted and drained. It was as if the pyloric sphincter muscle had cramped, as tension found its way into the upper digestive area.

Rashes—Skin outbreaks that are almost always undiagnosable as conventional skin conditions are TMS.

Raynaud's phenomenon (vasospastic attacks)—Bloodflow restriction to the hands and feet that stems from the same autonomic overreaction to external stimuli that encompasses TMS, causes the hands or feet to turn white or blue when they sense cold, while the ANS shuts down blood-carrying vessels to preserve heat for the core. It is harmless.

Repetitive Stress Disorder (RSD)—This is a new moneymaking label for TMS.

---

* From *The Divided Mind*, "There is a Latin phrase commonly quoted in scientific circles that refers to this particular kind of misdiagnosis: 'post hoc ergo propter hoc'. It means 'after this [i.e., polio] therefore because of this,' a classic error in logic leading to a dangerous and unscientific conclusion." [p. 17]

Restless leg syndrome (RLS, or Jimmy Legs)—As with leg cramps, this queasiness in the legs, or a floating or uncomfortable sensation of restlessness usually occurs while sleeping or resting. This is very similar to tinnitus, in that the more attention you give it, the more you bring it to you. Today television commercials are purposefully trying to get people to pay attention to it through conscious suggestion and the promise of medical $olution$. I found that relaxing the back of my neck along with observational breathing eliminated this symptom.

Rosacea—This refers to a redness in the face, often called red-mask. It is the opposite process of Raynaud's phenomenon. Instead of closing and constricting vessels, with rosacea they are expanding (dilating). This symptom reveals a level of hidden tension that thus far has gone unrecognized. It is symbolic of "red-in-the-face-angry." Ronald Reagan had it, and Bill Clinton has it.

Rotator cuff (tear)—Many of the so-called "rotator tears" were already existent but on viewing the imaging the surgeon often recommends unnecessary surgery. Soon after the surgery, the pain moves to the other shoulder, further proof that the surgery was unnecessary and that the tension needed a similar reservoir to hold the individual's attention. Partial tears are normally incidental findings and can almost always be ignored.

Scintillating scotoma—The loss of field of vision, often accompanied by zigzagging rainbow colors across the field of vision—these symptoms leave with TMS healing.

Scoliosis—An abnormal curvature of the spine is a condition that itself is not psychosomatic, but the resulting pain more often is. In Healing Back Pain, Dr. Sarno states, "It rarely causes pain in teenagers but is often blamed for back pain in adults."[325] Backs do not suddenly become crooked and painful, but tension does.

Seborrheic dermatitis—This is an inflammation of the skin that is characterized by oily red patches. In infants it is referred to as cradle cap. Anxiety and anger alter all and any autonomic functions that affect the skin. Anger often manifests on the epidermis—even in frightened babies.

Shin splints—Pounding feet on pavement is erroneously considered to be the cause of shin splints. The old wive's tale is that the muscle has pulled from the shin. Then somehow it miraculously reconnects again in a few days or weeks when the pain suddenly leaves. The foot hitting the pavement is merely the trigger for Phase 2 TMS. The inner self does not want to be running (demanding energy). Dr. Sarno called shin splints "TMS tendonitis."

Shiver-me-timbers (coldness)—The sensation of ice-water poured on the head or body is a symptom that leaves with TMS healing.

Shortness of breath—The inability to draw a satisfactory full breath, or the drawing of a painful breath is often rage-induced. There are many reasons for "unsatisfactory" or painful breathing and tension is one of the most common. There are other reasons that are not TMS of course, such as emphysema. Breathing is one of the autonomic functions and therefore susceptible to emotional influence.

Sinus infections—High tension levels often hide in the sinuses. These infections often start in childhood. They are much like colds, which occur when it is not acceptable to cry, and the infections replace the need to cry when the person is overwhelmed. Martin Rossman, MD, in Guided Imagery for Self-Healing, describes a patient, Ed, who suffered from recurrent sinus infections. Rossman gave him relaxation tapes with orders to listen to them twice daily. Ed reported in one week that he was 90 percent better. Soon after, his sinus infections ceased altogether and he has not had an occurrence in over ten years.[326]

> *Mary, twenty-four years old, had developed a sinus infection and was afraid that it would spread and get worse.... Mary asked Rose (Mary's Inner Advisor) about her illness and quickly became aware of the tension she'd been feeling between herself and her husband during the previous two weeks.... After the imagery session, Mary was greatly relieved, both emotionally and physically. Subsequently, she had a good talk with her husband during a quiet evening and found him supportive and responsive. They were able to share their concerns and hopes again, and her recovery was complete within two days.*
> — Martin Rossman, MD, *Guided Imagery for Self-Healing*[327]

Smoking—Anxiety needs to be calmed, and smoking is, unfortunately, one method people choose to cope and soothe that anxiety. There will be much more anxiety later when a deadly disease settles in due to the incessant pouring of toxins into the lungs.

Sore throat (acute or chronic)—Infections are often incidental findings. Most sore throats stem from stress and anxiety; the infections that creep in are secondary events. This may be hard to swallow for some, but sore throats don't come from infections—infections come from sore throats, which come from overstimulation.

Spasmodic dysphonia (laryngitis, both adductor and abductor)—People often report that they lose their voices under stress, such as before a speech. The vocal chords are common targets of tension since the voice is a mechanism of expressing self.

Spastic colon—I remember during finals week in college when many fellow students would tell me they were suddenly experiencing spastic colon symptoms. This supposedly feels like the proctologist is having a seizure during your rectal exam, "butt" it is simply TMS.

Stigmata—This is redness on certain body parts that reoccurs with triggers. The very first time I experienced rosacea (a stigmata effect) was right after my wife was paralyzed—it no doubt resulted from severe rage. Now, sometimes when I get angry or am under stress, it reappears as a conditioned response.

Stomachache—The solar plexus is a grouping of nerves located behind the stomach and is the largest group of autonomic nerves in the abdomen. Fear or worry, as well as love, are felt in the stomach, not in the brain. The brain is grey matter that thinks, but the solar plexus has a white outer layer that allows it to feel. This is where the term "gut feeling" comes from. Anxiety, stress, and anger are swallowed and digested by the stomach.

Stye (hordeolum)—People often report getting styes after arguing with people. Louise L. Hay writes in *You Can Heal Your Life* that a stye indicates being "angry at someone."

Sweating (excessive)—One symptom of TMS-anxiety is profuse sweating. But the ANS can also under-regulate its processes, as well as, over regulate them. It used to be that I rarely ever sweated, even in 100 degree weather. As I began to challenge my back pain, pre-and post-Sarno, I began to sweat normally for the first time as my ANS reregulated itself.

Swollen glands—There are many reasons for swollen glands and they should all be checked out with exams. I had multiple exams for my swollen throat glands but there was no apparent cause. If they can't find anything wrong, TMS is likely the culprit.

Tachycardia (rapid heart rate)—Former Callyfornyuh Governor Arnold Schwarzenegger was being heavily pressured as to whether to give clemency to former gang leader and convicted cop-killer Tookie Williams. Soon before the execution was to take place Arnold suffered from tachycardia and was admitted to the hospital. The Terminator attributed it to his heart valve replacement and a family history. But what the former governor doesn't know is that it has nothing to do with prior valve problems and everything to do with the massive public pressure he had been receiving from both sides of the death penalty argument. Even the medical director of the catheterization laboratory at Sutter Memorial Hospital in Sacramento, Dr. Miller, doubted the rapid heart rate had anything to do with his previous valve replacement. But the Terminator cannot show emotions; however, someday their effects "will be back," in the form of bodily symptoms.

Teeth grinding (bruxism)—As long as it's your own teeth you're grinding, then it is tension-related. If you're grinding someone else's teeth you may have more crunching issues to deal with.

Teeth sensitivity—Throbbing, or cold and hot sensitivity, is often the brain's strategy for distraction.

Telangiectasia—This is a generalized condition of flushing or redness caused by enlarging blood vessels, often seen on the face or the midline of the body. Telangiectasia tension "on the face" left unattended can lead to rhinophyma, a severe disfiguring of the nose and central face area, thus raising the importance of "potential" to a greater degree. Always get a check-up!

Tendonitis (inflammation of knee, shoulder, foot, etc., tendons)—I had all these pains and it was never from swelling or so-called tendonitis. It was always from tension-induced hypoxia—a.k.a. TMS.

Thirst—If you experience unquenchable thirst during self-imposed stress, check to see if you're diabetic first; if you are not, then it's probably an autonomic nervous system anxiety-related distraction.

Tinnitus—There may not be a better physical analogy for easing TMS symptoms than tinnitus. If you focus on the ear ringing, you give it strength. The back and neck pain are the same. If you give it attention you feed it. Treat tinnitus like joint pain and ignore it. Tinnitus is symbolic of not wanting to hear something. At the height of my back pain, my ear ringing was at its worst. The ringing left with TMS healing. Tinnitus also triggers the release of adrenaline in the body, elevating stress levels... *that vicious cycle....*

TMJ (or TMD) (Temporomandibular joint syndrome, or jaw pain)—This is caused by tension in the jaw that is often triggered by overextending the jaw (but not always). It can also be triggered by grinding of teeth from unconscious anxiety and anger, but not always. It often just suddenly begins, as in Phase 1 TMS.

TOS (Thoracic Outlet Syndrome)—Pain in the shoulders and arms is often mislabeled as TOS. "True" TOS impinges the blood vessels that serve the arms (through the thoracic outlet). However, this is extremely rare and so TMS arm and shoulder pain is often misdiagnosed as TOS when it is TMS.

Trichotillomania—Twisting of the hair with the fingers is a nervous habit. This is OCD-related and serves the same purpose as pain—an obsession that distracts the mind, as with all habits.

Trigeminal neuralgia (TN or prosopalgia, or facial nerve pain)—Characterized by pain in the facial area including teeth, jaw, nose, forehead, etc., it causes electric or lightning-like shocks when the face is touched during activities such as brushing teeth, eating, sleeping or putting on makeup, etc. Like many "itisus" or "algias," this is frequently misdiagnosed when it is simply TMS. It normally forms later in life and once again, more frequently in females.

Ulcerative colitis (IBD: inflammatory bowel disease)—This is inflammation of the lining of the colon, often combined with bleeding and infection. People have healed from this through relaxation and introspection. It is an unconscious tension-effect often resulting from trying to keep everyone happy; maintaining control under stress. From Andrew Weil, MD's *Spontaneous Healing*, "Diseases of the skin (and gastrointestinal tract) should be assumed to have an emotional basis until proved otherwise, because these systems are the most frequent sites of expression of stress-induced imbalances."[328]

Ulcers—Where have they gone? What was once very fashionable has now been replaced by newer, younger, more beautiful disorders.

Urinary tract infections (UTIs)—Urinary tract infections are the second most frequently occurring type of mindbody infection. Upper respiratory infections are numero uno.

Urination (frequent)—Anxiety and tension from perfectionistic desires often manifest themselves in the form of the need to urinate frequently as a distraction when the system is anxiously aroused, increasing kidney output. It is a TMS equivalent as focus shifts from madder to bladder. As with all ANS-functions and the mindbody, the process can also be reversed. People have also reported that they cannot urinate when they are anxious as the mind focuses on the fear of not being able "to go;" frozen bladder syndrome.

Ventricular premature beats (VPB)—This is the cause of most palpitations (disrupted heart rhythm, irregular pulse). Anxiety can strike the heart in many harmless ways, but don't take a chance ma'am, find a doctor and get an exam.

Vertigo (rapid bursts of dizziness, often labeled as BPPV: benign paroxysmal positional vertigo)—This can be the most frightening of TMS symptoms and should be medically tested first for more serious disorders. If all is well, then it's TMS hell.

Vision (varying changes)—As tension rises, vision often changes. The tension causes the eye to change its shape. On occasion people will no longer need corrective lenses after tensionalgia healing.

Warts—Many people have reported getting warts after or during tense times. They can also disappear after relaxation. They are outbursts of rage in the epidermis and are emotionally created and physically manifested.

Whiplash (chronic)—This can be seen in phases 2, 3 and 4 TMS. Characterized by Robert Scaer, MD, as "velocity-related injuries," a whiplash injury often ignites a post traumatic stress disorder (PTSD) that continually baffles physicians and patients due to the longevity and severity. Scaer cites the Gay and Abbott publishing of 1953, "Characteristically, these patients were more disabled and remained handicapped for longer periods than was anticipated, considering the mild character of the accident." The controversy stems from the discrepancy of the symptoms compared to the level of trauma experienced. Once again, with TMS, this is not due to people imagining or exaggerating. The symptoms are real but it is the unconscious forces and motivations that keep the pain ongoing—not a structural problem.

> *People will unconsciously choose symptoms that are in vogue and considered legitimate physical disorders by their doctors, which is why the syndromes of neck and back pain are of epidemic proportions in most of the Western world today.*
> — John E. Sarno, MD, *The Mindbody Prescription*[329]

Yawning—Yawning is a form of pandiculation,[330] akin to stretching, and is contagious, just like pain and many other symptoms. Yawning doesn't go away with TMS healing, and is actually good for you. I just wanted to use the word pandiculation somewhere. Yawning resets the mindbody and realigns mind, body, and consciousness—increasing self-awareness by increasing arousal.

Yeast infections—As with most chronic infections, they often have their basis in unconscious emotional upheaval.

And many more… anything that the autonomic and immune systems control can be affected unconsciously/emotionally.

Appendix B
TMS: A Healing Checklist

- Do you fully believe that your symptoms are from an unfelt psychological process?
- Do you realize that you have a hidden temper?
- Are you reflecting on what events may be triggering your pain?
- Have you set short-term physical goals?
- Have you forgiven any past grievances?
- Are you safely off any meds that may be triggering your pain through association?
- Are you decreasing your mental chatter through relaxation techniques?
- Are you excited about healing and good health?
- Are you actively imagining yourself as symptom-free and happy?
- Are you performing a daily transparent act for its own sake, and not for any other purpose?
- Have you changed your daily routine and habits?
- Do you understand that you have a demanding superego?
- Are you physically moving—oxygenating your system through healthy exercise?
- Are you eating healthily? Hydrating?
- Are you laughing each day at life's absurdities?
- Are you taking a moment each night to be appreciative of at least three things before sleep?
- Are you taking a moment before sleep to visualize a symptom-free vessel for the very next day?
- Are you consciously forcing your mind away from your symptom?
- Are you expanding your lung capacity through conscious breathing techniques?
- Did you get that physical exam in order to destroy any doubt in the TMS process?
- Have you slowed your negative internal language?
- Are you staying socially engaged?
- Have you stopped placating your pain with comfy pillows, chairs and self-crippling gadgets?

- Are you relaxing your healing time frame, ceasing trying too hard to heal too fast?
- Are you sticking to your goals?
- Do you want to heal?
- Are you acting on all of the information in this book?
- Are you practicing presence on a daily basis?
- Have you stopped trying to heal? Well… you should!

Appendix C
Healing Resources

www.SteveOzanich.com/ (Website for Steve Ozanich)

Organizations:

tmswiki.org/ (The Tension Myositis Syndrome Wiki, the Central-hub for TMS)

Medical Doctors

www.johnesarnomd.com/ (Official website for Dr. John Sarno)

www.gwozdzmd.com/ (Website for Dr. Paul Gwozdz)

drmiller.com/ (Website for Dr. Emmett Miller)

www.tms-mindbodymedicine.com/ (Website for Dr. Marc Sopher)

mindbodymedicine.com/ (Website for Dr. David Schechter)

www.thewellspring.com/ (Website for Dr. John W. Travis)

unlearnyourpain.com/ (Website for Dr. Howard Schubiner)

weillcornell.org/smann (Website for Dr. Samuel J. Mann)

irarashbaummd.com/ (Website for Dr. Ira Rashbaum)

healthy-mind-body.com/ (Website for Dr. Roger Gietzen)

gwcim.com/people/dr-andrea-leonard-segal-md/
    (Website for Dr. Andrea Leonard-Segal)

Therapists and Counselors:

drmargaretchan.com/ (Website for Dr. Margaret Chan)

www.painpsychologycenter.com/ (Website for Alan Gordon, LCSW at the
    Pain Psychology Center)

kirstenfliegler.com (Website for Dr. Kirsten Fliegler)

pathwaystopainrelief.com/about.html
    (Website for Dr. Frances Sommer Anderson & Dr. Eric Sherman)

lizwallensteintherapy.com/ (Website for Liz Wallenstein, LMHC)

laurelsteinberg.com/ (Website for Dr. Laurel Steinberg)

accessyoureverest.com (Website for Dr. Evana Hsiao-Henri)

www.thethingaboutchange.com/ (Website for Andrew Miller, LMFT)

arnoldbloch.com (Website for Arnold Bloch, LCSW)

www.colleenperry.com/ (Website for Colleen Perry, MFT)

pamelabenison.com/ (Website for Pamela Benison, MA)

www.wendynewmanlcsw.com (Website for Wendy Newman, LCSW)

www.jillsolomonmft.com/ (Website for Jill Solomon, MFT)

meaningoftruthbook.com/ (Website for Nicole Sachs, LCSW)

www.backpaincounseling.com (Website for Michele Lowenthal, MHC)

Coaches and Specialists:

louiselevy.co.uk/ (Website for Louise Levy, MA, DipCAH)

georgieoldfield.com/ (Website for physiotherapist, pain-specialist Georgie Oldfield)

abigailsteidley.com/ (Website for Abigail Steidley, coach)

www.tmspainrelief.com/ (Website for Andy Bayliss, coach)

Information:

www.podolsky.everybody.org/rsi/ (Rachel's RSI homage)

www.podolsky.everybody.org/rsi/audio/
     (Spring 2000 TMS Information Session Audiotape)

www.podolsky.everybody.org/rsi/stories.html (People's TMS stories)

psychologytoday.com/blog/crisis-knocks/201003/dealing-chronic-pain
     (Article in Psychology Today by Will Baum, LCSW)

www.tmshelp.com (Forum for TMS Help)

Bibliography

Ali, Majid. *Seven Core Principles of Integrative Medicine.* Capital University of Integrative Medicine, Washington, D.C.

American Tinnitus Association, [ata.org].

Amir, Fred. *Rapid Recovery from Back and Neck Pain.* Bethesda, Maryland: Health Advisory Group Publishing, 1999.

Arenson, Gloria. *Five Simple Steps To Emotional Healing.* New York: Fireside, 2001.

Armstrong, Lance. *It's Not About the Bike, My Journey Back to Life.* New York: GP Putnam's Sons, 2000.

Aron, Elaine N. *The Highly Sensitive Person.* New York: Broadway Books, 1998.

Aversa, Jeannine. *Debt hurts your body, too.* AP IMPACT: AP-AOL poll (March 24 to April 3 by Abt SRBI Inc.).

Bly, Robert. *The Night Abraham Called to the Stars, The Eel in the Cave.* New York: Harper Collins, 2001.

Bourne, Edmund. *The Anxiety and Phobia Workshop.* New York: MJF, 1995.

Bresler, David E., and Richard Trubo. *Free Yourself from Pain.* New York: Simon & Schuster, 1986.

Buchman, Dian Dincin. *Natural Sleep.* New York: Gramercy, 1997.

Captured Light and Lord of the Wind Films, *What The Bleep Do We Know?* 2004.

Cassels, Alan, and Ray Moynihan. *Selling Sickness: How the World's Biggest Pharmaceutical Companies Are Turning Us All into Patients.* New York: Nation Books, 2006.

Chopra, Deepak. *Quantum Healing.* New York: Bantam Books, 1989.

Chopra, Deepak. *The Soul of Healing, Body Mind & Soul.* Deepak Chopra and Haft Entertainment, 2003.

Chopra, Deepak. *The Way of the Wizard: Twenty Spiritual Lessons for Creating the Life You Want.* New York: Harmony, 1995.

Colbert, Don. *Deadly Emotions, Understand The Mind-Body-Spirit Connection That Can Heal or Destroy You.* Nashville Tennessee: Thomas Nelson Publishers, 2003.

Coldren, Jeffrey T., Steve Ellyson, William Rick Fry, Jane Kestner, and Peter A. Beckett. *General Psychology.* Dubuque Iowa: Kendall/Hunt Publishing Company, 2001.

Cousins, Norman. *Anatomy of an Illness as Perceived by the Patient: Reflections on Healing and Regeneration.* New York: WW Norton & Company, 1981.

Creighton, James L., Simonton Carl O., and Simonton, Stephanie Matthews. Getting Well Again

Dawkins, Richard. *The Selfish Gene: 30th Anniversary Edition* 3rd ed. New York: Oxford University Press, 2006.

Eddy, Mary Baker. *Science and Health, with Key to the Scriptures:* Boston: The Christian Science Board of Directors, 1994.

Finley, Guy. *The Secret of Letting Go.* St. Paul: Llewellyn, 2003.

Fox, Michael J. *Lucky Man: a Memoir.* New York: Hyperion, 2003.

Freud, Sigmund, and Peter Gay. *Inhibitions, Symptoms and Anxiety (Standard Edition of the Complete Psychological Works of Sigmund Freud).* New York: W. W. Norton & Company, 1990.

Freud, Sigmund. *Dora: An Analysis of a Case of Hysteria (Collected Papers of Sigmund Freud).* New York: Touchstone, 1997.

Freud, Sigmund. *The Ego and the Id.* New York: WW Norton & Company, 1960.

Freud, Sigmund. *The Standard Edition of the Complete Psychological Works of Sigmund, Freud, Some Thoughts on Development and Regression—Aetiology.* trans. James Strachey, 24 vols. London: Hogarth, 1953-74.

Friedman, Meyer and Ray Rosenman. *Type A Behavior and Your Heart.* New York: Knopf, 1974.

Fulford, Robert. *Dr Fulford's Touch of Life: The Healing Power of the Natural Life Force.* New York: Pocket, 1997.

Gordon, Rochelle. *Body Talk.* New York: International Rights, 1997.

Groddeck, Georg. *The Book of The It.* New York: Random House, 1949.

Hall, Edward T. *The Hidden Dimension.* New York: Doubleday Anchor, 1990.

Hamblin, Henry T. *The Power of Thought.* Electronic edition: Cornerstone Publishing, 2001.

Hanh, Thich Nhat. *Anger, Wisdom for Cooling the Flames.* Boston: Riverhead Trade, 2002.

Hanh, Thich Nhat. *Going Home: Jesus and Buddha as Brothers.* New York: Riverhead Trade, 2000.

Hanh, Thich Nhat. *Living Buddha, Living Christ.* New York: Riverhead Books, 1995.

Hay, Louise L. *You Can Heal Your Life.* 21st ed. Carlsbad: Hay House, 2007.

Horney, Karen. *Neurosis and Human Growth: The Struggle Toward Self-Realization.* New York: WW Norton, 1970.

Horney, Karen. *Our Inner Conflicts: A Constructive Theory of Neurosis.* New York: WW Norton, 1945.

Horney, Karen. *Self-Analysis.* New York: WW Norton, 1968.

Horney, Karen. *The Neurotic Personality of Our Time.* New York: WW Norton, 1937.

Hurte, Marcellous. "Back in Shape," *Guideposts*, October, 2003. pp. 40-45.

Hutschnecker, Arnold A. *The Will to Live.* New York: Perma Books, 1956.

Jacobson, Edmund. *Progressive Relaxation.* Chicago: University of Chicago Press, 1938.

Jampolsky, Gerald G. *Love Is Letting Go of Fear.* Berkeley: Ten Speed Press, 1979.

Jung, Carl, and Campbell, Joseph. *The Portable Jung.* New York: Penguin Books, 1976.

Jung, Carl. *Analytical Psychology: Its Theory & Practice* (The Tavistock Lectures). New York: Vintage, 1970.

Jung, Carl. *Contributions to Analytical Psychology.* New Haven: Kegan Paul, 1948.

Jung, Carl. *Jung on Evil.* Princeton: Princeton University Press, 1995.

Jung, Carl. *Modern Man in Search of a Soul.* London: Kegan Paul, 1933.

Jung, Carl. *Psychiatric Studies.* Princeton: Princeton University Press, 1975.

Jung, Carl. *Psychological Reflections. A New Anthology of His Writings.* Princeton: Princeton University Press, 1973.

Jung, Carl. *Psychology and Alchemy.* New York: Routledge, 1980.

Jung, Carl. *Psychology and Religion.* New Haven: Yale University Press, 1960.

Kalb, Claudia. "End Your Back Pain," *Reader's Digest:* March 2005, 141-145.

Kalb, Claudia. "The Great Back Pain Debate," *Newsweek:* April 26, 2004.

Kaufman, Leslie. "A Superhighway Bliss," *New York Times*: May 25, 2008.

King, Kahili Serge. *Instant Healing.* New York: St. Martin's Press, 2000.

Kolata, Gina. "Cancer Society, in Shift, Has Concerns on Screenings," *New York Times:* October 21, 2009.

Kramer, Diane Dunaway and Jonathan Kramer. *Losing the Weight of the World: Spiritual Diet to Nourish the Soul.* New York: Newleaf, 1997.

Kushner, S Harold. *How Good Do We Have to Be? A New Understanding of Guilt and Forgiveness.* Boston: Back Bay Books, 1997.

Lee, John. *Facing the Fire: Experiencing and Expressing Anger Appropriately.* New York: Bantam, 1993.

Losier, Michael J. *Law of Attraction: The Science of Attracting More of What You Want and Less of What You Don't.* Victoria, BC Canada: Michael J Losier, 2003.

Marsden, Paul. Memetics and Social Contagion: Two Sides of the Same Coin? *Journal of Memetics—Evolutionary Models of Information Transmission,* Volume 2, 1998.

Miller J., L. Lewis and J. Bayse Sander, *Heavenly Miracles.* New York: Harper Collins, 2000.

Miller R. and R. Funk. *The Complete Gospels.* San Francisco: Harper Collins, 1994.

Miller, Emmett E. *Deep Healing, The Essence of Mind/Body Medicine.* Carlsbad, CA: Hay House, 1997.

Miller, Emmett E. *Easing into Sleep.* Hay House, 1996 (audio recording).

Miller, Emmett E. *I Am*. Hay House, 1996 (audio recording).

Miller, Emmett E. *The 10-Minute Stress Manager,* Hay House, 1997 (audio recording).

Murphy, Joseph. *The Power of Your Subconscious Mind*. London: Createspace, 2010.

Myss, Caroline. *Why People Don't Heal and How They Can*. New York: Three Rivers Press, 1998.

Napoli, Maryann. "Cholesterol Skeptics: Conference Report, Cholesterol Skeptics and the Bad News about Statins." [Originally posted on MedicalConsumers.org, June 2003].

Newman, Susan. *The Book of NO, 250 Ways to Say It—and Mean It and Stop People Pleasing Forever*. New York: McGraw-Hill, 2005.

Pennebaker, James W. *Opening Up: The Healing Power of Confiding in Others*. New York: Avon Books, 1991.

Pennebaker, James W. *Opening Up: The Healing Power of Expressing Emotions*. New York: The Guilford Press, 1997.

Popper, Karl. *The Logic of Scientific Discovery* (Routledge Classics). New York: Routledge, 2002.

Preeclampsia Foundation [preeclampsia.org/].

Pukui, Kawena Mary. *Nana I Ke Kumu. Look To The Source*. Honolulu: Hui Hanai, 1976.

Ratcheson, Robert A. Deposition of Robert A. Ratcheson (S. Ozanich, et. al., v. D. Bitonte, DO et. al.) Cleveland, Ohio: April 1987.

Rogers, Carl. *On Becoming a Person: A Therapist's View of Psychotherapy*. New York: Mariner Books, 1995.

Romano, Ray. *Face to Face with Ray Romano*. Reader's Digest. February 2004.

The National Rosacea Society, 2001. Retrieved from [www.rosacea.org/rr/2001/summer/article_3.html].

Rossman, Martin L. *Guided Imagery for Self-Healing*. 2nd ed. Novato, CA: HJ Kramer/New World Library, 2000.

Sapolsky, Robert M. *Why Zebras Don't Get Ulcers*. New York: WH Freeman, 1998.

Sapolsky, Robert. "Stress Is a Pain." Lecture at Ohio University Memorial Auditorium, *The Athens News:* April 24, 2003.

Sarno, John E. *Healing Back Pain: The Mind-Body Connection*. New York: Warner Brothers, 1991.

Sarno, John E. *Mind Over Back Pain: A Radically New Approach to the Diagnosis and Treatment of Back Pain*. New York: Berkley Pub Group, 1999.

Sarno, John E. *The Divided Mind: The Epidemic of Mindbody Disorders*. 1st ed. New York: Harper Collins, 2007.

Sarno, John E. *The Mindbody Prescription: Healing the Body, Healing the Pain*. New York: Warner Brothers, 1998.

Sarno, John. Larry King Live, CNN, aired 8/12/99.

Selye, Hans. *From Dream to Discovery: On Being a Scientist*. New York: McGraw-Hill, 1964.

Sha, Gang Zhi. *Power Healing*. San Francisco: Harper Collins, 2002.

Shook, Victoria E. *Ho'oponopono: Contemporary Use of a Hawaiian Problem-Solving Process*. Honolulu: University of Hawai'i Press, 2002.

Siegel, Bernie S. *Love Medicine and Miracles*. New York: Harper and Row, 1986.

Silverman, Linda, and Jeffrey N. Freed. "The Visual Spatial Learner." *The Dyslexic Reader*. Issue No. 4, Winter, 1996.

Simonton, Carl O., James L Creighton, and Stephanie Matthews Simonton, *Getting Well Again*. New York: Bantam, 1992.

Sopher, Marc D. *To Be or Not To Be... Pain-Free: The Mindbody Syndrome*. Boston: 1st Books Library, 2003.

Stossel, John. *Give Me A Break*. New York: Perennial Currents, 2004.

Tanner, Lindsey. "Despite Tests, Many Consumers Swear by Remedies," AP, February 2006.

Taylor, Sir Henry, David Lewis Schaefer, and Roberta Rubel Schaefer. *The Statesman,* Revised Edition. Westport, CT: Praeger Publishers, 1992.

Tolle, Eckhart. *A New Earth: Awakening to Your Life's Purpose*. New York: Penguin, 2008.

Tolle, Eckhart. *The Power of Now: A Guide to Spiritual Enlightenment*. Novato, CA: New World Library, 2004.

Churchwell, Gordon. *Pregnant Man: How Nature Makes Fathers Out of Men*, New York: Harper Paperbacks, 2001.

Walker, Eugene C. *Learn to Relax*. New York: John Wiley and Sons, 2001.

Warren, Rick. *The Purpose-Driven Life*. Grand Rapids MI: Zondervan, 2002.

Weil, Andrew. *Spontaneous Healing: How to Discover and Embrace Your Body's Natural Ability to Maintain and Heal Itself*. New York: Random House, 1995.

Zweig, Connie and Jeremiah Abrams. *Meeting the Shadow*. New York: Tarcher/Putnam, 1991.

Zweig, Connie and Steve Wolf. *Romancing the Shadow: Illuminating the Dark Side of the Soul*. Chicago: Ballantine Books, 1997.

Research Studies

Al'abadie, M.S., G.G. Kent and D.J. Gawkrodger. "The relationship between stress and the onset and exacerbation of psoriasis and other skin conditions," *British Journal of Dermatology*, 1994; 199(130):199-203.

Arden, N.K., C. Price, I. Reading, J. Stubbing, J. Hazelgrove, C. Dunne, M. Michel, P. Rogers, C. Cooper. "A multicentre randomized controlled trial of epidural corticosteroid injections for sciatica: the WEST study," *Rheumatology*, 2005; 44: 1399-406.

Cherkin, D.C., R.A. Deyo, J.D. Loeser, T. Bush, G. Waddell. "An international comparison of back surgery rates," *Spine*, 1994; 19:1201-6.

Hackney, A.C. and A. Viru. "Twenty-four-hour cortisol response to multiple daily exercise sessions of moderate and high intensity," *Clinical Psychology*, 1999; 19(2):178.

Cohen, B.G.F., M.J. Colligan, W. Wester II, M.J. Smith. "An investigation of job satisfaction factors in an incident of mass psychogenic illness at the workplace," *Occupational Health Nursing*, 1978 January:10-16.

Colligan, M.J., J.W. Pennebaker, L.R. Murphy. "A review of mass psychogenic illness in work settings." In *Mass psychogenic illness: a social psychological analysis*. Hillsdale, NJ: L. Erlbaum Associates, 1982.

Eisenberg, D.M., R.C. Kessler, C. Foster, F.E. Norlock, D.R. Calkins, T.L. Delbanco. "Unconventional medicine in the United States—Prevalence, costs, and patterns of use," *New England Journal of Medicine*, 1993; 328:246-52.

Fassbender, H.G., K. Wegner. "Morphologie und pathogenese des weichteilrheumatismus," *Z Rheumaforsch*, 1973; 32:355-74.

Gatherer, D. "Identifying cases of social contagion using memetic isolation: comparison of the dynamics of a multisociety simulation with an ethnographic data set," *Journal of Artificial Societies and Social Stimulation*, 2002; 5(4).

Holmes, T.H., R.H. Rahe. "The social readjustment scale," *Journal of Psychosomatic Research*, 1967; 11:213-8.

Jensen, M.C., M.N. Brant-Zawadzki, Nancy Obuchowski, Michael T. Modic, Dennis Malkasian, and Jeffrey Ross. "Magnetic resonance imaging of the lumbar spine in people without back pain," *New England Journal of Medicine*, 1994; 331(2):69-73.

Kharabsheh, S., H. Al-Otoum, J. Clements, A. Abbas, N. Khuri-Bulos, A. Belbesi, T. Gaafar and N. Dellepiane. "Mass psychogenic illness following tetanus-diphtheria toxoid vaccination in Jordan," *Bull World Health Organization,* 2001; 79(8):764-70.

Langewitz, W., J. Izakovic, J. Wyler, C. Schindler, A. Kiss, A.J. Bircher. "Self-hypnosis on hay fever symptoms—a randomised controlled intervention study," *Psychotherapy and Psychosomatics,* 2005; 74(3).

Lund N., A. Bengtsson, and P. Thorborg. "Muscle tissue oxygen pressure in primary fibromyalgia," *Scandinavian Journal of Rheumatology,* 1986; 15(2):165-173.

Moseley, Bruce J., K. O'Malley, N.J. Petersen, T.J. Menke, B.A. Brody, D.H. Kuykendall, J.C. Hollingsworth, C.M. Ashton, and N.P. Wray. "A controlled trial of arthroscopic surgery for osteoarthritis of the knee," *New England Journal of Medicine,* 2002; 347(2):81-88.

Rahe, Richard H., M. Meyer, M. Smith, G. Kjaer, T.H. Holmes. "Social stress and illness onset," *Journal of Psychosomatic Research,* 1964; 8(1):35-44.

Surgical vs Nonoperative Treatment for Lumbar Disk Herniation, Vol. 296 No. 20, November 22/29, 2006. Acute Low Back Pain Problems. [Publication No. 95-0644 (Rockville, MD: December 1994.

Weinstein, J.N., T.D. Tosteson, J.D. Lurie, A.N. Tosteson, B. Hanscom, J.S. Skinner, W.A. Abdu, A.S. Hilibrand, S.D. Boden, R.A. Deyo. "Surgical vs nonoperative treatment for lumbar disk herniation: The Spine Patient Outcomes Research Trial (SPORT): a randomized trial," *JAMA,* 2006; 296:2441-2450.

Weinberger Daniel A., G.E. Schwartz, R.J. Davidson. "Low-anxious, high-anxious, and repressive coping styles: Psychometric patterns and behavioral and physiological responses to stress," *Journal of Abnormal Psychology,* 1979; 88(4):369-380.

Index

Notes

1 J. Sarno, *Healing Back Pain* (New York: Warner Brothers, 1991), pp. 62-63.

2 J. Sarno, *The Mindbody Prescription* (New York: Warner Brothers, 1999), p. 141.

3 J. Sarno, *Dr. Sarno's Cure*, ABC 20/20, 7/25/99.

4 J. Sarno, *The Mindbody Prescription* (New York: Warner Brothers, 1999), p. 143.

5 R. Rogers. New York Times, Feb. 25, 1985.

6 J. Sarno, *The Mindbody Prescription* (New York: Warner Brothers, 1999), p. 57.

7 J. Sarno, *Healing Back Pain* (New York: Warner Brothers, 1991), p. 51.

8 *Ibid.*, p. 55.

9 *Ibid.*, p. 101.

10 *Ibid.*

11 A. Weil, *Spontaneous Healing* (New York: Random House, 1995), p. 120.

12 *Ibid.*, p. 121.

13 *Ibid.*, p. 121.

14 *Ibid.*, p. 120.

15 J. Sarno, *Healing Back Pain* (New York: Warner Brothers, 1991), p. 99.

16 Hanscom, David. (2018, April 18). "The Perils of Back Surgery: A Spine Surgeon's Roadmap" [Video; at 33:10]. *Talks at Google*. Retrieved from [https://www.youtube.com/watch?v=B5cwZ2iu8jU]

17 *Ibid.*, p. 100.

18 *Ibid.*, p. 105.

19 *Ibid.*, p. 78.

20 J. Pennebaker, *Opening Up: The Healing Power of Confiding in Others* (New York: Avon Books, 1991), pp. 41-47.

21 *Ibid.*, p. 49.

22 J. Sarno, *Healing Back Pain* (New York: Warner Brothers, 1991), p. 130.

23 *Ibid.*, p. 4.

24 *Ibid.*, p. 5.

25 *Ibid.*, p. 77.

26 *Ibid.*, p. 79.

27 *Ibid.*, p. 52.

28 F. Amir, *Rapid Recovery from Back and Neck Pain* (Bethesda, Maryland: Health Advisory Group Publishing, 1999), p.102.

29 H. Taylor, *The Statesman* (Westport, CT: Praeger Publishers, 1992), p. 88.

30 S. Freud, *The Standard Edition of the Complete Psychological Works of Sigmund Freud, Inhibitions, Symptoms, and Anxiety*, translated by James Strachey (London: Hogarth, 1953-74).

31 *Ibid.*, p. 9.

32 J. Coldren et al., *General Psychology* (Dubuque Iowa: Kendall/Hunt, 2001), p. 563.

33 C. Rogers, *On Becoming a Person* (New York: Mariner Books, 1995), pp. 11-12.

34 J. Coldren et al., *General Psychology* (Dubuque Iowa: Kendall/Hunt, 2001), p. 563.

35 C. Zweig and J. Abrams, *Meeting The Shadow, The Hidden Power of the Dark Side of Human Nature* (New York: Tarcher/Putnam, 1991), p. XVII.

36 *Ibid.*, p. XVIII.

37 *Ibid.*, p. 4.

38 K. Horney, *Our Inner Conflicts* (New York: WW Norton, 1945), p. 103.

[39] J. Sarno, *Mind Over Back Pain: A Radically New Approach to the Diagnosis and Treatment of Back Pain* (New York: Berkley Pub Group, 1999), p. 68.

[40] Retrieved from [www.rosacea.org/rr/2001/summer/article_3.html].

[41] D. Colbert, *Deadly Emotions, Understand The Mind-Body-Spirit Connection That Can Heal or Destroy You* (Nashville: Thomas Nelson Publishers, 2003), p. 21.

[42] Retrieved from [preeclampsia.org].

[43] *Ibid.*

[44] S. Ozanich Plaintiff, et. al. v. David Bitonte, DO et al., defendants, (deposition of Robert A. Ratcheson, MD, April 10, 1987), pp. 15-16.

[45] *Ibid.*, pp. 20-24.

[46] R. Traci, plaintiff's attorney, S. Ozanich, et al. v. D. Bitonte, et al., (Case# 86 CV 73, March 17-19 1988), p. 727.

[47] W. Shaffer, testimony, S. Ozanich, et al. v. D. Bitonte, et al., (Case# 86 CV 73, March 17-19 1988), p. 634.

[48] R. Ratcheson, S. Ozanich et al., v. D. Bitonte, DO et al., defendants (deposition of Robert A. Ratcheson, MD, April 10, 1987), p. 13.

[49] J. Sarno, *Healing Back Pain* (New York: Warner Brothers, 1991), p. 55.

[50] S. Ozanich v. D. Bitonte, et al., Case# 86 CV 73, March 17-19 1988), p. 565.

[51] J. Sarno, *The Mindbody Prescription* (New York: Warner Brothers, 1999), p. 112.

[52] L. Haye, *You Can Heal Your Life* (Carlsbad: Hay House, 2007), p. 204.

[53] J. Sarno, *Mind Over Back Pain: A Radically New Approach to the Diagnosis and Treatment of Back Pain* (New York: Berkley Pub Group, 1999), p. 46.

[54] J. Sarno, *Healing Back Pain* (New York: Warner Brothers, 1991), pp. 17-18.

[55] D. Chopra, "The Soul of Healing." *Body, Mind & Soul* DVD set.

[56] J. Lee, *Facing the Fire: Experiencing and Expressing Anger Appropriately* (United States and Canada: Bantam, 1993), p. 5.

[57] *Ibid.*, p. 28.

[58] Alexithymia is "the inability to talk about feelings due to a lack of emotional awareness," but is not considered to be a disorder or disability. Retrieved from [www.angelfire.com/al4/alexithymia/].

[59] With alexithymia, *"There is just pain, nausea and discomfort."* Retrieved from [www.emotionallystunted.co.uk/alexithymia/isnt.html].

[60] J. Sarno, *Healing Back Pain* (New York: Warner Brothers, 1991), p. 51.

[61] *Ibid.*, p. 83.

[62] *Ibid.*, p. 81.

[63] *Ibid.*, p. 42.

[64] *Ibid.*, p. 79.

[65] *Ibid.*, p. 15.

[66] *Ibid.*, p. 100.

[67] C. Jung, *Modern Man in Search of a Soul* (London: Harvest Books, 1955), p. 229.

[68] M. Sopher, *To Be or Not To Be... Pain-Free: The Mindbody Syndrome* (Boston: 1st Books Library, 2003), p. 35.

[69] K. Horney, *Our Inner Conflicts* (New York: WW Norton, 1945), p. 102.

[70] J. Sarno, *Healing Back Pain* (New York: Warner Brothers, 1991), p. 81.

[71] *Ibid.*, p. 15.

[72] *Ibid.*, p. 126.

[73] *Ibid.*, p. 80.

[74] *Ibid.*, p. 83.

[75] *Ibid.*, p. 21.

[76] J. Sarno, *Healing Back Pain* (New York: Warner Brothers, 1991), p. 79.

[77] M. Sopher, *The Divided Mind: The Epidemic of Mindbody Disorders* (New York: Harper Collins, 2007), p. 341.

[78] J. Sarno, *Healing Back Pain* (New York: Warner Brothers, 1991), p. 138.

[79] J. Stossel, *Give Me a Break* (New York: Harper Collins, 2004), p. 230.

[80] K. Popper, *The Logic of Scientific Discovery* (New York: Routledge, 2002), p. 281.

[81] M. Ali, *Seven Core Principles of Integrative Medicine, J Integrative Medicine 1998; 2:77-81.*

[82] D. Colbert, *Deadly Emotions, Understand The Mind-Body-Spirit Connection That Can Heal or Destroy You* (Nashville: Thomas Nelson Publishers, 2003), p. 34.

[83] A. Hutschnecker, *The Will To Live* (New York: Permabooks, 1956), p. 71.

[84] R. Sapolsky, "Stress: Portrait of a Killer." National Geographic Television, 2008.

[85] A. Weil, *Health and Healing: The Philosophy of Integrative Medicine and Optimum Health* (New York: Houghton Mifflin, 2004), p. 56.

[86] L. Creighton and O. Simonton and S. Simonton-Matthews, *Getting Well Again* (United States and Canada: Bantam, 1992), p. 67.

[87] N. Cousins, *Anatomy of an Illness* (New York: WW Norton & Company, 1981), p. 56.

[88] *Ibid.*, p. 56.

[89] B. Moseley et al. "A Controlled Trial of Arthroscopic Surgery for Osteoarthritis of the Knee," *New England Journal of Medicine* 2002; 347: 81-8.

[90] Retrieved from [www.webmd.com/osteoarthritis/news/20020710/popular-knee-surgery-may-be-useless].

[91] *Ibid.*

[92] Retrieved from [naturalnews.com/023656_body_cancer_health.html], 7/11/2002.

[93] A. Kirkley et al., "A Randomized Trial of Arthroscopic Surgery for Osteoarthritis of the Knee," *New England Journal of Medicine* 2008; 359:1097-1107.

[94] *Understanding Acute Low Back Pain Problems.* Publication No. 95-0644 (Rockville, MD, December 1994).

[95] G. Kolata, "Arthritis Surgery In Ailing Knees Is Cited as Sham," New York Times, 7/11/2002.

[96] D.C. Cherkin et al., "An international comparison of back surgery rates," *Spine.* 1994; 19:1201-6].

[97] J. Sarno, *Healing Back Pain* (New York: Warner Brothers, 1991), p. 121.

[98] *Ibid.*, p. 121.

[99] The WEST Group. "A multicentre randomized controlled trial of epidural corticosteroid injections for sciatica," *Rheumatology* 2005; 44: 1399-406.

[100] J. Weinstein et al., "Surgical vs. Nonoperative Treatment for Lumbar Disk Herniation," *Journal of the American Medical Association* 2006; 296 2441-50.

[101] G. Groddeck, *The Book of The It* (New York: Random House, 1949), Chapter 32, German version.

[102] J. Sarno, *Healing Back Pain* (New York: Warner Brothers, 1991), p. 120.

[103] J. Sarno, *The Divided Mind: The Epidemic of Mindbody Disorders* (New York: Harper Collins, 2007), p. 31.

[104] M. Sopher, *To Be or Not To Be... Pain-Free: The Mindbody Syndrome* (Boston: 1st Books Library, 2003), p. 117.

[105] *Ibid.*, p. 113.

[106] *Ibid.*, p. 114.

[107] *Ibid.*, p. 113.

[108] Retrieved from [naturalnews.com/023656_cancer_health_immune_system.html], July 19, 2008.

[109] F. Amir, *Rapid Recovery from Back and Neck Pain* (Bethesda, Maryland: Health Advisory Group Publishing, 1999), p. 72.

[110] M. Sopher, *To Be or Not To Be... Pain-Free: The Mindbody Syndrome* (Boston: 1st Books Library, 2003), p. 59.

[111] Retrieved from [www.msnbc.msn.com/id/10242034/].

[112] F. Benedetti et al., "Neurobiological Mechanisms of the Placebo Effect," *The Journal of Neuroscience*, 2005; 25(45):10390-10402.

[113] Retrieved from [www.msnbc.msn.com/id/10242034/].

[114] C. McRae et al., "Effects of Perceived Treatment on Quality of Life and Medical Outcomes in a Double-blind Placebo Surgery Trial," *Arch Gen Psychiatry.* 2004; 61(4):412-420.

[115] Retrieved from [www.medicalnewstoday.com]. Mind-body connection in placebo surgery trial studied by University of Denver researcher, April 8 2004.

[116] C. McRae. et al., "Effects of Perceived Treatment on Quality of Life and Medical Outcomes in a Double-blind Placebo Surgery Trial," *Arch Gen Psychiatry.* 2004; 61(4):412-420.

[117] Kristen Dahlgren, NBC Today Show, "Acupuncture—Real or fake-best for back pain," AP, 7/24/07.

[118] J. Sarno, *Healing Back Pain* (New York: Warner Brothers, 1991), p. 29.

[119] Retrieved from [pespmc1.vub.ac.be/memerep.html].

[120] P. Marsden, "Memetics & Social Contagion: Two Sides of the Same Coin?" *Journal of Memetics* 1998; 2:2.

[121] *Ibid.*, p. 4.

[122] R. Dawkins, *The Selfish Gene* (New York: Oxford University Press, 2006), p. 200.

[123] *Ibid.*, p. 196.

[124] Retrieved from [www.pobox.com/~r/rsi].

[125] R. Cabot, *St. Louis Medical Review,* Editor Loeb, HW, March 21, 1903, Volume XLVII, p. 208.

[126] Retrieved from [naturalhealthperspective.com].

[127] C. Zweig and J. Abrams, *Meeting The Shadow, The Hidden Power of the Dark Side of Human Nature* (New York: Tarcher/Putnam, 1991), p. 110.

[128] *Ibid.*, p. 110.

[129] [www.youtube.com/watch?v=lPMYdalCyA0].

[130] Retrieved from [familydoctor.org/648.xml].

[131] S. Kharabsheh et al., *Bull World Health Organ.* 2001; 79(8):764-70.

[132] H. Gold, *Cornell Conferences on Therapy*, vol. 1. Edited by H. Gold with others. (New York: Macmillan, 1946).

[133] R. Fulford, *Dr. Fulford's Touch of Life: The Healing Power of the Natural Life Force* (New York: Pocket, 1997), p. 88.

[134] F. Amir, *Rapid Recovery from Back and Neck Pain* (Bethesda, Maryland: Health Advisory Group Publishing, 1999), p.55.

[135] J. Sarno, *Healing Back Pain* (New York: Warner Brothers, 1991), p. 54.

[136] M. Rossman, *Guided Imagery for Self-Healing* (Novato, CA: HJ Kramer/New World Library, 2000), p. 207.

[137] D. Eisenberg, et al., "Unconventional Medicine in the United States — Prevalence, Costs, and Patterns of Use," *New England Journal of Medicine* 1993; 328:246-252.

[138] *Ibid.*

[139] F. Amir, *Rapid Recovery from Back and Neck Pain* (Bethesda, Maryland: Health Advisory Group Publishing, 1999), p.54.

[140] J. Sarno, *Healing Back Pain* (New York: Warner Brothers, 1991), p. 72.

[141] G. Kolata, "Cancer Society, in Shift, Has Concerns on Screenings," *The New York Times*, October 21, 2009.

[142] Otis Brawley, editorial, *Journal Of The National Cancer Institute Advance Access* originally published online on August 31, 2009 *JNCI Journal of the National Cancer Institute* 2009 101(19):1295-1297.

[143] *Ibid.*, p. 211.

[144] M. Losier, *The Law of Attraction* (Victoria, BC Canada: Michael J. Losier, 2003), p. 8.

[145] R. Sapolsky, "Stress Is a Pain," *The Athens News*, 4/24/2003.

[146] M. Losier, *The Law of Attraction* (Victoria, BC Canada: Michael J. Losier, 2003), p. 18.

[147] M. Eddy, *Science and Health* (Boston: The First Church of Christ, 1994), p. 168.

[148] *Ibid.*, p. 169.

[149] G. Jampolsky, *Love is Letting Go of Fear* (Berkeley, CA: Ten Speed Press, 1979), p. 79.

[150] J. Sarno, *The Divided Mind: The Epidemic of Mindbody Disorders* (New York: Harper Collins, 2007), p. 44.

[151] Retrieved from [www.cbssports.com/golf/story/13368425/neck-problem-another-low-point-in-a-lousy-six-months-for-tiger].

[152] Retrieved from [www.buzzle.com/editorials/11-25-2002-31037.asp].

[153] *Ibid.*

[154] Retrieved from [www.thegolfchannel.com/core.aspx?page=15101&select=1445].

[155] G. Beratlis, *CNN*, 12/13/2004.

[156] R. Rahe, et al., "Social Stress and Illness Onset, Relationships of Environmental Variables to the Onset of Illness," *Journal of Psychosomatic Research*, 1964; 8:35-44.

[157] J. Smolowe, et al., "Dana Reeve Brave To The End" (*People*: March, 27 2006).

[158] S. Freud, *Standard Edition of the Collected Works of Sigmund Freud,* translated by James Strachey (London: Hogarth, 1953-74), p. 357.

[159] M. Watts, "The Poets: Cat Stevens" in *The Melody Maker File,* IPC Specialist and Professional Press Ltd, 1974).

[160] G. Groddeck, *The Book of The It* (New York: Random House, 1949), p. 101.

[161] J. Lee, *Facing the Fire: Experiencing and Expressing Anger Appropriately* (United States and Canada: Bantam, 1993), p. 91.

[162] F. Amir, *Rapid Recovery from Back and Neck Pain* (Bethesda, Maryland: Health Advisory Group Publishing, 1999), p.143.

[163] Retrieved from [web.jet.es/lheglar/catharsis.pdf].

[164] J. Sarno, *Healing Back Pain* (New York: Warner Brothers, 1991), p. 166.

[165] J. Sarno, *The Mindbody Prescription* (New York: Warner Brothers, 1999), p. 184.

[166] R. Gordon, *Body Talk* (New York: International Rights, 1997), p. XVII-XVIII.

[167] A. Weil, *The Mindbody Prescription* (New York: Warner Brothers, 1999), inside cover review.

[168] M. Sopher, *To Be or Not To Be... Pain-Free: The Mindbody Syndrome* (Boston: 1st Books Library, 2003), pp. 106-107.

[169] J. Pennebaker, *Opening Up: The Healing Power of Confiding in Others* (New York: Avon Books, 1991), p. 49.

[170] *Ibid.*, p. 49.

[171] J. Sarno, *The Divided Mind: The Epidemic of Mindbody Disorders* (New York: Harper Collins, 2007), p. 112.

[172] E. Tolle, *The Power of Now: A Guide to Spiritual Enlightenment* (Namaste Publishing, 2004), p. 4

[173] J. Sarno, *Healing Back Pain* (New York: Warner Brothers, 1991), pp. 22-23.

[174] Retrieved from [www.dfwcfids.org/medical/limbcsys.repatterning.htm].

[175] J. Sarno, *Healing Back Pain* (New York: Warner Brothers, 1991), p. 22.

[176] R. Scaer, *The Trauma Spectrum: Hidden Wounds and Human Resiliency* (New York: WW Norton, 2005), p. 197.

[177] J. Sarno, *Healing Back Pain* (New York: Warner Brothers, 1991), pp. 80-81.

[178] J. Sarno, *Mind Over Back Pain: A Radically New Approach to the Diagnosis and Treatment of Back Pain* (New York: Berkley Pub Group, 1999), p. 51.

[179] *Ibid.*, p. 24.

[180] J. Sarno, *Healing Back Pain* (New York: Warner Brothers, 1991), p. 126.

[181] *Ibid.*, p. 130.

[182] J. Sarno, *Mind Over Back Pain: A Radically New Approach to the Diagnosis and Treatment of Back Pain* (New York: Berkley Pub Group, 1999), p. 50.

[183] C. Jung, *Psychology and Religion* (New Haven and London: Yale University Press, 1960), p. 93 and p. 101.

[184] J. Sarno, *Mind Over Back Pain: A Radically New Approach to the Diagnosis and Treatment of Back Pain* (New York: Berkley Pub Group, 1999), p. 53.

[185] C. Jung, *The Essential Jung* (Princeton: Princeton University Press; Revised ed., 1999), p. 142.

[186] C. Jung, Psychological Reflections. *A New Anthology of His Writings* (Princeton: Princeton University Press, 1973), p. 281.

[187] K. Horney, *Our Inner Conflicts* (New York: WW Norton, 1945), p. 91.

[188] *Ibid.,* pp. 50-52.

[189] J. Sarno, *Healing Back Pain* (New York: Warner Brothers, 1991), p. 142.

[190] K. Horney, *Our Inner Conflicts* (New York: WW Norton, 1945), pp. 51-52.

[191] J. Sarno, *The Mindbody Prescription* (New York: Warner Brothers, 1999), pp. 12-13.

[192] Retrieved from [www.stress.org/topic-heart.htm?AIS=a7072510dea2b512fd2472011a1df4a9].

[193] Retrieved from [www.stress.org/interview-TypeA_CoronaryDisease.htm].

[194] J. Sarno, *Healing Back Pain* (New York: Warner Brothers, 1991), p. 151.

[195] *Ibid.*, p. 152.

[196] Retrieved from [www.stress.org].

[197] J. Sarno, *Mind Over Back Pain: A Radically New Approach to the Diagnosis and Treatment of Back Pain* (New York: Berkley Pub Group, 1999), p. 54.

[198] Retrieved from [www.webster.edu/~woolflm/horney.html].

[199] Retrieved from [webspace.ship.edu/cgboer/jung.html].

[200] T. Hanh, *Going Home, Jesus and Buddha as Brothers* (New York: Riverhead Trade, 2000), p. 58.

[201] Retrieved from [webspace.ship.edu/cgboer/horney.html].

[202] S. Freud, "Dora: An Analysis of a Case of Hysteria," *Collected Papers of Sigmund Freud* (New York: Touchstone, 1997), p. 37.

[203] C. Jung, "Analytical Psychology, It's Theory and Practice," *The Tavistock Lectures* (New York: Vintage, 1970), p. 188.

[204] Retrieved from [www.webster.edu/~woolflm/horney.html].

[205] *Ibid.*

[206] *Ibid.*

[207] C. Jung, *The Portable Jung* (New York: Viking, 1971), p. 209.

[208] J. Lee, *Facing the Fire: Experiencing and Expressing Anger Appropriately* (United States and Canada: Bantam, 1993), p. 28.

[209] E. Tolle, *The Power of Now: A Guide to Spiritual Enlightenment* (Novato, CA: New World Library, 2004), p. 122.

[210] C. Jung, "Analytical Psychology, It's Theory and Practice," *The Tavistock Lectures* (New York: Penguin Books, 1976), p. 20.

[211] Retrieved from [golf.about.com/b/a/172831.htm].

[212] [http://staging.thegolfchannel.com/tour-insider/bad-forces-amiee-corning-16297/].

[213] K. Wilber, *Meeting The Shadow, The Hidden Power of the Dark Side of Human Nature* (New York: Tarcher/Putnam, 1991), p. 273.

[214] C. Jung, *The Portable Jung* (New York: Viking, 1971), p. xii.

[215] E. Aron, *The Highly Sensitive Person* (Broadway Books, 1997), p. 120.

[216] *Ibid.*, p. 126.

[217] M. Hurte, *Back In Shape* (Guideposts: October, 2003), p. 45.

[218] E. Aron, *The Highly Sensitive Person* (Broadway Books, 1997), p. 190.

[219] J. Sarno, *The Divided Mind: The Epidemic of Mindbody Disorders* (New York: Harper Collins, 2007), p. 77.

[220] H. Stone and S. Winkleman, *Meeting The Shadow, The Hidden Power of the Dark Side of Human Nature* (New York: Tarcher/Putnam, 1991), p. 286.

[221] S. Freud, *Sigmund Freud: The Ego and the ID* (New York: WW Norton & Company, 1960), p. 61.

[222] Retrieved from [www.fact-index.com/s/sc/scenario_analysis.html].

[223] J. Aversa, "Debt hurts your body, too" AP-AOL Health poll conducted March 24 to April 3 by Abt SRBI Inc.

[224] E. Hall, *The Hidden Dimension* (New York: Doubleday Anchor, 1990), p. 5.

[225] D. Kadagian, *Portrait of a Radical: The Jesus Movement*, Four Seasons Productions, 2000.

[226] R. Moynihan and A. Cassels, *Selling Sickness: How the World's Biggest Pharmaceutical Companies Are Turning Us All Into Patients* (New York: Nation Books, 2006), p. 4

[227] *Ibid.*, p. ix.

[228] M. Napoli, "Cholesterol Skeptics: Conference Report," *Cholesterol Skeptics and the Bad News About Statins*, 6/1/2003.

[229] *Ibid.*

[230] Retrieved from [stress.org].

[231] P. Rosch, "An interview with Ray H. Rosenman," *Health and Stress*, June 2004.

[232] F. Benedetti. et al., "Neurobiological Mechanisms of the Placebo Effect," *The Journal of Neuroscience*, 2005, 25(45):10390-10402.

[233] J. Lee, *Facing the Fire: Experiencing and Expressing Anger Appropriately* (United States and Canada: Bantam, 1993), p. 32.

[234] L. Tanner, Alternative remedies fail government tests. Retrieved from [www.azcentral.com/health/wellness/articles/0226altremedies.html], 2/26/2006.

[235] M. Rossman, *Guided Imagery for Self-Healing* (Novato, CA: HJ Kramer/New World Library, 2000), p. 3.

[236] *Ibid.*, p. 2.

[237] C. Jung, *The Portable Jung* (New York: Viking, 1971), p. 4.

[238] M. Fox, *Lucky Man* (New York: Hyperion, 2003), p. 6.

[239] L. Creighton and O. Simonton and S. Simonton-Matthews, *Getting Well Again* (United States and Canada: Bantam, 1992), pp. 133-134.

[240] Retrieved from [www.infinityinst.com/articles/cell_conscious.html].

[241] C. Jung, *Contributions to Analytical Psychology* (New Haven CT: Kegan Paul, 1948), p. 193.

[242] M. Rossman, *Guided Imagery for Self-Healing* (Novato, CA: HJ Kramer/New World Library, 2000), p. 122.

[243] *Ibid.*, p. 122.

[244] *Ibid.*, p. 123.

[245] *Ibid.*, p. 122.

[246] T. Hanh, *Going Home, Jesus and Buddha as Brothers* (New York: Riverhead Trade, 2000), p. 124.

[247] T. Hanh, *Anger, Wisdom for Cooling the Flames* (Boston: Riverhead Trade, 2002), p. 95.

[248] E. Tolle, *A New Earth: Awakening to Your Life's Purpose* (New York: Penguin, 2008), p. 102.

[249] J. Lee, *Facing the Fire: Experiencing and Expressing Anger Appropriately* (United States and Canada: Bantam, 1993), p. 13.

[250] *Ibid.*, p. 14.

[251] G. Groddeck, *The Book of The It* (New York: Random House, 1949), p. 101.

[252] J. Lee, *Facing the Fire: Experiencing and Expressing Anger Appropriately* (United States and Canada: Bantam, 1993), p. 16.

[253] *Ibid.*, p. 32.

[254] T. Hanh, *Anger, Wisdom for Cooling the Flames* (Boston: Riverhead Trade, 2002), p. 44.

[255] *Ibid.*, p. 115.

[256] J. Pennebaker, *Opening Up, The Healing Power of Expressing Emotions* (New York: The Guilford Press, 1997), p. 116.

[257] *Ibid.*, p. 49.

[258] B. Lipton, *The New Biology—Where Mind and Matter Meet*, Spirit, 2000, Inc. Retrieved from [www.veoh.com/collection/AgriculturalNews/watch/v378751X35FGG5H].

[259] S. Newman, *The Book of NO, 250 Ways to Say It—and Mean It and Stop People Pleasing Forever* (New York: McGraw-Hill, 2005), p. 2.

[260] *Ibid.*, pp. 5-6.

[261] J. Sarno, *Healing Back Pain* (New York: Warner Brothers, 1991), p. 80.

[262] *Ibid.*, p. 79.

[263] D. Colbert, *Deadly Emotions, Understand The Mind-Body-Spirit Connection That Can Heal or Destroy You* (Nashville: Thomas Nelson Publishers, 2003), p. 168.

[264] *I Won't Grow Up: The Causes of Psychogenic Dwarfism*, Biology 202, 2001.

[265] R. Romano, "Face to Face with Ray Romano," *Reader's Digest*, Feb. 2004, p. 115.

[266] Retrieved from [www.online.pacifica.edu/dissertations/stories/storyReader$183].

[267] Retrieved from [www.worldwideschool.org/library/books/phil/psychology/ FreudandHisSchoolNewPathsofPsychology/Chap1.html].

[268] Retrieved from [www.anaturalcure.com/a-snapshot-of-fibromyalgia/].

[269] A. Weil, *Spontaneous Healing* (New York: Random House, 1995), p. 31.

[270] L. Creighton and O. Simonton and S. Simonton-Matthews, *Getting Well Again* (United States and Canada: Bantam, 1992), p. 186.

[271] F. Amir, *Rapid Recovery from Back and Neck Pain* (Bethesda, Maryland: Health Advisory Group Publishing, 1999), p.195.

[272] C. Myss, *Why People Don't Heal and How They Can* (New York: Three Rivers Press, 1998), p. 202.

[273] M. Rossman, *Guided Imagery for Self-Healing* (Novato, CA: HJ Kramer/New World Library, 2000), p. 23.

[274] S. Rama, *Conscious Living: A Guidebook for Spiritual Transformation* (Lotus Press, 2007), p. 28.

[275] M. Rossman, *Guided Imagery for Self-Healing* (Novato, CA: HJ Kramer/New World Library, 2000), p. 79.

[276] W. Langewitz, "Effect of self-hypnosis on hay fever symptoms: A Randomised controlled intervention study," *Int. Arch Allergy Immunology*, 2004; 135(1):44-53.

[277] C. Reeve, *A Remembrance of actor Christopher Reeve*, Charlie Rose, PBS, 10/2/02.

[278] M. Rossman, *Guided Imagery for Self-Healing* (Novato, CA: HJ Kramer/New World Library, 2000), p. 35.

[279] J. Pennebaker, *Opening Up: The Healing Power of Confiding in Others* (New York: Avon Books, 1991), p. 44.

[280] *Ibid.*, p. 44.

[281] J. Sarno, *Healing Back Pain* (New York: Warner Brothers, 1991), p. 41.

[282] V. Shook, *Ho'oponopono* (Honolulu: University of Hawaii Press, 1986), p. 6.

[283] *Ibid.*, p. 11.

[284] *Ibid.*

[285] C. Jung, *Collected Works : Psychology and Alchemy*, Vol. 12 (London: Routledge, 1953), p. 24.

[286] J. Murphy, *The Power of Your Subconscious Mind* (London, UK: CreateSpace, 2010), p. 18.

[287] L. Marsa, *Health Magazine*, March 2004, p. 132.

[288] J. Sarno, *Healing Back Pain* (New York: Warner Brothers, 1991), p. 81.

[289] H. A. H. D'haenen, *Biological Psychiatry* (West Sussex, England: John Wiley and Sons, Ltd, 2002), p. 1318.

[290] C. Jung, *Psychology and Alchemy* (New York: Routledge, 1980), p. 51.

[291] M. Rossman, *Guided Imagery for Self-Healing* (Novato, CA: HJ Kramer/New World Library, 2000), p. 18.

[292] *Ibid.*, pp. 18-20.

[293] *Ibid.*, p. 19.

[294] *Ibid.*

[295] L. Silverman and J. Freed, *The Dyslexic Reader*, Issue No. 4, Winter 1996.

[296] *Ibid.*

[297] C. Myss, *Why People Don't Heal and How They Can* (New York: Three Rivers Press, 1998), p. ix.

[298] *Ibid.*, p. 130.

[299] D. Bresler, *Free Yourself From Pain* (New York: Simon & Schuster, 1986), p. 102.

[300] B. Lipton, *The New Biology—Where Mind and Matter Meet*, Spirit, 2000, Inc. Retrieved from [www.veoh.com/collection/AgriculturalNews/watch/v378751X35FGG5H].

[301] C. Myss, *Why People Don't Heal and How They Can* (New York: Three Rivers Press, 1998), p. 80.

[302] *Ibid.*, p. 81.

[303] *Ibid.*, p. 81.

[304] *Ibid.*, p. 39.

[305] *Ibid.*, p. 12.

[306] *Ibid.*, p. 12.

[307] *Ibid.*, p. 13.

[308] C. Zweig, and S. Wolf, *Romancing The Shadow* (Chicago: Ballantine Books, 1997), p. 12.

[309] *Ibid.*, p. 12.

[310] M. Losier, *The Law of Attraction* (Victoria, BC Canada: Michael J. Losier, 2003), p. 69.

[311] A. Leonard-Segal, *The Divided Mind: The Epidemic of Mindbody Disorders* (New York: Harper Collins, 2007), p. 270.

[312] G. Groddeck, *The Book of The It* (New York: Random House, 1949), p. xii.

[313] *Ibid.*, pp. vi-vii.

[314] *Ibid.*, pp. xi-xii.

[315] D. Colbert, *Deadly Emotions, Understand The Mind-Body-Spirit Connection That Can Heal or Destroy You* (Nashville: Thomas Nelson Publishers, 2003), p. 118.

[316] *Ibid.*, p. 119.

[317] *Ibid.*, p. 118.

[318] G. Jampolsky, *Love is Letting Go of Fear* (Berkeley, CA: Ten Speed Press, 1979), pp. 73-74.

[319] M. Eddy, *Science and Health* (Boston: The First Church of Christ, 1994), p. 400.

[320] J. Lee, *Facing the Fire: Experiencing and Expressing Anger Appropriately* (United States and Canada: Bantam, 1993), p. 11.

[321] Bob Greene and Oprah Winfrey, *Make The Connection* (New York: Hyperion, 1996), pp. 46-48.

[322] Retrieved from [www.ichelp.com/whatisic/AnIntroductionToIC.html].

[323] J. Sarno, *Healing Back Pain* (New York: Warner Brothers, 1991), p. 51.

[324] D. Colbert, *Deadly Emotions, Understand The Mind-Body-Spirit Connection That Can Heal or Destroy You* (Nashville: Thomas Nelson Publishers, 2003), p. 29.

[325] J. Sarno, *Healing Back Pain* (New York: Warner Brothers, 1991), p. 112.

[326] M. Rossman, *Guided Imagery for Self-Healing* (Novato, CA: HJ Kramer/New World Library, 2000), pp. 36-37.

[327] *Ibid.*, pp. 100-101.

[328] A. Weil, *Spontaneous Healing* (New York: Random House, 1995), p. 229.

[329] J. Sarno, *The Mindbody Prescription* (New York: Warner Brothers, 1999), p. 92.

[330] Retrieved from [faculty.washington.edu/chudler/yawning.html].